The Chemistry of CEREAL PROTEINS

Second Edition

Radomir Lásztity, D.Sc.
Professor
Department of Biochemistry and Food Technology
Technical University
Budapest, Hungary

CRC Press
Boca Raton New York London Tokyo

Library of Congress Cataloging-in-Publication Data

Lásztity, Radomír.
The chemistry of cereal proteins / author, R. Lásztity. -- 2nd ed.
p. cm.
Includes bibliographical references and index.
ISBN 0-8493-2763-6 (alk. paper)
1. Plant proteins. 2. Grain. I. Title.
TP453.P7L37 1995
664′.7--dc20 95-22630
CIP

Direct all inquiries to CRC Press, Inc., 2000 Corporate Blvd., N.W., Boca Raton, Florida 33431.

International Standard Book Number 0-8493-2763-6
Library of Congress Card Number 95-22630
Printed in the United States of America 1 2 3 4 5 6 7 8 9 0
Printed on acid-free paper

The Author

R. Lásztity, D.Sc., is Professor of the Department of Biochemistry and Food Technology at the Technical University, Budapest, Hungary. Dr. Lásztity received his M.Sc. degree in chemical engineering in 1951 and his D.Sc. degree in chemical sciences in 1968 from Technical University.

After receiving his M.Sc., Dr. Lásztity began work in the Department of Food Chemistry (later changed to the Department of Biochemistry and Food Technology) at the Technical University as an assistant. In 1963 he was promoted to Associate Professor and in 1969 to University Professor. He was Head of the Department in the period 1972 to 1993. From 1970 to 1976 he was acting Vice Rector of the University.

Dr. Lásztity's main research activities are chemistry and biochemistry of cereal proteins, rheology of food, and food analysis. The results of his research work have been published in more than 550 scientific papers in Hungarian and foreign scientific journals. He is Chairman of the Food Protein Working Group of the Hungarian Academy of Sciences, Deputy Technical Director and a member of the Executive Committee of the International Association for Cereal Science and Technology (ICC). He was Chairman of the Codex Committee on Methods of Analysis and Sampling of the FAO/WHO Food Standards Program from 1975 to 1988.

Preface

In the last decade or so since the first edition of this book appeared, the field of chemistry of cereal proteins has continued to grow. New, powerful separation techniques, such as reverse phase high performance chromatography and capillary electrophoresis, have been introduced and there has been dramatic progress in the application of achievements of molecular biology and genetic engineering of proteins. Thanks to the development in methods of study on the structure of proteins, our knowledge concerning interactions in protein systems has increased enormously.

Although the central role of investigation of wheat proteins remains the same, more rapid progress may be observed in the field of proteins of other cereals. Particularly in some industrial countries (e.g., Western Europe) — due to the standing surplus of cereal production — growing interest has focused on the nonfood uses of cereals, including the protein preparations made from cereals.

The objective of this edition is the same as the first edition. The book gives an overview on the present status of our knowledge of cereal proteins and about recent trends in this field.

The structure of the book also remains unchanged, but all the chapters are revised and additions and corrections have been made. The chapters dealing with cereals, other than wheat, are substantially enlarged, including newer results of investigations. Particular attention has been given to the progress made in molecular biology of cereal proteins and also to some aspects of nonfood uses of cereal proteins.

I would like to thank those who expressed their views and comments regarding the first edition; this has been a help in improving the second edition.

Table of Contents

Chapter 4

Chapter 5

Chapter 9

Chapter 10

Chapter 11

1 Introduction

The growing of cereals plays the major role in the agricultural production of the majority of countries. This fact is connected first of all with the importance of some cereals in nutrition. The majority of wheat, rice, rye, sorghum, and millet is used for food; they contribute an important source of protein in the diet in different countries of the world. In many developing countries cereal proteins form 70 to 90% of the total protein consumption. Maize, barley, and growing parts of other cereals are used in animal feed, especially in developed countries.

The great nutritional importance of cereals, the deficiency of some essential amino acids, and the efforts to increase the efficiency of the feeding, enhanced by severe shortages of foods in parts of the world, have stimulated the investigation of the genetics and biosynthesis of the cereal proteins. In the last decade significant advances have been made in the biochemical and genetic studies of individual cereal protein components. A number of genes were isolated and sequenced. The results of these completed investigations, along with the results of the morphological investigation of cereal grains, have led to new methods and possible means of breeding and production of cereals. At the same time, these results are also interesting with regard to the cereal processing, nutrition, feeding, and industrial uses of cereals.

A relatively new field of investigation of cereal proteins involves the connection of the preparation of cereal protein concentrates with the biological (nutritive) value of proteins, as well as with the possible nonfood uses of these proteins. Recently some new results were published concerning the biological value of food proteins, especially protein mixtures. In light of these results it seems that our views concerning the nutritive value of plant proteins must be reevaluated because the role of animal proteins was in many cases overestimated. From the point of view of the nutritive value of cereals, the problem of the inhibitors of the proteolytic enzymes is also very interesting. The existence of trypsin inhibitors in soya has been known for many years, and due to the intensive study of them the primary structures of some compounds are also known. The isolation and characterization of some protein inhibitors from wheat, rye, triticale, and barley show that the problem of proteolytic inhibitors is probably a general problem of all the cereals.

Besides the relatively new fields of investigation — mentioned above — the traditional desire of cereal chemists to understand the contributions of the protein to the milling, dough forming, and baking properties of wheat and some other cereals remained unaltered.

Making a comparison between the different cereals, it can be stated that the main efforts of scientists were concentrated on wheat and that the investigation of proteins of the other cereals was not so developed. Recently an increasing interest in maize, barley, rye, triticale, rice, and sorghum protein investigation has been evident.

Although extensive reviews covering the storage proteins[1] — and particularly prolamins[2] — have been published in some monographs, and also some reviews concerning wheat[3] and maize[4] proteins as well as the chemistry of triticale,[5] rice,[6] barley,[7] oats,[8] sorghum, and millet,[9] no monograph is available giving a general review of the more recent results on the protein chemistry of all important cereal grains.

In the framework of this book, based on the analogies between the different cereal proteins, a new general approach to the chemistry and biochemistry of these proteins will be given. A very important element of this approach is the separation of the storage proteins and metabolically active proteins, which have in many cases quite different character, composition, and technological value.

Great attention was given to the interpretation of the bread-making function and other technological properties of cereal proteins at the molecular level.

It is hoped that this book will provide new information about the progress in the chemistry of cereal proteins and also on some new forms of interpretation for all who are involved in any aspect of cereal research and technology.

REFERENCES

1. Shewry, P. R. and Miflin, B. J., Seed storage proteins of economically important cereals, in *Advances in Cereal Science and Technology,* Vol. 7, Pomeranz, Y., Ed., American Association of Cereal Chemists, St. Paul, MN, 1986, 1.
2. Tatham, A. S., Shewry, P. R., and Belton, P. S., Structural studies of cereal prolamins, including wheat gluten, in *Advances in Cereal Science and Technology,* Vol. 10, Pomeranz, Y., Ed., American Association of Cereal Chemists, St. Paul, MN, 1990, 1.
3. Kasarda, D. D., Bernardin, J. E., and Nimmo, C. C., Wheat proteins, in *Advances in Cereal Science and Technology,* Vol. 1, Pomeranz, Y., Ed., American Association of Cereal Chemists, St. Paul, MN, 1976, 155.
4. Mossé, J. and Landry, J., Recent research on major maize proteins: zeins and glutenins, in *Cereals for Food and Beverages. Recent Progress in Cereal Chemistry,* Inglett, G. E. and Munck, L., Eds., Academic Press, New York, 1980, 255.
5. Larter, E. N., Gustafson, J. P., Kaltsikes, P. J., and Bushuk, W., Twenty-Five Years of Triticale Research at the University of Manitoba, Department of Plant Science, University of Manitoba, Winnipeg, 1980.
6. Juliano, B. O., Ed., *Rice Chemistry and Technology,* American Association of Cereal Chemists, St. Paul, MN, 1986.
7. Cameron-Mills, V., Brandt, A., and Ingversen, J., The molecular biology of barley storage protein synthesis, in *Cereals for Food and Beverages. Recent Progress in Cereal Chemistry,* Inglett, G. E. and Munck, L., Eds., Academic Press, New York, 1980, 33.
8. Webster, F. H., Ed., *Oats: Chemistry and Technology,* American Association of Cereal Chemists, St. Paul, MN, 1986.
9. Dendy, A. D. V., Ed., *Sorghum and Millets: Chemistry and Technology,* American Association of Cereal Chemists, St. Paul, MN, 1994.

2 The Importance and General Characterization of Cereal Proteins

I. INTRODUCTION

Cereals have been important crops for thousands of years. In most countries of the world the proportion of land devoted to cereals is the highest among cultivated plants. According to statistical data,[1] the world production of cereals was estimated at 1815 million tonnes (see Table 1). In the last period (1986 to 1990) both the area under cereal crops and the production increased. The most marked increases were observed in the production of wheat, maize, rice, and barley. A decreasing tendency was characteristic for oats and rye. The majority of the cereals produced is used for human consumption. The most important other forms of use are animal feed, industrial uses, and seed corn. The total protein consumption of the world population is estimated at more than 100 million tonnes. Cereal proteins provide more than half of the total protein production of the world. If we consider that the production of milk and meat is also based on feed containing cereals, it is clear that in the provision of protein requirements the cereal proteins play the most important role.

II. GENERAL CHARACTERISTICS OF CEREAL PROTEINS

The chemical composition of cereals is characterized by a high content of starch, a relatively significant protein content, and a relatively low lipid content. The differences between different cereal grains are significant, as they are between different varieties of the same cereal. The average chemical compositions of the cereals are demonstrated in Table 2.

It can be seen that among the cereals the protein content of wheat is the highest. Some Russian spring wheats may have a protein content over 20%. The lowest protein content is observed in rice.

According to the comprehensive studies of Osborne,[2] the wheat proteins were divided into four classes on the basis of solubility: albumins, soluble in water; globulins, soluble in salt solutions (10% NaCl solution was frequently used), but insoluble in water; gliadins, soluble in 70 to 90% ethanol; and glutenins, insoluble

TABLE 1
World Production of Cereals[1] (10^6 t)

Kind of Cereal	Period 1971–1975	1976–1980	1981–1985	1986–1990
Total cereals	1420	1550	1680	1815
Wheat	420	455	506	523
Rice	360	392	441	484
Maize	350	395	423	467
Barley	170	168	162	160
Rye	34	30	24	24
Oats	56	48	44	43
Sorghum	54	61	74	82
Millet	32	29	30	33
Triticale[a]	0.4	0.5	0.6	1

[a] Estimated data.

TABLE 2
Average Gross Composition of Cereal Grains (% Dry Weight Basis)

Cereal Grains	Protein	Fat	Starch	Fiber	Ash
Wheat	12.2	1.9	71.9	1.9	1.7
Rye	11.6	1.7	71.9	1.9	2.0
Barley	10.9	2.3	73.5	4.3	2.4
Oats	11.3	5.8	55.5	10.9	3.2
Maize	10.2	4.6	79.5	2.3	1.3
Millet	10.3	4.5	58.9	8.7	4.7
Sorghum	11.0	3.5	65.0	4.9	2.6
Rice	8.1	1.2	75.8	0.5	1.4

in neutral aqueous solutions, saline solutions, or alcohol, but soluble in acids and bases. The terms gliadin and glutenin are usually reserved for preparations from wheat. Osborne suggested the generic names prolamin and glutelin for the equivalent protein fractions of other cereal grains.

The fractionation of the cereal proteins on the basis of solubility has retained its importance to the present time. It gives relatively reproducible results that provide some information about the proteins. However, the fractions obtained are mixtures of different proteins. Each group has subgroups, and none of the groups consists of a single pure protein. There are also proteins that do not appear to fall into any of the four groups; e.g., some proteins remain insoluble (residue protein) after the extraction procedure of Osborne.

Thus, it is understandable that better classification schemes are needed. Biologists and biochemists suggest classification according to biological function. According to this proposition, proteins of cereal grains can be divided into two classes: metabolically active or cytoplasmic proteins and storage proteins. The former correspond roughly to the group consisting of albumins and globulins (according to Osborne's classification), and the latter are comprised of the prolamins and glutelins. However, some overlapping of properties and function is possible. In addition — due to our lack of knowledge — the biological role of many proteins is not yet known.

On the basis of the morphology of cereal grains the proteins may be divided into three groups: endosperm proteins, proteins of the aleurone layer, and proteins of the embryo (or germ). The different classification possibilities are summarized in Table 3. The cytoplasmic protein group includes the most important metabolically active proteins, the membrane proteins, nonenzymic regulatory proteins, proteins of organelles, etc.

TABLE 3
Possibilities for the Classification of Cereal Proteins

On the Basis of Morphology	On the Basis of Biological Function	According to Solubility (Osborne)	On the Basis of Chemical Composition
Endosperm proteins	Metabolically active cytoplasmic proteins	Albumins	Simple proteins
Proteins of the aleurone layer		Globulins	Complex proteins
Proteins of the embryo	Enzymes	Prolamins	Lipoproteins
	Membrane proteins	Glutelins	Glycoproteins
	Proteins of ribosomes	Residue proteins	Nucleoproteins
	Regulatory proteins		Metalloproteins
	Other proteins		Chromoproteins
	Storage proteins		Phosphoproteins
	Low molecular weight proteins		
	High molecular weight proteins		

Storage proteins are typically endosperm proteins. Nevertheless, smaller amounts of storage proteins also may be found in the aleurone layer and in the embryo.

From the chemical point of view the existence of complex proteins is also interesting. In Osborne's classification the complex proteins were not taken into account. The newer investigations show that the protein-lipid and protein-carbohydrate interactions and the lipo- and glycoproteins play a very important role in the properties and technological value of different cereals.

Cytoplasmic and storage proteins differ considerably in physical properties and amino acid composition. Generally the cytoplasmic proteins are easily soluble in water or salt buffer solutions, their molecular weight is relatively small, and the molecules have a globular form. The storage proteins of the endosperm are generally insoluble in water and salt solutions. It is characteristic for the endosperm storage proteins to include two types of proteins: a low molecular weight protein consisting of single polypeptide chains and having only intramolecular disulfide bonds, and high molecular weight proteins consisting of many polypeptide chains cross-linked by intermolecular disulfide bonds. Many of the polypeptides of storage proteins have repeated sequences of amino acids. This suggests that the genes encoding them evolved initially by tandem duplication of short sequences of DNA. Reviews of the structure and evolution of cereal grain proteins are given by Kreis et al.[3] and Tatham et al.[4]

The differences in amino acid composition of cytoplasmic and storage proteins are relatively great and influence the nutritive value of the two types of proteins. The storage proteins contain a large proportion of glutamic acid and proline and only a small proportion of lysine, arginine, threonine, and tryptophan. The metabolically active proteins, containing considerably lower glutamic acid and proline content and a higher proportion of lysine and arginine, have a higher biological (nutritive) value.

Concerning the distribution of metabolically active and storage proteins it can be stated that the proteins of the aleurone layer and germ belong mainly to the group of metabolically active proteins, and the storage proteins are presumably located in the endosperm. Modern milling procedures allow a comparatively clean separation of the embryo (or germ), pericarpaleurone layer (or bran), and endosperm (or flour). Therefore the differences in amino acid composition — demonstrated in Table 4 — approximately represent the differences between the storage and cytoplasmic proteins.

The protein concentration in the different morphological parts (endosperm, aleurone layer, embryo) of the cereal grains shows big variations. The protein content of the germ is the highest (about 30%); a relatively high concentration (about 20%) may be observed in the aleurone layer; and the lowest protein concentration is evident in endosperm. The ultrastructure of the endosperm of different cereal grains is similar. The storage proteins form a matrix and/or protein granules surrounding the starch granules. It has been observed by many research workers that the protein concentration varies from the inner to the outer endosperm parts. Hinton[5] investigated soft wheats and found a protein concentration range from 6.2% in the innermost endosperm cells through 8.8% in the middle endosperm to 13.7% in the outer (subaleurone) endosperm cells. In high-protein hard wheat types the uneven distribution may be even more marked. As a consequence of the differences in protein concentration and amino acid composition, the nutritive value of the whole grain is generally higher than that of the endosperm. Finally, the total content of essential amino acids depends on the mass ratio of the main morphological parts of the grain. The aleurone layer and germ have higher protein content than the endosperm and a higher ratio of essential amino acids; therefore, the higher mass ratio of the aleurone layer and germ results in a higher protein content and essential amino acid content in the grain kernal. Differences in the proportion of the different proteins (including

TABLE 4
Amino Acid Composition of Wheat Grain, Flour (Extraction Grade 72%), Wheat Germ, and Wheat Aleurone Proteins (g/100 g Protein)

Amino Acid	Wheat Grain	Flour	Whole Germ[a]	Aleurone[b]
Alanine	3.40	2.91	7.00	6.5
Arginine	4.61	3.20	8.96	12.3
Aspartic acid	4.71	4.10	10.21	9.3
Cystine	2.24	1.69	0.66	—
Glutamic acid	31.52	36.86	15.45	18.3
Glycine	3.89	3.39	6.54	7.0
Histidine	2.20	1.83	2.63	4.3
Isoleucine	3.59	3.61	3.91	3.2
Leucine	6.79	6.74	6.79	6.7
Lysine	2.52	1.95	7.76	5.9
Methionine	2.11	1.49	1.88	0.4
Phenylalanine	4.75	4.68	4.07	4.2
Proline	10.44	11.38	4.37	4.6
Serine	4.53	4.40	4.62	5.0
Threonine	2.87	2.31	4.82	3.8
Tryptophan	1.32	1.15	—	—
Tyrosine	3.20	2.31	3.12	2.8
Valine	4.22	3.94	5.65	5.5

[a] From Pomeranz et al.[6] (g/100 g amino acids).
[b] From Fulcher et al.[7]

different types of storage proteins) may have a similar effect. This is the situation in some mutants of corn and barley, where changes in the proportion of prolamins and glutelins (i.e., lower quantity of prolamins) result in a higher lysine content and higher nutritive value. The problem of the mutants with high lysine content will be discussed later in Chapters 6 and 7.

Researchers have observed the negative correlation between yield and protein content of cereals. The theoretical basis for these observations has also been considered, and generally the following explanation is accepted. The energy needed to produce proteins is approximately twice that required for starch synthesis. Therefore, an increase in protein concentration at a constant yield level will require either a higher photosynthetic rate and duration or more efficient partitioning of assimilates into grain (higher harvest index). Application of nitrogen fertilizer leads to an increase in yield and protein content. Low-protein cultivars did not necessarily give a greater protein response to nitrogen fertilizer than high-protein cultivars.

The wide variation in protein content is not only dependent on genetic factors; it may be a result of environmental effects. Protein is synthesized throughout the fruiting period of the plant. Starch synthesis, on the other hand, starts later during fruiting and accelerates as maturity approaches. If growing conditions in the late fruiting period are good, starch yield will be good and grain yields high, but protein content will be relatively low. The availability of nitrogen throughout the growing period is of course of major importance, as mentioned above. Other environmental factors that might result in high protein are drought and certain diseases. The protein content of cereals is important for two reasons. First, cereal protein is an important nutrient. Second, the amount and type of protein are important in the functional uses of the flour. When the protein content of a cereal grain changes, the relative proportions of the various protein classes also change. Generally at a low protein content the amount of metabolically active proteins (albumins and globulins), expressed as a percentage of total protein, is much higher than at a higher protein content. In contrast, a relative decrease in the ratio of storage proteins might be observed. This appears logical if we remember the biological roles of the two groups of proteins. As the plant produces more protein, less is required for physiological functions and more is available as storage protein.

In this book the proteins of the individual cereals will be discussed based on classification according to biological role. Although this classification also has disadvantages, it may be justified by the fact that the technological role, functionality, nutritive value, physical properties, etc. of the two groups differ considerably. In many cases the roles of different groups are well defined (e.g., enzymes, natural enzyme inhibitors), the individual protein components may be isolated in pure form, or, based on the knowledge of corresponding DNA sequences, their primary structure may be determined.

III. THE BIOSYNTHESIS OF CEREAL PROTEINS

In the last decade much progress has been made in determining the molecular biology of cereal proteins. This progress is based on the growing knowledge about the genomes of cereal plants, the location of protein-coding genes, the isolation, sequencing, and cloning of these genes, and the involvement of improved techniques used in the morphological study of cereal grains.

It is not the author's intention to cover this field in any detail; rather, the subject will be outlined and the reader referred to other sources from which more details may be obtained.

Different types of cereal proteins have been studied in recent years; nevertheless, research on synthesis and deposition of storage proteins has predominated.

In a review on seed storage proteins, Shewry and Miflin[8] give a good summary about synthesis of cereal grain proteins, particularly that of storage proteins. Storage proteins are tissue specific, only being synthesized in the corresponding storage organ. They accumulate relatively late in development after cessation of cell division. The amount of storage proteins is highly dependent on the nutritional status of the plant. Under conditions of low nutritient availability, the seed synthesizes mainly metabolically active proteins. With more available nutrients the proportion of storage proteins increases.

An excellent review on protein synthesis in the developing wheat endosperm has been published by Kasarda et al.[9] Simmonds and O'Brien[10] published a good review on the morphological and biochemical development of the wheat endosperm. Concerning the storage proteins of barley the review of Cameron-Mills et al.[11] may be mentioned.

The results of the research work in biosynthesis of storage proteins of maize were summarized by Mosse and Landry.[11a]

On the basis of the observations made on wheat during the different stages of endosperm development, three mechanisms of protein biosynthesis appear to be operating.[15] These three mechanisms, which may be observed and postulated at different stages of development by electron microscopy are

1. Synthesis on polyribosomes which are abundant in the cytoplasm surrounding the large central vacuole
2. Synthesis on ribosomes bound to or associated with protein bodies, which may be seen developing within the vacuoles between 12 and 20 days postanthesis (p.a.); in an alternative mechanism, the protein may be synthesized in the cytoplasm and transported to the vacuole either through the lumen of the endoplasmic reticulum or by a process akin to pinocytosis
3. Synthesis on the endoplasmic reticulum-bound ribosomes and accumulation within the lumen of this organelle

The results of the investigation of other cereals show that these statements probably may be generalized for all cereal grains.

Concerning the biosynthesis of the different classes of proteins several studies were performed by research workers. On the basis of these investigations it can be generally stated that the metabolically active (cytoplasmic) proteins (belonging to the group consisting of albumins and globulins) are synthesized rapidly in the early stages of kernel development. It is likely that this takes place on the polysomal aggregates present in the cytoplasm. The results show that the cytoplasmic proteins are present in a significant amount even at the earliest stages at which the material can be analyzed. On the basis of the observation that high-protein wheats have a greater proportion of their total protein as acetic acid-soluble storage protein, it has been suggested that after the developing wheat kernel has satisfied its requirements for cytoplasmic proteins any additional nitrogen is channeled into the synthesis of storage proteins.

Storage protein first appears in the developing endosperm about 10 days p.a. in the form of membrane-bound spherical bodies generally closely associated with the endoplasmic reticulum. A clear distinction should be made between the protein bodies of the aleurone layer and those of the starchy endosperm cells. These two groups of organelles differ in composition, structure, and to some extent function. The endosperm cells have only a storage function. The aleurone layer possesses synthetic and secretory functions as well. Aleurone protein bodies are typically 2 to

4 μm in diameter and contain globoid and crystalline inclusions. The former inclusions store phytic acid and the latter contain protein, carbohydrate, and niacytin.[16]

Protein bodies in the starchy endosperm, on the other hand, have a homogeneous structure without inclusions, except for certain intensively osmiophilic zones. Protein bodies in the developing wheat endosperm cells are typically spherical, about 0.5 to 0.15 μm in diameter, and ranging up to 20 μm in the mature tissue. In mature tissue, however, their shapes are extensively distorted due to the dehydration of the kernel and compression by starch granules. Many smaller protein bodies are fused during growth, so the storage protein matrix of the mature wheat grain tends to be a continuum within which the starch granules are embedded. Wheat differs from most other cereals in that its protein bodies cannot be recognized at maturity because of the compression and fusion which have occurred. In barley, rice, maize, millet, and sorghum individual protein bodies may be recognized. A good summary about the morphology of cereal grains has been published by Simmonds.[15] In some cereals it was shown by differential extraction that the individual protein bodies contain exclusively the prolamin fraction. The matrix, on the other hand, contains only glutelins.[17]

Many data have been collected concerning the mechanisms of synthesis, transport, and deposition of storage proteins. Nevertheless, further investigations are needed for the total elucidation of these processes. It is generally accepted and has been experimentally confirmed that proteins synthesized on the rough endoplasmic reticulum (RER) are made first as precursor molecules with an extension at the N-terminus. This signal sequence, rich in hydrophobic amino acids, causes binding of the ribosomes to the RER membrane and assembly of a protein "tunnel" through the membrane. This signal sequence followed by the remainder of the polypeptide then passes through the RER into the lumen. The signal peptide is then cleaved off by a specific protease within the lumen. A review about mechanisms for the incorporation of proteins in membranes and organelles is given by Sabatini et al.[18]

The final site of deposition of the storage proteins and the route by which this is reached are not yet fully elucidated. It seems that the site of deposition and the transport mechanism are not uniform; there are differences between cereals, and even in the same kernel more mechanisms may exist, with different types of protein bodies being formed in some cases. Deposits associated with RER are most typical, but storage proteins are deposited also in vacuoles.

In recent years, immunocytochemical techniques have been used to elucidate the morphogenesis and structure of protein bodies.[12,14] Studies done on different cereals strongly support the involvement of the Golgi apparatus in prolamin body formation.[19,20]

IV. GERMINATION (SPROUTING)

The germination of cereal grains is of interest for several reasons. Rapid and even germination are important properties of malting barleys. On the other hand, germination (sprouting) during the harvesting or the storage of grains is a very disadvantageous process causing big losses and deterioration of the technological value of cereals.

Seeds of cultivated cereal plants germinate when they are morphologically mature and are placed under optimal conditions of moisture, temperature, and oxygen concentration. However, even when provided with such conditions seeds of many species may fail to germinate. This stage is described as dormancy. Seed quiescence is an environmentally imposed temporary suspension of growth and reduction of metabolic activity in viable seeds which occurs under conditions that are unfavorable for germination. On the other hand, the dormancy of seeds is an endogenously controlled and/or environmentally imposed temporary suspension of growth which is independent of immediate environmental conditions. Consequently, dormant seeds — until the end of this stage — do not germinate under conditions which may be favorable for normal growth. The cereal growers, especially in countries with rain during harvest, prefer grain with some dormancy to resist field sprouting. The biochemical process of germination may be divided into three steps:[22] (1) initiation or "wake up" period, (2) a period of intensive biosynthesis of proteins, and (3) degradation of the storage proteins and other macromolecules in the endosperm.

The "wake up" period is relatively short (0.5 to 1 h). After placing the dormant seed under optimal conditions its ribosomes, mitochondria, DNA, and mRNA molecules are rapidly activated by a regulatory mechanism not yet known in detail. Some of the enzymes preexisting in the seed are also activated (enzymes of glycolysis, respiration, and synthesis of NAD, UDP, ADP, ATP). By deamination of some amino acids, α-keto acids are formed which take part in the processes of the citric acid cycle. The low rate of respiration — characteristic of the dormant seed — increases rapidly.

In the second stage a very intensive synthesis of nucleic acids and proteins may be observed. During this period the enzymes taking part in the degradation of the reserve nutrients of the endosperm and also the enzymes catalyzing the biochemical processes of the new plant growth are synthesized. It has been known for a relatively long time that the enzymes involved in the degradation of the reserve nutrients in the endosperm are synthesized in the aleurone layer. This synthesis is induced by gibberellic acid formed in the embryo. In this stage of germination liberation or activation of preexisting hydrolases such as β-amylase occurs first. The activation and *de novo* synthesis of the major enzymes (α-amylases, proteases) of the degradation process follow the processes mentioned above. Hydrolytic enzymes such as β-amylase and carboxypeptidase are found in the starchy endosperm and are activated, possibly by endoproteases or reducing substances, during malting.[22]

In the first stage of the degradation of the reserve proteins the structure of the protein bodies will be broken down, and after that the proteolysis begins. The initial changes of the storage proteins may be controlled by investigation of the changes in solubility. An increase in the proportion of the albumin and globulin fractions occurs. A more detailed picture may be obtained using gel electrophoresis. The quantity of free amino acids is increased in the first period of degradation, and it later remains at a constant level. The effects of germination (sprouting) on the technological value of cereals are discussed in a review by Meredith and Pomeranz.[21]

V. THE NUTRITIVE VALUE OF CEREAL PROTEINS

Characteristic of the cereal endosperm storage proteins is the high proportion of the amino acids glutamic acid and proline and the low proportion of lysine, methionine, and tryptophan. The essential amino acid content in cereal grains plus that of cysteine, tyrosine, arginine, and histidine is demonstrated in Table 5. The data summarized in Table 5 show that the highest lysine content is characteristic for oats and rice; the protein of maize is the poorest in tryptophan content. The biological value of cereal proteins (expressed by chemical indexes) lies between 50 and 60.

TABLE 5
Amino Acid Contents of Cereals (g/100 g Protein)

Amino Acid	Wheat	Rye	Triticale	Rice	Maize	Barley	Millet	Sorghum	Oats
			References						
			27	26	26	25	26	23	24
Arginine	4.71	4.93	5.25	8.26	4.19	4.40	4.70	3.19	6.98
Cystine	2.19	1.90	2.97	1.07	1.55	2.50	2.19	1.73	1.73
Histidine	2.02	2.20	2.40	2.49	2.72	2.10	2.35	1.71	2.46
Isoleucine	4.70	4.26	3.70	3.71	3.68	3.80	4.55	3.77	3.90
Leucine	6.72	6.68	6.98	8.22	12.43	6.90	10.30	13.11	7.55
Lysine	2.79	3.42	3.31	3.69	2.67	3.50	3.05	2.24	4.51
Metionine	1.30	1.68	1.63	2.32	1.92	1.60	1.85	1.23	1.65
Phenylalanine	4.96	4.82	4.94	5.15	4.88	5.10	4.91	4.89	4.93
Threonine	2.84	3.70	3.20	3.91	3.60	3.50	3.19	3.64	3.64
Tryptophan	1.28	1.13	1.11	1.15	0.70	1.40	1.40	1.20[a]	1.70[a]
Tyrosine	3.72	3.27	2.84	3.49	3.83	2.50	3.70	3.41	3.61
Valine	4.48	5.21	4.52	5.51	4.85	5.40	5.31	4.51	5.24

[a] Unpublished measurements of the Department of Biochemistry and Food Technology, Technical University of Budapest.

Because of their more favorable amino acid composition the biological value of the proteins of the germ and aleurone layers is higher than that of the storage proteins of the endosperm. Generally, high-protein cereal grains contain a higher proportion of endosperm storage proteins and have a lower biological value.

Because of the facts mentioned above, breeding efforts to improve the nutritive value of cereal grains have concentrated on increasing protein content without decreasing (and eventually increasing) the protein quality. The amino acid composition of each of the different proteins of cereal grains is genetically determined. Therefore, a change in the overall amino acid composition is only possible in this case if the proportions of different types of protein fractions are change. For example, a new variety having a greater germ or a thicker aleurone layer may have a higher essential amino acid content because of the more favorable amino acid composition of these proteins. Also, a change in the proportion of the different storage proteins of the endosperm may be advantageous from the point of view of nutritional value. Some new varieties of high-lysine maize, barley, etc. are characterized by a lower content of prolamins and higher amount of other proteins. Maize variety Opaque-2 has a 50% higher lysine content than the normal maize varieties. Opaque-2 maize has a higher ratio of germ to endosperm and a much lower zein content than other maize varieties. In wheat and other cereals used for bread making the disproportionately low storage protein content means a lowering of protein quality for bread making. Therefore a number of specialists are of the opinion that a more scientifically attractive approach to the improvement of the nutritional quality of wheat in terms of lysine content would be to select for higher protein content. The additional protein content more than offsets the slight decrease in the nutritional and bread-making quality of the protein.[28] The solution for the contradictory needs of nutrition and bread-making technology in the future may be the practical use of gene engineering in cereal grain production.

During evaluation of the nutritional value of cereal proteins it is necessary to keep in mind some newer results concerning the biological value of protein mixtures. As was shown, the biological value of the protein mixtures may not be characterized by the arithmetic mean of the values of the protein components. Because of possible complementation the biological value of the mixtures may be higher than that of any components. For example, in a mixture of wheat and yeast proteins the high lysine content of yeast proteins and relatively high cystine content of wheat proteins compensate for the lower lysine content of the former and the lower content of sulfur-containing amino acids in the latter. As a result the biological value of the mixtures of optimal composition is much higher than that of yeast or wheat proteins.

VI. EXTRACTION OF CEREAL GRAIN PROTEINS

Any knowledge of grain protein composition, structure, and properties requires the separation and extraction of these proteins; the proteins must be dissolved under conditions as mild as possible using solvents. The effective and total extraction (separation) of the different protein fractions can involve great difficulties. There are several reasons behind the difficulties associated with extraction.[29]

1. The almost anhydrous state of the cereal grain, the development of which arises from possible aggregation, partially due to desiccation
2. The strong chemical heterogeneity of the grain, which contains so many biochemical components: lipids, carbohydrates, enzymes, nucleic acids, polyphenols, etc.
3. The biological heterogeneity of grain tissues, with the presence of at least two distinct parts, embryo and endosperm
4. The relatively small size of the grains
5. The unfortunate frequent confusion between solubility and extractability, which do not have the same characteristics; because of the multiplicity of components, it is possible to extract a pool of seed proteins with a solvent mixture in which they may not be soluble, or vice versa.

The extraction can be performed either in order to study a limited group of proteins or in order to put them all in solution by an exhaustive procedure. In many cases the extraction is not "total" and we can wonder whether unextracted proteins are really similar to the already extracted ones. It is possible that a few fractions having a very significant function still remain unextracted.

Recent work concerning improvement of the methods of extraction has focused on newer solvents or the combination of solvents having a powerful dispersing or disrupting effect. It has been emphasized that a well-planned combined extraction is a necessary tool in obtaining well-defined fractions.

The main solvents, used more or less in combination one with another, may be summarized as follows:

1. Alcohols, mainly ethanol and propanol
2. Detergents (sodium dodecyl sulfate [SDS], acetyltrimethylammonium bromide, etc.)
3. Fatty acid salts, the use of which is perhaps the most recent[30]
4. Reducing agents (mercaptoethanol, dithiothreitol)
5. Weak acids (acetic acid, lactic acid)
6. Urea (having a powerful disrupting effect upon hydrogen bonds)

One of the problems discussed connected with extraction is the preliminary defatting of cereal grain (meals) before extraction. The defatting of flours before extraction may prevent the later formation of lipid-protein complexes in the natural grain. On the other hand, some denaturation of proteins has been classified on the basis of solubility. There are some protein components (e.g., lipothionines) which may be extracted by lipid solvents. The problems of defatting were exhaustively discussed by Jankiewicz.[31] Summarizing the results and views of different research workers, the author is of the opinion that whether or not defatting should be used is dependent on the purposes of the extraction.

The dry methods of classification are relatively rarely used in research work. The air classification (the process depends upon differences between starch and proteins in both density and particle size) is well known in the milling industry as a tool for producing fractions enriched in proteins. The flotation technique developed by Hess[32] (separating the flour components on the basis of their particle density) is also not commonly used. The separation of protein bodies of the endosperm seems to be a very promising dry method of separation, especially in the research work concerning distribution and biosynthesis of proteins and structure of the endosperm.[33]

REFERENCES

1. *Statistical Yearbook* (in Hungarian), Statiqum Kiado, Budapest, 1992.
2. Osborne, T. B., *The Proteins of the Wheat Kernel,* Carnegie Institute, Washington, D.C., 1907.
3. Kreis, M., Shewry, P. R., Forde, B. G., Forde, J., and Miflin, B. J., Structure and evolution of seed storage proteins and their genes with particular reference to those of wheat, barley and rye, in *Oxford Surveys of Plant Molecular and Cell Biology,* Vol. 2, Miflin, B. J., Ed., Oxford University Press, Oxford, 1985, 253.
4. Tatham, A. S., Shewry, P. R., and Belton, P. S., Structural studies of cereal prolamins, including wheat gluten, in *Advances in Cereal Science and Technology,* Vol. 10, Pomeranz, Y., Ed., American Association of Cereal Chemists, St. Paul, MN, 1990, 1.
5. Hinton, J. J. C., The distribution of vitamin B1 and nitrogen in the wheat grain, *Proc. R. Soc. London Ser. B.,* 134, 418, 1947.
6. Pomeranz, Y., Carvajal, M. I., Hoseney, R. C., and Ward, A. B., Wheat germ in bread making. I. Composition of germ lipids and germ protein fractions, *Cereal Chem.,* 47, 373, 1970.
7. Fulcher, R. G., O'Brien, T. P., and Simmonds, D. H., Localization of arginine-rich proteins in mature seeds of some members of Gramineae, *Austr. J. Biol. Sci.,* 25, 487, 1972.
8. Shewry, P. R. and Miflin, B. J., Seed storage proteins of economically important cereals, in *Advances in Cereal Science and Technology,* Vol. 7, Pomeranz, Y., Ed., American Association of Cereal Chemists, St. Paul, MN, 1985, 1.
9. Kasarda, D. D., Bernardin, J. E., and Nimmo, C. C., Wheat proteins, in *Advances in Cereal Science and Technology,* Vol. 1, Pomeranz, Y., Ed., American Association of Cereal Chemists, St. Paul, MN, 1976, 158.
10. Simmonds, D. H. and O'Brien, T. P., Morphological and biochemical development of the wheat endosperm, in *Advances in Cereal Science and Technology,* Vol. 4, Pomeranz, Y., Ed., American Association of Cereal Chemists, St. Paul, MN, 1980, 5.
11. Cameron-Mills, V., Brandt, A., and Ingversen, J., The molecular biology of barley storage protein synthesis, in *Cereals for Food and Beverages. Recent Progress in Cereal Chemistry,* Inglett, G.E. and Munck, L., Eds., Academic Press, New York, 1980, 339.

11a. Mossé, J. and Landry, J., Recent research on major maize proteins, zeins and glutelins, in *Cereal for Food and Beverages. Recent Results in the Cereal Chemistry,* Inglett, G.E. and Munck, L., Eds., Academic Press, New York, 1980, 255.

12. Lending, C. R., Kriz, A. L., Larkins, B. A., and Bracker, C. E., Structure of maize protein bodies and immunochemical localization of zeins, *Protoplasma,* 143, 51, 1988.
13. Oparka, N. and Harris, N., Rice protein body formation: all types are initiated by dilatation of the endoplasmic reticulum, *Planta,* 154, 184, 1982.

14. Krishnan, H. B., White, J. A., and Pueppke, S. G., Immunocytochemical analysis of protein body formation in seeds of *Sorghum bicolor* (L.) Moench. *Can. J. Bot.*, 67, 2850, 1989.
15. Simmonds, D. H., Structure, composition and biochemistry of cereal grains, in *Cereals '78; Better Nutrition for the World Millions,* Pomeranz, Y., Ed., American Association of Cereal Chemists, St. Paul, MN, 1978, 105.
16. Fulcher, R. G. and Wong, S. I., Inside cereals — a fluorescence microchemical view, in *Cereals for Food and Beverages, Recent Progress in Cereal Chemistry,* Inglett, G.E. and Munck, L., Eds., Academic Press, New York, 1980, 1.
17. Wolf, M. J., Knov, V., and Seckinger, H. L., Subcellular structure of endosperm protein in high-lysine and normal corn, *Science,* 157, 556, 1967.
18. Sabatini, D. D., Kreibiach, G., Morimoto, T., and Adesnik, G., Mechanisms of the incorporation of proteins in membranes and organelles, *J. Cell Biol.*, 92, 1, 1982.
19. Krishnan, H. B., White, J. A., and Pueppke, S. G., Immunocytochemical evidence for the involvement of the Golgi apparatus in the transport of the vacuolar protein γ-secalin in rye *(Secale cereale)* endosperm, *Cereal Chem.*, 67, 360, 1990.
20. Kim, N. T., Franceschi, V. R., Krishnan, H. B., and Okita, T. V., Formation of wheat protein bodies: involvement of the Golgi apparatus in gliadin transport, *Planta,* 176, 173, 1988.
21. Meredith, P. and Pomeranz, Y., Sprouted grain, in *Advances in Cereal Science and Technology,* Vol. 7, Pomeranz, Y., Ed., American Association of Cereal Chemists, St. Paul, MN, 1985, 239.
22. Zsigmond, A., Investigation of the Changes of Wheat Proteins during Germination, Ph.D. thesis, Technical University of Budapest, Budapest, Hungary, 1982.
23. Hoseney, R. C., Davis, A. B., and Harbers, L. H., Pericarp and endosperm structure of sorghum grain shown by scanning electron microscopy, *Cereal Chem.,* 51, 552, 1974.
24. Lasztity, R., Berndorfer Kraszner, E., and Huszar, M., On the presence and distribution of some bioactive agents in oats varieties, in *Cereals for Food and Beverages, Recent Progress in Cereal Chemistry,* Inglett, G.E. and Munck, L., Eds., Academic Press, New York, 1980, 429.
25. Tkachuk, R. and Irvine, G. N., Amino acid composition of cereals and oilseed meals, *Cereal Chem.,* 46, 206, 1969.
26. Barber, S. and Barber, C. B., Chemical and biological data of rice proteins for nutrition and feeding, in *Amino Acid Composition and Biological Value of Cereal Proteins,* Lasztity, R. and Hidvegi, M., Eds., Reidel, Dordrecht, 1985, 481.
27. Golenkov, V. F., Comparative amino acid composition of proteins of wheat, rye and triticale grain, in *Amino Acid Composition and Biological Value of Cereal Proteins,* Lasztity, R. and Hidvegi, M., Eds., Reidel, Dordrecht, 1985, 349.
28. Lookhart, H. B. and Nesheim, R. O., Nutritional quality of cereal grains, in *Cereals '78, Better Nutrition for the World Millions,* Pomeranz, Y., Ed., American Association of Cereal Chemists, St. Paul, MN, 1978.
29. Lásztity, R. and Mossé, J., Extraction and composition of wheat proteins, *Ann. Technol. Agric.,* 29(2), 101, 1980.
30. Kobrehel, K., Extraction of wheat proteins with salts of fatty acids and their electrophoretic characterization, *Ann. Technol. Agric.,* 29(2), 125, 1980.
31. Jankiewicz, M., *Proteins in Cereal Technology* (Bialka w technologii zboz), Wydawnictwo Przemyslu Legkiego i Spozywczego, Warszawa, 1968.

32. Hess, K., Recent work on the constitution of wheat grain protein and the practical application of the results to new methods of manufacturing flours having high protein content, *Ind. Aliment. Agric.,* 78, 221, 1961.
33. Miflin, B. J., Byers, M., Field, J. M., and Faulks, J. A., The isolation and characterization of proteins extracted from whole milled seed, gluten and developing protein bodies of wheat, *Ann. Technol. Agric.,* 29(2), 133, 1980.

3 Wheat Proteins

I. INTRODUCTION

As a result of intensive investigations in the last 90 years the wheat proteins are the best known among the proteins of cereal grains. Many results of these investigations are summarized in some extensive reviews covering different wheat protein properties.[1-6] Nevertheless, the more in-depth investigations of wheat proteins using new techniques for separation and isolation show the complexity of these proteins. As an example it may be mentioned that only the gliadin fraction of the endosperm proteins of a single wheat variety may be separated into 46 components by a combination of gel isoelectric focusing and gel electrophoresis.[7] This fact means that in the storage protein group alone, we must work with more than 100 different proteins, not to mention the enormous number of metabolically active proteins, such as enzymes, regulatory proteins, transport proteins, etc. This great complexity of the wheat protein pool suggests that approaching the problems on the basis of solubility is not sufficient for understanding at the molecular level, the relationships of the different protein fractions to the dough properties, to indicate the significance of the varietal and agrotechnical factors in determining the properties of wheat, to find new methods in the development of baking technologies, or to solve many other problems connected with the production and processing of cereals.

The rapid growth in knowledge of molecular biology and in the development of new biochemical techniques provides new opportunities and methodologies for understanding, i.e., solving the problems mentioned above. A new approach based on biological function and biochemical development, especially genetic control, seems to be very fruitful and promising. The investigation of the genetics and biosynthesis of wheat proteins at the beginning was stimulated by the importance of wheat proteins in human nutrition and by severe shortages of foods in parts of the world. It later became clear that the knowledge of the biochemical mechanism of wheat protein biosynthesis and, generally, that of the development of cereal grains is interesting not only from the point of view of the quantity and nutritional value of the wheat proteins, but also in the understanding of some traditional problems of wheat protein investigations concerning the contribution of the wheat proteins to milling, dough forming, and baking properties of wheat and in the elaboration of more objective methods of determination of baking value. So it is understandable that in recent work on wheat proteins the investigations mentioned above play an important role.

New, improved methods for the separation of wheat proteins were developed recently, and important steps were realized in the elucidation of the structure of protein complexes of gluten. In separation and identification of specific proteins and in the study of their structural homology, immunochemical methods are of great importance.[34] Concerning the metabolically active components of the wheat grain, important new results were achieved by the investigation of enzymes, natural enzyme inhibitors, and some specific groups of minor proteins such as purothionins, ligolin, agglutinins, friabilin, etc.

This chapter is intended to provide a review of the most important developments in this area with no claims to complete the interpretation of the literature.

II. NOMENCLATURE, EXTRACTION

As was mentioned in the previous chapter, at this time an internationally accepted system for classification and nomenclature of the cereal proteins does not exist. This is also true for the wheat proteins, with the exception of enzymes and some well-defined specific proteins such as natural enzyme inhibitors or purothionines. In this and forthcoming chapters the proteins will be divided into two main groups: (1) storage proteins and (2) cytoplasmic (metabolically active) proteins. In the case of wheat, storage proteins will be treated as low molecular weight (LMW) proteins (covering practically all of the gliadins of Osborne's classification) and high molecular weight (HMW) proteins (glutenins).

Gliadin is treated as a protein according to the definition proposed by Kaczkowski and Tkachuk:[8] "proteins of wheat endosperm soluble in alcohol such as 70/100 ethanol (v/v) at room temperature, and which migrate in polyacrylamide and starch gels without reduction as reasonable discrete bands, and which are not excluded during gel filtration on Sephadex-G-100." For gliadin components the nomenclature based on gel electrophoretic mobility and proposed by Woychik et al.[9] and Jones et al.[10] (α-, β-, γ-, and ω-gliadins) will be used.

The name glutenin will be used for the high molecular weight storage protein components not soluble at room temperature in ethanol and being composed of more polypeptide chains bonded by intermolecular disulfide bonds. The polypeptides obtained after reduction of glutenin will be named as subunits of glutenin.

With regard to metabolically active proteins for enzymes, generally the widely used trivial names will be used, and in the case of minor components the names proposed by the authors of publications will be presented.

Any other specific questions about nomenclature will be discussed together with the individual proteins in corresponding chapters.

General aspects of cereal protein extraction were discussed in the previous chapter. In practice two approaches are generally used for extraction and fractionation of wheat proteins. In the first, differential extraction methods are used to achieve a preliminary fractionation based on solubility or molecular weight. The components of the fractions obtained may be further examined by other techniques possessing high resolution power. In the other (total solubility methods), an attempt is made to dissolve completely all proteins and to resolve the complex mixture obtained by differential precipitation and other effective new techniques of separation.

The use of the differential solubility method of Osborne or one of its modifications leads to relatively high quantities of insoluble "residue" proteins which remain behind.

Extraction with progressively increasing concentrations of urea has been used by Lee and McRitchie[12] and Simmonds and Wrigley,[120] among others. The first 2 *M* urea extracts contained almost exclusively low molecular weight gliadin-type proteins as judged by gel filtration. By progressively increasing the urea concentration a mixture of gliadin and glutenin and, finally, glutenin was extracted. Storage protein from which lipid had been removed during the course of its preparation was almost entirely soluble in 4 to 6 *M* urea. The residue (3 to 5% by mass) was mainly composed of organelle remnants such as small pieces of endoplasmic reticulum and small starch granules. On the basis of these results a solubility separation chart may be developed[13] (see Figure 1).

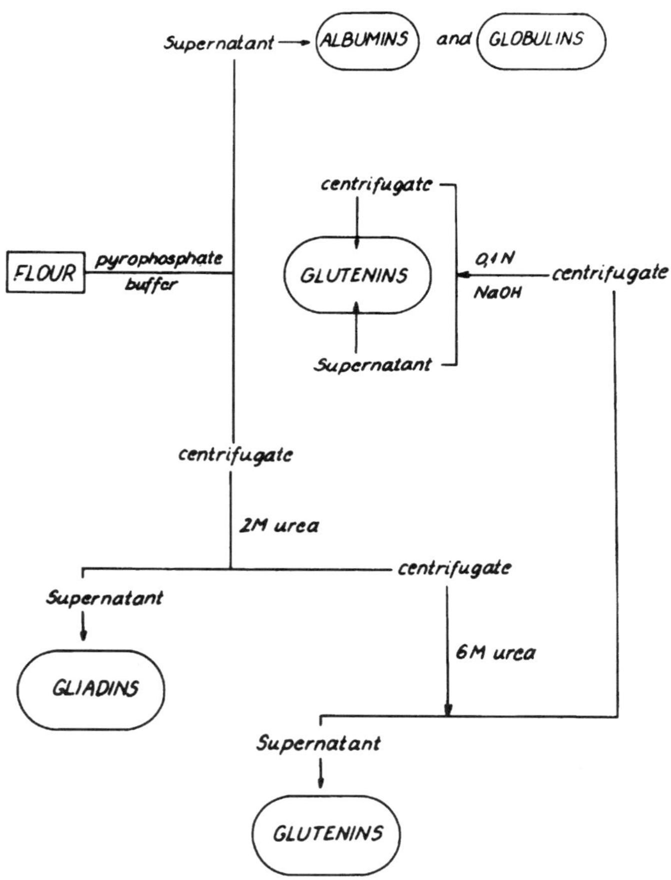

FIGURE 1 Extraction and separation of wheat protein using increasing concentrations of urea.[11-13]

In the total solubility methods group, the extraction by acetic acid[14] and the acetic acid-urea-cetyltrimethylammonium bromide (AUC) method[15,16] are widely used. When acetic acid is used, a significant fraction of the proteins remains undissolved as a gel-like residue. This protein is therefore excluded from further consideration, and this causes some uncertainty because it is not certain that the residual fraction has the same properties as the extracted glutenin; the AUC method is preferred for preparation of glutenin since it dissolves a higher proportion of the flour proteins.

Good results were achieved with the recently elaborated techniques of extraction using salts of fatty acids. It has been shown by different authors[17-20] that glutenin can be solubilized in distilled water in the presence of sodium salts of fatty acids. It has also been stated[19,20] that this method of extraction does not disrupt disulfide bonds. The solubilization of glutenin can be explained by the hydrophobic interactions between the soap molecules and the polypeptide chains.[17,19] Kobrehel[21] exhaustively investigated factors influencing the effectiveness of solubilization. On the basis of the investigations it was stated that the wheat flour proteins could be quantitatively solubilized with distilled water containing sodium salts of fatty acids. The wheat flour protein pool seems to be composed of proteins solubilized with higher or lower soap concentrations depending on the quality of the variety. The easily solubilized proteins would be albumins, globulins, and some of the gliadins, namely ω-gliadins. Protein aggregates would be composed mainly of glutenin and α-, β-, γ-gliadins.

A method combining extraction and centrifugation was elaborated by Graveland et al.[22] The purpose of this new separation method was to obtain more insight into the behavior and composition of gluten and its components. Three principles were kept in mind at the elaboration of this procedure: (1) during extraction and fractionation no cleaving of the disulfide bonds must take place; (2) fractions obtained by fractionation must be of uniform composition; and (3) characterization of the fractions must be done by more than one technique. The procedure was later improved,[23,24] especially from the point of view of the characterization and nomenclature of the different fractions to be separated. The procedure for the extraction and separation is shown in Figure 2. With the aid of sodium dodecyl sulfate (SDS) solution, the proteins of wheat flours could be separated into SDS-soluble and SDS-insoluble fraction. The SDS-soluble fraction may be fractionated with the aid of ethanol precipitation and gel filtration chromatography into albumins, globulins, gliadins, glutenins II and III, and glutelins I, II, III, and IV. The SDS-insoluble material may be separated by centrifugation into glutenin and glycoproteins.

The work of Graveland et al.[24] mentioned above is also interesting from the point of view of nomenclature of the wheat storage proteins. The terms, *soluble and residual glutenin,*[25] *glutenin I and II,* and *glutelin I, II, III, and IV,* proposed by Graveland et al.,[24] Feillet et al.,[26] and other authors are not yet widely used. The terms, *glutenin I, II, and III,* are also used for the preparations of maize proteins obtained by the method of Landry and Moureaux[29] and have been adapted for wheat glutenins by Ryadchikow et al.[30] According to this procedure, after the extraction of salt-soluble proteins and zeins by the classical Osborne method, 2-mercaptoethanol is systematically added to solvents used for glutenin subgroup extraction. The

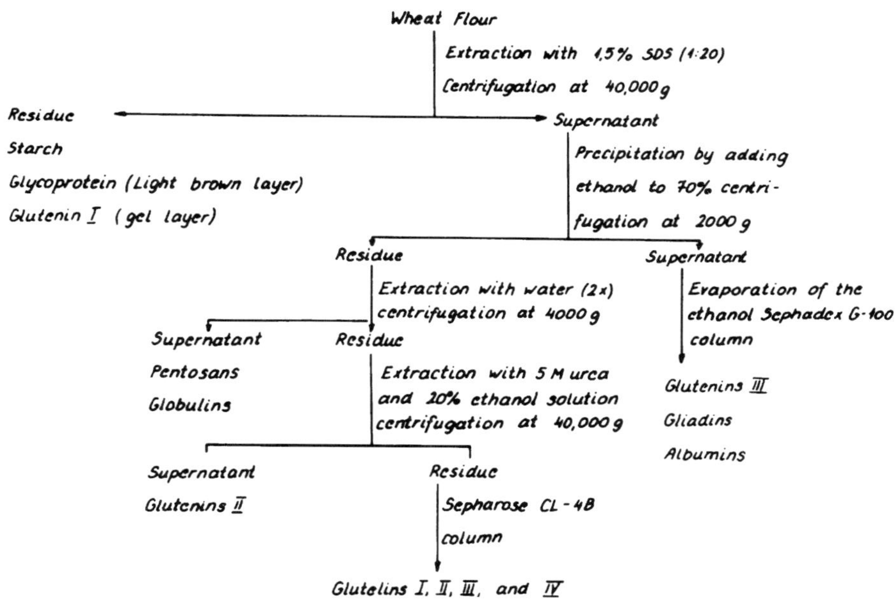

FIGURE 2 Scheme for separating SDS-insoluble and SDS-soluble wheat flour proteins.[22-24]

glutenin I is extracted by an alcohol-water mixture. The two other subgroups are then extracted by an alkaline buffer solution (pH = 10) containing either some salt (0.5 *M* NaCl) for glutenin II or some detergent (0.5% SDS) for glutenin III. The subunits of glutenin separated by gel electrophoresis are commonly divided into groups A, B, and C. The problem with the nomenclature of glutenin and its subfractions, i.e., insoluble residual proteins, probably may be solved after the more detailed investigations of the subunits by gel electrophoresis and the elucidation of the genetic background of glutenin biosynthesis.

III. STORAGE PROTEINS OF THE ENDOSPERM

A. Low Molecular Weight Storage Proteins (Gliadins)

1. Separation, Nomenclature, and Identification of Varieties

In the fractionation of gliadins extracted from the endosperm, gel filtration chromatography is known to be a useful technique. Especially in purification and preliminary fractionation the different gel columns play an important role. Also, for the comparison of different varieties (elution profile) or the investigation of the effect of agrotechnical parameters on the rough distribution of fractions this technique may be useful. On the other hand, the long separation time and the relatively poor resolution power (generally the fractions to be separated contain many individual components as revealed by gel electrophoresis) are limiting factors in the use of gel filtration. Improvement of the technique and elimination of the disadvantages could lead to a wider application. Some improvement was achieved by use of alkyl dextrans cross-linked with *N,N′*-methylene bisacrylamide (Sephacryl). These gels, introduced some years ago,[31] have relatively "rigid" properties and can withstand fairly high flow rates. They include Sephacryl S-200, which has a molecular mass fractionation range similar to that of Sephadex G-150, and Sephacryl S-300, which has a fractionation range similar to that of Sephadex G-200. The former gel has been used with formamide[32] to fractionate prolamins from wheat and corn and the latter for gel filtration of gluten proteins.[33]

Since the late 1970s a new chromatographic technique, high-performance liquid chromatography (HPLC), has become widely used also in separation of cereal proteins. Most HPLC columns are based on uniform silica spheres, which are modified to permit size exclusion (SE-HPLC) or ion exchange. Reversed-phase high performance liquid chromatography (RP-HPLC) was also developed. This technique complements most electrophoretic and chromatographic methods which separate proteins by size or charge, being based on surface hydrophobicity of individual protein components. HPLC techniques were successfully used for separation,[35,36,39] detection of quality differences,[37,38] and variety identification.[39] RP-HPLC is a particularly powerful separation technique: it reveals generally 30 to 40 components in a typical preparation of gliadin.[39]

At this time the most powerful techniques for the fractionation of proteins are gel electrophoresis and gel electrofocusing. These methods, alone or combined, thus far offer the highest resolving power of any technique yet applied to cereal proteins. Since the pioneering work of Elton and Ewart,[40,41] Woychik et al.[42] (starch gel electrophoresis), Wrigley[43,44] (electrofocusing), Bietz and Wall,[45] and Orth and Bushuk[46] (SDS-polyacrylamide gel electrophoresis [SDS-PAGE]), the various electrophoretic techniques have been widely used in different fields of study of wheat and other cereal proteins. Two-dimensional electrophoresis procedures are capable of achieving the highest resolution of wheat proteins, as approximately 418, 344, 112, and 398 protein spots were obtained from the analysis of albumins, globulins, gliadins, and glutenins, respectively, while the two-dimensional analysis of total wheat kernel proteins yielded over 1300 protein subunits.[47]

Recently a newer electrophoretic technique has been utilized in wheat protein research: capillary electrophoresis. This procedure has recently yielded excellent separations of many low and high molecular weight compounds, including proteins. A review on the applicability of capillary electrophoresis in wheat gluten investigations was recently published by Bietz.[48,49]

Gliadins are the protein group most exhaustively studied by electrophoresis. This fact is strongly correlated with efforts to find a reliable method for variety identification and to explore the genetic background of gliadin proteins, including correlations between the quality of wheat and the distribution of individual polypeptides coded in the genome of wheat.

Three main protein fractions of wheat grain — albumin, gliadin, and glutenin — have been assessed in terms of their suitability for variety identification. The gliadin proteins are clearly the best and are used most often. They are readily extracted and fractionated, and the genetic control of their synthesis is well understood.[3,4,50] On the basis of investigations it has also been stated that the gliadin electropherogram is not affected by the growth conditions of the grain, by its protein content, by sprouting, by dusting or fumigation of the grain, or by heat treatment up to and beyond that required to destroy baking quality. Significant changes occur in the relative intensities of gliadin bands only when sulfur is severely deficient during growth.[51] This condition rarely, if ever, exists in commercial crops.

Extracts used in gel electrophoretic investigation may be prepared with different solvents. The water-ethanol (1:2) mixture — used in the classical Osborne fractionation of cereal proteins — is a good solvent for gliadin, but after extraction its composition must be altered by dilution, and sucrose must be added to make the preparation suitable for electrophoresis.[52,53] Aqueous 2-chloroethanol is also widely used.[34,55] The technique for identification of varieties was recently reviewed by Wrigley.[386]

Among the methods used most commonly for the electrophoretic separation of gliadins, the starch gel electrophoresis methods are the oldest. Effective procedures for variety identification were elaborated and used in France,[56] Australia,[57] and the former Soviet Union,[58] and they were employed in modified form in many other countries.[59,60] In the most widely used methods, electrophoresis is done in acidic buffered starch gel. At such a pH, gliadin proteins are positively charged and in the applied electric field they migrate toward the cathode and separate into individual bands according to electric charge density and molecular size. After electrophoresis, the gel is stained to reveal the location of the protein bands (see Figure 3). The electropherograms obtained in this way are related to genetic constitution and are the "fingerprints" of varieties. Because most wheat varieties have specific, characteristic, unique gliadin patterns, the variety of an unknown sample can be identified by its gliadin electropherogram. If the sample is suspected to be heterogeneous, grains must be examined individually, and the result must be analyzed statistically. This "single kernel technique" has been elaborated and used to determine the varieties in the mixture and to obtain information about its composition.

By evaluating the starch gel electrophoresis technique as the first procedure effective enough for variety identification, it can be stated that the starch gel method has several advantages. Simple equipment is used that does not require cooling; the fastest moving bands of gliadins have good resolution and the support material (starch) is nontoxic.

Some disadvantages of the method were summarized by Autran et al.[61] Resolution is influenced by stirring and heating conditions of the starch slurry, and resolution of the slowest moving bands of gliadin is poor. Uniform and reproducible gels are difficult to make because the consistency of commercial batches varies. Densitometer scans are of questionable accuracy. Nevertheless, starch gel electrophoresis is routinely used in many European laboratories.

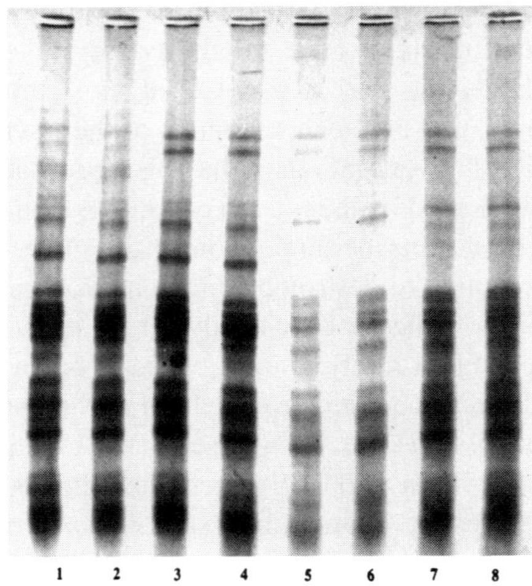

FIGURE 3 Characteristic gel electropherograms of some wheats grown in Hungary. 1 and 2, GK Pusztaszer; 3 and 4, GK Boglar; 5 and 6, Besostaya 1; 7 and 8, GK Orsi.

The PAGE procedure for separation of gliadins is also widely used in America and in many countries in Europe.[53,62-66] One-dimensional PAGE on a uniform gel is most commonly used. The procedure gives good, reproducible results under standard conditions. A disadvantage that may be mentioned is that the acrylamide monomer is a toxic chemical that is absorbed directly through the skin, and so caution should be exercised when handling the crystalline powder, the solution, or the gel. In recent years the uniform gel procedure in some cases was replaced by gradient gel electrophoresis. In gradient gel electrophoresis the concentration of polyacrylamide gel increases from the top point of sample application to the bottom. The protein zones are consequently sharpened and resolution is enhanced. Gradient gel electropherograms for the systematic identification of Australian wheats have been published by Du Cros.[68] For identifying these varieties gradient gels were preferred over starch or uniform-pore polyacrylamide gels.[62]

Gel isoelectric focusing also may be used for the separation of gliadins. The information about protein composition provided by gel isoelectric focusing is likely to differ from that obtained with gel electrophoresis because the separation principles are different: whereas gel electrophoresis gives a separation on the basis of size and charge, the protein molecules in isoelectric focusing are focused within a pH gradient to the point at which each protein loses its overall charge. Gel isoelectric focusing has not proved popular for routine identification of wheat cultivars. This is partly because differences in gliadin composition tend to be obscured by the presence of the water-soluble proteins that are extracted with the gliadins in the simple extraction procedures. On the other hand, the combination of isoelectric focusing with gel electrophoresis is useful in distinguishing between closely related wheats.[62] In this application, isoelectric focusing has revealed differences in gliadin composition that would be marked during electrophoresis in only one dimension by other components of similar electrophoretic mobility.

In practice, different systems of nomenclature and variety identification were used. The system of Konarev et al.[64,69,70] is based on the Greek letter-Arabic numeral system. Four groups of gliadins (α, β, γ, and ω-gliadins) have been distinguished on the basis of electrophoretic mobility as proposed by Woychik et al.[9] The bands within the four main zones mentioned above are identified by Arabic numbers. On the basis of the investigation of wheat in Russia the possible number of bands in the four groups are the following: α-zone, 7; β-zone, 5; γ-zone, 5; and ω-zone, 12. The composite electropherogram of hexaploid (common) wheat has the following formula, α, 1 to 7; β, 1 to 5; γ, 1 to 5; and ω, 1 to 12.

In the formula used by Konarev for characterization of wheat varieties, the numbers representing bands that stain intensively are underlined and those that stain weakly are written in parentheses. Doublets are identified with two dots above the number. A minor deviation in mobility (not considered as a different component) of a β- or ω-band is indicated by a subscript 1 if the displacement is in the direction of the faster neighboring band and by a subscript 2 if the deviation is in the direction of the slower neighboring band. An example of the formula generated by this procedure for the variety Kharkovskaja 46 is

$$\alpha 5\ (6)\ 7\ \beta(2)\ 3_2\ 4\ 5\ \gamma 2\ 5\ \omega\ 3\ \dot{4}\ \dot{6}\ \dot{7}$$

This nomenclature is used extensively in the published catalogs of the gliadin electropherogram formula of Soviet hard and durum wheats.[71,72]

In the system developed at the University of Manitoba by Bushuk et al.[53,67] each band in the electropherogram is represented by two numbers: the first represents the relative mobility, and the second represents relative intensity. Both numbers are derived by comparison with the values for an arbitrary reference band in the electropherogram of the Canadian hard red spring wheat variety Marquis. This system of nomenclature based on the relative mobilities referred to well-characterized wheat protein standards (characteristic bands of gliadin or other wheat proteins) and might be used successfully for practical purposes. The derivation of the varietal formula for Marquis according Bushuk et al.[67] is shown in Figure 4. The Marquis reference band, readily identified because it is followed by a distinct doublet, is assigned an arbitrary relative mobility of 50, and its migration distance is measured to the nearest millimeter. Similarly, the migration distances of all other visible bands are measured, and the relative mobility values are calculated to the nearest half unit (right). With an appropriate linear scale based on 50 for the reference band, the relative mobilities can be read directly. Next the band intensities are quantified subjectively by a number from one to five, with five representing the most intensely stained bands. This can be done by a visual examination of electropherograms, with one "intensity reference band" chosen to represent each relative intensity. The varietal formula for Marquis can be written in the following way: the relative mobility of each band is represented by the first number and the relative intensity of the band is shown in parentheses.

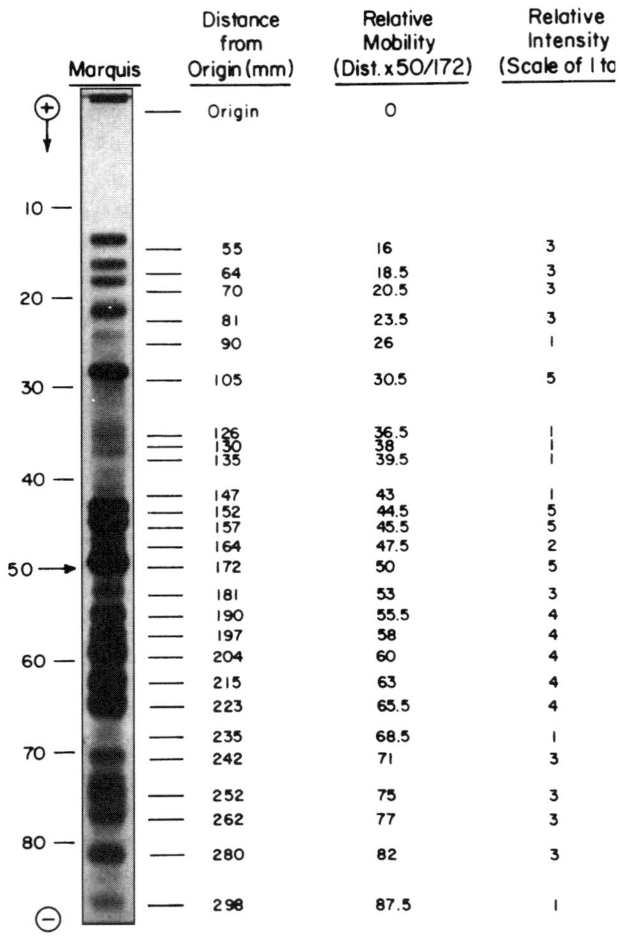

FIGURE 4 Derivation of the varietal formula from the gliadin electropherogram for the variety Marquis. (From Bushuk, W., Rerie, W., and Zillman, R.R., Procedure Manual for Polyacrylamide Gel Electrophoresis of Gliadins as a Basis for Wheat Cultivar Identification, Department of Plant Science, University of Manitoba, Winnipeg. With permission.)

16.0 (3) 18.5 (3) 20.5 (3) 23.5 (3) 26.0 (1) 30.5 (5)
36.5 (1) 38.0 (1) 39.5 (1) 43.0 (1) 44.5 (5) 45.5 (5)
47.5 (2) 50.0 (5) 53.0 (3) 55.5 (4) 58.0 (4) 60.0 (4)
63.0 (4) 65.5 (4) 68.5 (1) 71.0 (3) 75.0 (3) 77.0 (3)
82.0 (3) 87.5 (1)

The distribution and intensity of characteristic bands may be registered by an automatic recording densitometer. For variety identification different computer procedures have also been developed.[73]

An improved method for standardizing polyacrylamide gel electrophoresis of wheat gliadin proteins was published by Lookhart et al.[74] This standardized method — as reported by the authors — should reduce the deleterious effects of the variables (purity and concentration of aluminum lactate, the type of gel former, and the method of gel preparation) and enhance the day-to-day reproducibility of the gliadin separations. The method was successfully used for the identification of wheat cultivars most commonly grown in the U.S.[75] A characteristic densitogram and a summary of electrophoretic formulas of gliadins of hard red winter wheats grown in the U.S. are given in Figure 5 and Table 1, respectively.

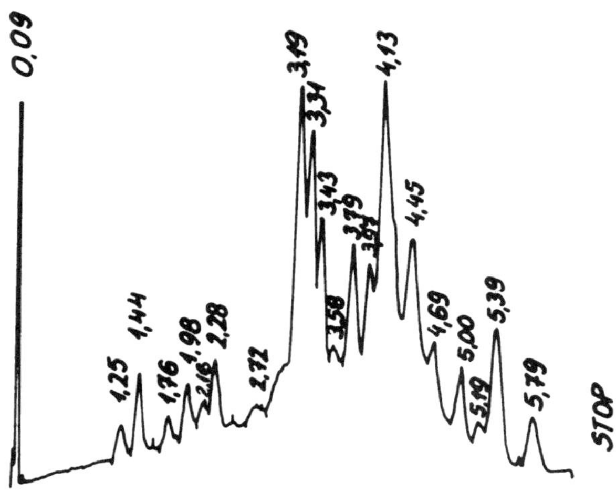

FIGURE 5 Densitometer scan of the Tascosa gliadin electropherogram. The numbers above the peaks indicate the times, in minutes, that bands were encountered by the densitometer. (From Jones, B.L., Lookhart, G.L., Hall, S.E., and Finney, F.K., *Cereal. Chem.*, 59, 181, 1982. With permission.)

A third approach to nomenclature is used by some Australian specialists.[76] Electrophoretic patterns were first reduced to a series of numbers to facilitate systematic comparison. Sufficient band positions were allocated to provide for all bands in the patterns being considered. These positions were numbered 1 to 31. Later consideration of other cultivars necessitated the allocation of band position 32. For each band position a number was given to indicate band intensity. Absence was indicated by number 1; light, medium, and dark intensities were designated by 2, 3, and 4, respectively. Diagrams of electrophoretic patterns for some Australian wheats, including a numerical formula, according to Wrigley[65] and Wrigley and McCausland[77] are shown in Figure 6.

A completely different system for genetic classification of storage proteins of wheat and for variety characterization was elaborated by Sozinov and Poperelya.[58] The analysis of monosomic and segregating lines of the gliadin electropherogram indicated to these researchers that gliadin bands were inherited in linked groups or

TABLE 1
Electrophoretic Formulas of Gliadins of Some Hard Red Winter Wheats Grown in the U.S.[75]

Cultivar	Mobility of Bands Relative to Marquis Standard Band
Agent	17(2), 20(2), 25(2), 30(1), 33(2), 36(1), 40(1), 42(5), 47(4), 49(1), 52(3), 54(2), 55(2), 60(2), 61(2), 63(2), 65(2), 71(1), 73(2), 77(3), 80(2), 81(1), 85(1)
Centurk	13(1), 17(1), 19(1), 22(2), 32(2), 43(1), 45(5), 48(2), 52(2), 55(3), 57(2), 58(3), 62(2), 65(1), 69(1), 72(1), 75(4), 78(2)
Cheyenne	13(1), 16(1), 18(1), 22(1), 30(1), 32(2), 44(4), 45(4), 50(2), 52(1), 56(3), 59(3), 62(2), 65(1), 69(1), 73(1), 76(4), 79(2)
Eagle	13(1), 16(2), 18(1), 21(2), 25(1), 29(1), 31(2), 33(1), 40(1), 42(1), 45(5), 48(1), 49(2), 52(1), 55(3), 57(1), 59(4), 62(3), 65(1), 69(1), 72(2), 75(3), 79(1), 81(1)
Lancota	13(1), 16(1), 18(1), 21(1), 25(1), 30(1), 38(1), 42(1), 45(5), 49(1), 51(3), 53(1), 56(3), 60(3), 63(2), 66(2), 71(2), 75(2), 77(2), 83(2), 88(1)
Parker	13(1), 16(2), 18(1), 22(2), 28(2), 30(1), 33(1), 38(1), 39(1), 44(1), 46(4), 48(5), 53(2), 56(3), 58(2), 60(3), 63(2), 70(2), 73(2), 76(3), 80(2), 82(1)
Scout 66	13(1), 16(26), 18(1), 21(2), 25(1), 29(1), 31(2), 33(1), 40(1), 42(1), 45(5), 48(1), 49(2), 51(1), 54(3), 59(4), 62(3), 65(1), 69(1), 72(1), 75(3), 77(1)
Triumph 64	13(1), 16(2), 18(1), 21(3), 25(2), 27(1), 29(1), 33(2), 36(1), 38(1), 40(1), 42(5), 44(1), 46(4), 49(1), 51(1), 53(1), 55(1), 58(2), 60(3), 63(1), 65(2), 73(3), 77(3), 80(1), 83(1), 86(1)

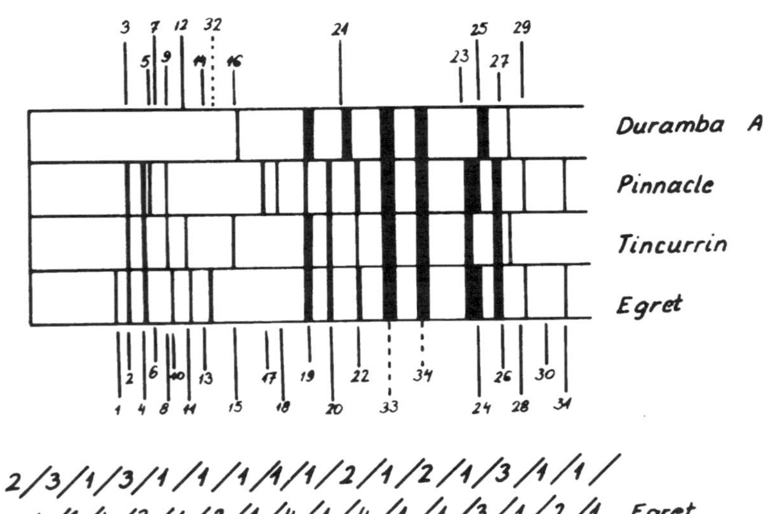

FIGURE 6 Diagrams of electrophoretic patterns and gliadin band positions used for computer-based comparisons. The electropherogram of Egret is shown in the numerical form used for computer-based comparison.[80,81]

blocks controlled by genes on specific chromosomes. When electropherograms of different wheat varieties were examined, it was noted that the same chromosome could give rise to different blocks, called allelic blocks. Each allelic block is identified by the chromosome and the block number. This approach has been developed to the extent that the varietal electropherogram can be represented by an allelic block formula. Allelic blocks of some Russian wheat varieties are given in Table 2.[78] On the basis of the allelic block analysis, varietal formulae for the first two varieties in Table 2 can be written as Alabasskaja-1A1, 1B1, 1D5, 6A3, 6B1, and 6D1, and Uljanovka-1A2, 1B1, 1D5, 6A3, 6B1, and 6D2.

TABLE 2
Genetic Formulas of Gliadin in Several Russian (Soviet) Wheat Varieties[78]

	Gliadin Formula According to Blocks Controlled by Chromosomes					
Variety	1A	1B	1D	6A	6B	6D
Alabasskaja	1	1	5	3	1	2
Uljanovka	2	1	5	3	1	2
Odesskaya 16	1+2	1	5	3	2	1
Kharkhovskaja 159	1	1	5	3	1	1
Mironovskaja 808	3	1	5	3	1	2
Jubileynaya	4	1	5	3	1	2
Byelotserkovskaja 198	5	1	5	3	1	2
Krasnodarskaya 39	1	1+2	1	3	1	2
Dneprovskaya 521	1	2	1	1	1	1
Besostaya 1	4	1	1	1	1	1
Kavkaz	4	3	2	1	1	1

This genetic classification of storage and gliadin proteins is relatively complex for routine variety identification. On the other hand, the method has great potential in the solving of many theoretical and practical problems of plant breeding and seed production. The relationships between the allelic blocks and variation in traits such as technological (baking) value, low temperature tolerance, disease resistance, spike, color, etc. are not quite clear. However, the accumulating data suggest that prolamin allelic blocks are markers of gene blocks or nonrecombinant parts of the chromosomes that play an important role in the formation of some characteristics.

Recently a RP-HPLC technique has also been successfully used for variety identification, as reported by Lookhart et al.,[79] Marchylo et al.,[80] Bietz,[81] and Bietz and Cobb.[82] Capillary electrophoresis is also suggested for such purposes.[49,387]

2. Composition and Structure

The investigation made by high resolution power techniques of separation showed the complexity of the gliadin group of proteins. Since there are many differences in gliadin components among different wheat varieties, there are probably hundreds of different gliadin components that can be distinguished by electrophoresis and electrofocusing. In addition, some data from the amino acid sequencing indicated that heterogeneity might occur at positions in the sequence corresponding to neutral amino acids; such heterogeneity would not be distinguishable by most physical methods. Because of the complexity of the gliadins the isolation of totally homogeneous components is very difficult. Mostly preparations containing some components very similar in amino acid composition and structure are obtained, showing only one major band upon gel electrophoresis. Most of the single bands separated by SDS-PAGE or electrophoresis at low pH can be separated into two or more components by two-dimensional electrophoresis.[83]

As mentioned earlier, on the basis of electrophoretic mobility at low pH the wheat gliadins may be separated into the slowest group, named the ω-gliadins, and three faster groups, named the α-, β-, and γ-gliadins. Due to the differences in cysteine content the gliadin components may be divided into S-rich (α-, β-, and γ-gliadins) and S-poor (ω-gliadins) components.

The amino acid compositions of isolated α-, β-, γ-, and ω-gliadin preparations (containing more or less individual polypeptides) were determined and published. Some of these results are summarized in Tables 3 and 4. All data are transformed on a uniform basis of residues per 100,000 g protein to make it easier for the reader to compare compositions. A comparative evaluation of the amino acid compositions of the gliadins of *Triticum vulgare* was published by Charbonnier et al.[89] The amino acid content ranges presented are summarized in Table 5. The data, given in residues per 1000 residues, were transformed to residues per 100,000 g protein using the factor 8.55 (assuming an average amino acid weight of 117).

On the basis of the data collected in Tables 3 to 5, it can be stated that all gliadin components have an extremely high glutamic acid content. In some ω-gliadins the glutamic acid content is higher than 50%. Almost all of the glutamic acid content of the gliadins is present as glutamine. Investigations of a large number of Hungarian wheat samples showed an amidation degree of 88.8%. These data are supported also by the low free carboxyl group content in the whole gliadin content determined on the basis of titration curves or esterification of free carboxyl groups. Since glutamine provides a concentrated source of nitrogen that can be used readily by the germinating seed, it seems that the cereal grains, such as wheat, have a highly concentrated glutamine reserve in the form of gliadins and other storage proteins. It also may be mentioned that the nitrogen reserve in the form of glutamine is the most economical from the perspective of biochemical pathways. As is known to occur in plants, glutamic acid (i.e., glutamine) is directly formed from α-keto-glutaric acid and ammonia produced by the nitrate reductase system via reduction of nitrates. The ω-gliadins contain the highest proportion of glutamine. The aspartic acid and asparagine contents of all gliadins are relatively low.

The gliadins have a high proline content. Proline may be present in such large proportions for the same reason that glutamine is present in large quantities — it has a close connected pathway of biosynthesis to glutamic acid. The high proline content has an effect on the secondary structure of gliadin polypeptides because the formation of α-helices is hindered by the presence of proline side chains.

TABLE 3
Amino Acid Composition of Gliadin and Gliadin Subfractions

	Residues per 100,000 g Protein				
Amino Acid	Whole Gliadin[a]	A_2-Gliadin HRW Mixture[b]	A_{1b}-Gliadin[b]	A_2-Gliadin[b]	G_1-Gliadin[c]
Lysine	5.0	3.2	5.3	3.1	Trace
Histidine	16.3	17.5	17.2	17.5	13.1
Arginine	17.4	14.7	15.9	14.7	12.5
Aspartic acid	24.8	25.1	24.1	25.0	25.0
Threonine	21.3	12.6	12.8	12.5	16.9
Serine	53.6	46.3	46.9	46.3	46.9
Glutamic acid	301.1	336	314	339	344
Proline	142.0	127	125	127	133
Glycine	26.8	21.5	21.3	21.6	21.3
Alanine	28.6	23.0	21.9	23.1	29.4
Cysteine	29.0	16.3	18.8	16.3	18.1
Valine	41.6	38.3	40.3	38.4	38.1
Methionine	10.9	8.7	6.3	8.8	6.9
Isoleucine	38.0	38.4	37.5	38.1	40.6
Leucine	60.6	69.1	72.2	69.1	61.9
Tyrosine	16.0	26.5	26.9	26.6	24.4
Phenylalanine	37.5	30.7	30.6	30.6	31.9
Tryptophan	3.8	3.3	3.4	3.4	1.9
Amide	298.7	307	ND	ND	ND

Note: ND, not determined.

[a] From Ewart.[388]
[b] From Platt and Kasarda.[85]
[c] From Huebner et al.[86]

Gliadins are poor in basic amino acids, especially lysine. From the nutritional point of view, lysine is the limiting essential amino acid in the storage proteins (and also in the whole grain) of wheat. The low levels of lysine, arginine, and histidine, along with the low levels of free carboxyl groups, place the gliadins among the least charged proteins known.

The ω-gliadins have relatively high levels of phenylalanine in addition to their high content of glutamine and proline. Phenylalanine residues make up about 10% of the total residues in ω-gliadins. Low amounts of S-containing amino acids are typical for ω-gliadins. Some fractions do not contain cysteine and methionine; they have been named "atkins" by Booth and Ewart.[90]

On the basis of molecular weight the gliadin components may be divided into two groups. The α-, β-, and γ-gliadins have molecular weights of about 30 kDa. The molecular weights of ω-gliadins, determined as well by ultracentrifugation as

TABLE 4
Amino Acid Composition of Some Gliadin Components (Residues Per 100,000 g Protein)

	Gliadins			
Amino Acid	β_3 ("Wichita")[a]	γ_3 ("Ponca")[b]	ω_{42} ("Capelle")[c]	Gliadin ("Ponca")[d]
Lysine	4.4	5.6	2.6	5.0
Histidine	14.0	12.2	4.5	14.5
Arginine	14.1	10.6	2.2	15.0
Aspartic acid	25.3	15.0	0.7	20.0
Threonine	15.6	18.9	13.5	18.0
Serine	50.1	38.1	46.5	38.0
Glutamic acid	313	343	386	317
Proline	146	163	255	148
Glycine	22.9	23.3	7.2	25.0
Alanine	28.2	28.9	2.5	25.0
Cysteine	19.6	16.7	0.0	10.0
Valine	40.6	36.1	2.8	43.0
Methionine	5.2	9.4	0.0	12.0
Isoleucine	40.7	39.4	15.4	37.0
Leucine	62.4	55.6	30.3	62.0
Tyrosine	27.7	3.3	9.7	16.0
Phenylalanine	32.1	48.9	75.3	38.0
Tryptophan	5.5	6.7	1.5	5.0
Amide	ND	ND	ND	301

Note: ND, not determined.

[a] From Booth.[87]
[b] From Huebner et al.[86]
[c] From Charbonnier et al.[88]
[d] From Wu and Dimler.[155,156]

by SDS-PAGE or gel filtration, are approximately twice as high as those of α-, β-, and γ-gliadins.

The investigations of the primary structure (amino acid sequence) of gliadin components began in 1974 with the work of Kasarda et al.[91] The N-terminal sequence of the α-gliadin components was determined. Later N-terminal sequences of other gliadins were also investigated.[92-94] The results support the theory that the large number of gliadins is believed to be due to genetic mutation of a common precursor during the natural evolution of bread wheats. It is supposed that mutations affecting the storage proteins of the cereals may be less critical to their survival than those affecting metabolically active proteins. Such mutations, since they are not lethal, have persisted to the present time. Most of the α- and β-gliadins and also some γ-gliadins have the following N-terminal sequence:[91,93]

TABLE 5
Ranges of Gliadin Amino Acid Contents (Residues per 100,000 g Protein)[89]

Amino Acid Groups	Gliadins α	β	γ	ω_1	ω_2	ω_3
Basic amino acids	50–35	37–28	28–25	27	20–21	8–12
Glutamic acid and glutamine	282–333	291–342	321–342	422	475–476	386–400
Proline	124–137	128–145	133–162	168	167–169	214–255
Cysteine	17–22	19–22	17–21	8	0	0
Methionine	6–9	5–12	7–14	3	0	0
Phenylalanine	30–34	29–42	32–47	73	81–88	75–80

1 2 3 4 5 6 7 8 9 10
Val–Arg–Val–Pro–Val–Pro–Glu–Leu–Glu–Pro

This sequence was called an "α-type" N-terminal sequence by Autran et al.[92] This α-type sequence is common not only to most of the α- and β-constituents and some of the γ-gliadins of a given wheat variety, but also to the α- and β-constituents of different varieties.

The N-terminal amino acid sequences of two γ-gliadins of Ponca wheat[93] were found to be different:

1 2 3 4 5 6 7 8 9 10
γ2 Asn–His–Gly–Val–Asp–Pro–Trp–Gly–Glu–Val
Pro Glu Val Glu Leu

γ3 Asn–Met–Gly–Val–Asp–Pro–Trp–Gly–Glu–Val
Pro Glu Glu Val Glu Glu

This type of sequence was called a γ-type N-terminal sequence. The few known sequences of ω-gliadins cannot be connected with any of these sequences.

The most highly characterized gliadin fraction is the aggregable α-gliadin of Bernardin et al.,[95] also called A-gliadin. This protein is composed of a number of very similar protein components. The multiplicity of the A-gliadin components is probably connected with multiple genes. This problem was discussed by Kasarda.[84] This author proposed a hypothesis concerning the ancestral A-gliadin gene. The possible mechanism for formation of this ancestral gene is based on the following amino acid sequence observed in an ω-gliadin from the wheat variety Justin:

–PRO–GLN–GLN–PRO–TYR–PRO–GLN–GLN–PRO–TYR

The predominance of glutamine and proline in gliadins, combined with the observation of the repeated five-member sequence shown above, leads to the speculation that reiteration of a short DNA sequence similar but not necessarily identical to the ω-gliadin repeat provided the basis for the ancestral A-gliadin gene. Introduction of transcription controls at appropriate points in the sequence completed this process. This mechanism is similar to that proposed for the origin of genes for many other proteins that include highly repetitive sequences. In addition, Thompson and Murray[96] have concluded from a consideration of the considerable variations in genome size that occur, even within a single genus, among higher plants that DNA sequence amplifications, rearrangements, and deletions are frequent events during evolution.

To illustrate the hypothesis the author calculated the composition of A-gliadin on the basis of the expected mutation of the ancestral gene by using a single model based on the following assumption:

1. The reiterated DNA sequence consisted of five codons (CAG, CAG, CAG, CCA, TAC) corresponding to the sequence –GLN–GLN–GLN–PRO–TYR; this sequence was chosen on the basis of trial calculations.
2. The only changes in amino acids resulted from single base changes of the fundamental codons; these are illustrated in Figure 7.
3. The extent of mutation that occurred was equivalent to the change in the proportion of glutamine going from the unmutated protein to A-gliadin (43%); proline and tyrosine changed in the same proportion.
4. Only those changes that produced neutral amino acids became fixed; changes that produced charged amino acids disappeared. The entire 43% change in glutamine resulted only in the production of two amino acids, leucine and proline, in equal amounts.
5. There were no functional constraints on mutation (except in the implied constraint of the fourth assumption).

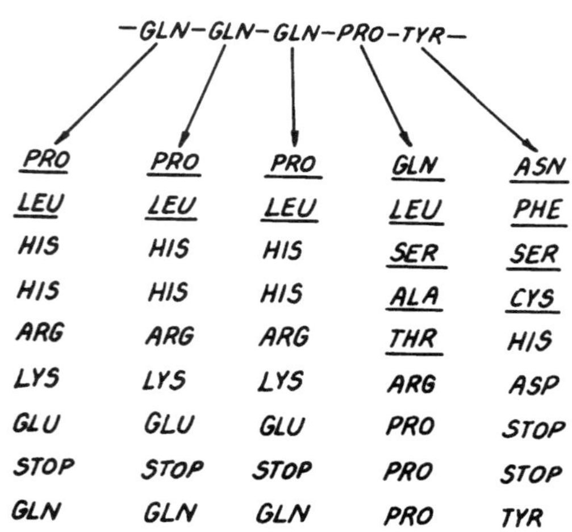

FIGURE 7 Transformations resulting from single-base changes in the codons of the fundamental repeating unit. Allowed amino acid changes are underlined. (From Kasarda, D.D., *Ann. Technol. Agric.*, 29, 151, 1980. With permission.)

The results of the calculation showed good agreement between the hypothetical A-gliadin composition and the actual amino acid composition. Kasarda suggests that it is possible that the ancestral gene for A-gliadins was also the ancestral gene for all other gliadins, which have diverged from one another by way of duplications and mutations.

In the last decade major progress was made in genetic analysis of wheat storage proteins. Investigations of gliadin polypeptides showed that genes coding for gliadin polypeptides are located on the short arm of chromosomes 1A, 1B, 1D, 6A, 6B, and 6D.[97] Structural genes for the ω-gliadins (S-poor prolamins) are located on the short arm of chromosomes 1A, 1B, and 1D. Most of the γ-gliadins and a few β-gliadins are encoded by genes tightly linked to those for ω-gliadins at the Gli-A1 and Gli-D1 loci. The remaining γ- and β-gliadins and all the α-gliadins are encoded by additional loci present on the short arm of chromosomes 6A, 6B, and 6D (Gli-A2, Gli-B2, Gli-D2).[83] The knowledge of gliadin-coding genes and their isolation and sequencing opened new pathways for studying the amino acid sequence and structure of individual gliadin polypeptides. As a result of more recent investigations the amino acid sequences of a number of α-type and β-type gliadins are known, most of which have been deduced from genomic and cDNA sequences.[98-100] These results confirm the suggested general characteristics of sequences (variability, presence of repeating units with high glutamic acid and proline content, relatively higher cysteine-cystine content comparing to ω-gliadins) suggested in earlier publications.

In all cases the α-gliadins contain six cysteines and the γ-gliadins eight cysteines. Comparison of the sequence contexts of the cysteine residues in the two types of proteins demonstrate that all six cysteines present in the α-type gliadins are also present in the γ-type gliadins, but that the latter contain two additional cysteines. Only partial sequences of ω-gliadins are known. Nevertheless, the main features of these polypeptides (repetitive domains, low cysteine content) are confirmed.

Structural studies of gliadin polypeptides have been limited by the difficulty of preparing adequate amounts of single homogeneous components. Progress in molecular biology has provided possibilities for solving these problems. *In vitro* synthesis of proteins,[102] expression of gliadin polypeptides in *Saccharomyces cerevisiae* yeast,[101,103] and expression of wheat seed protein genes in transgenic tobacco[104] are examples of realization of the possibilities mentioned above.

In earlier studies Lásztity[105] suggested that the molecular structure of the gliadin components is generally globular. The proportion of α-helical parts is relatively low due to the high proline content. Disulfide bonds are in every case intramolecular. The proposed structure is demonstrated in Figure 8.

The conformation of A-gliadins was exhaustively studied by Kasarda[84] using circular dichroism (CD) and spectropolarimetry. A-gliadins are a group of α-type gliadins encoded by genes on chromosome 6A. They aggregate to form fibrils under certain conditions of pH (approximately 5.0) and ionic strength (0.005 *M*) and can be prepared in a form that is substantially pure. The results indicate that A-gliadin has a significant amount of α-helical structure; about 33% of its polypeptide chain is α-helical in structure. Because of the large number of proline residues (which cannot participate in α-helices) in A-gliadin, it seems likely that many of the

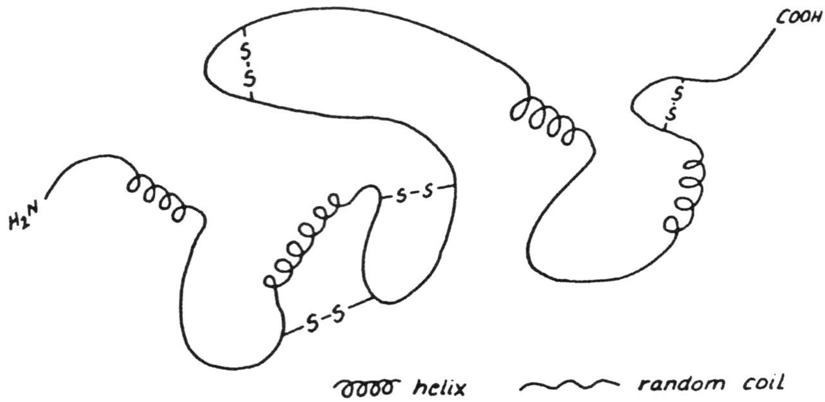

FIGURE 8 Structure of the low molecular weight gluten protein.

α-helical segments of A-gliadin will be short. Optical measurements also show the presence of a stable conformational structure. The tyrosine, tryptophan, phenylalanine, and cysteine residues are involved in the fixed conformational structure. It was also stated that conformational changes occur in the A-gliadin molecule when it goes from aqueous solution to alcohol-water solution, although the optical activity indicates that the new conformation is a stable one. The optical characteristics of tyrosine and tryptophan side chains have diminished, and new bands near 260 and 268 μm may result from stable structures involving phenylalanine side chains, insofar as similar bands have been observed in a protein that has no tyrosine or tryptophan.[107] For the A-gliadin components it is characteristic that the A-gliadin monomers aggregate, forming microfibrils. The possible mechanism of aggregation proposed by Kasarda[84] is shown in Figure 9.

At pH 3 A-gliadin dissociates and partially unfolds as a consequence of excess positive charges. As the pH is increased, free carboxyl groups ionize, which decreases the net charge of the molecule. The subunits become compactly folded and aggregate in a specific way to form microfibrils. This aggregation is enhanced by increased ionic strength. Hydrophobic interactions may also play a role in formation of A-gliadin aggregates.[84,108,109]

More recent investigations concerning the structure of α-gliadins have shown that the molecular structure of these proteins is more complicated that was suggested on the basis of earlier studies. A recent review about the molecular structure of cereal prolamins has been published by Tatham et al.[3] The general features of an α-gliadin protein[114] and the domain structure of α-gliadin[115] are shown in Figure 10. All the cysteine groups are involved in intrachain disulfide bond formation and are located in the C-terminal nonrepetitive domains.

The N-terminal portion contains the repetitive domain and the first polyglutamine region. The contents of different types of secondary structure in the A-gliadin and α-gliadins are shown in Table 6, which is based on data of Purcell et al.[116] and Tatham et al.[117] The predicted secondary structure of the A-gliadin sequence published by Kasarda et al.[98] is shown in Figure 11.

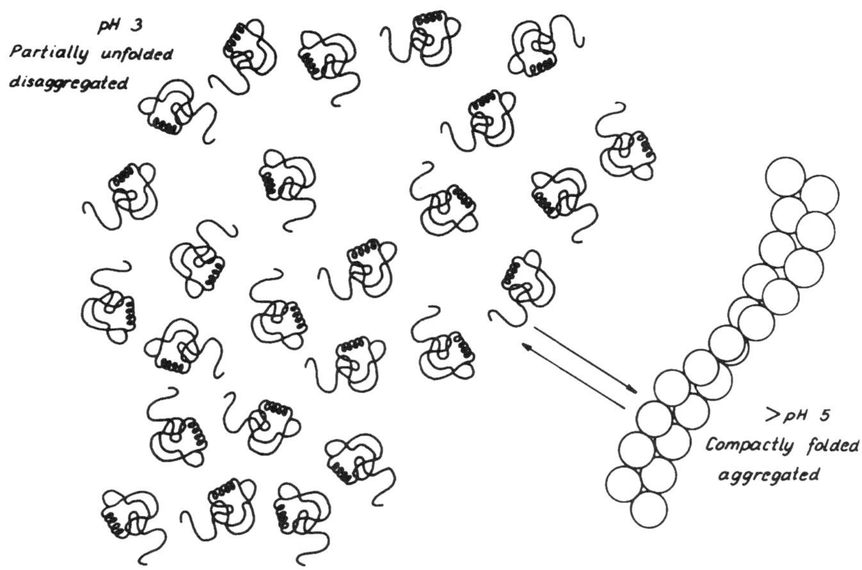

FIGURE 9 Schematic representation of the aggregation of A-gliadin protein subunits into fibrillar form. (From Kasarda, D.D., *Ann. Technol. Agric.*, 29, 151, 1980. With permission.)

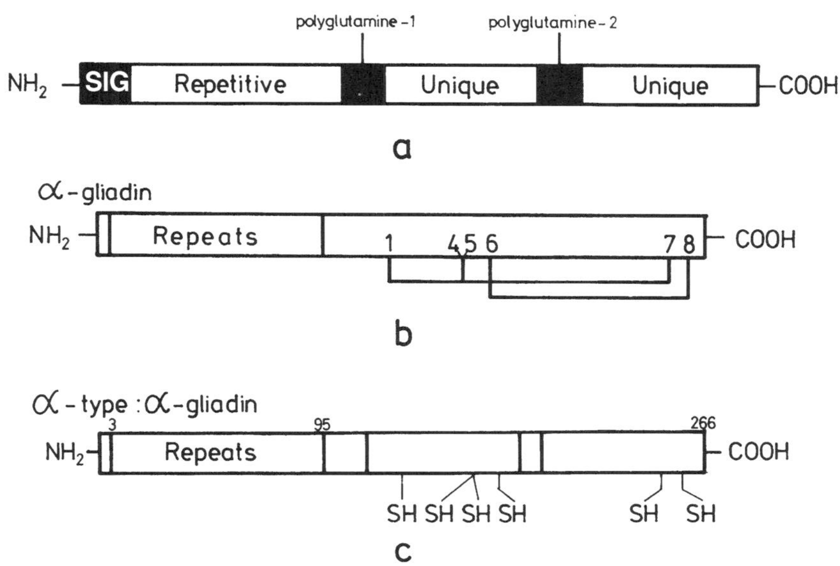

FIGURE 10 (a) General features of an α-gliadin protein.[114] The signal sequence (SIG) is cleaved during posttranslational processing. (b) Location of disulfide bridges. (c) Location of SH groups in α-gliadins.[115]

TABLE 6
Secondary Structure Contents of Gliadins Determined from the Deconvolution of Circular Dichroism Spectra

	Secondary Structure			
Protein	**α-Helix**	**β-Sheet**	**β-Turn**	**Random Coil**
A-Gliadins[116]				
pH = 3, 20°C	24	33	1	43
pH = 5, 20°C	28	38	0	34
α-Gliadins[117]				
70% ÉtOH, 20°C	36–37	11–12	52–53	52–53
70% ÉtOH, 80°C	29–30	8–9	61–62	61–62

Note: Values are content (%).

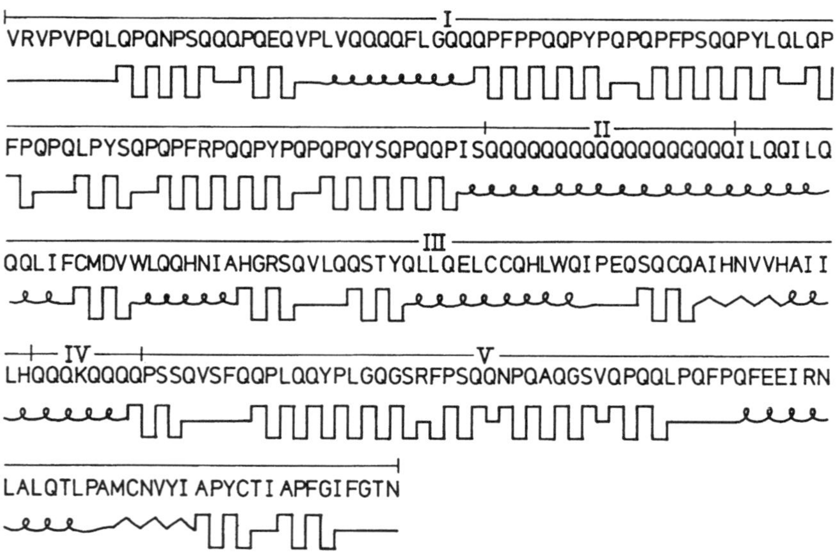

FIGURE 11 Predicted secondary structure of the A-gliadin sequence α-helix (ℓℓℓℓ), random coil (⎍⎍⎍), nucleic acid (cDNA), and amino acid sequences of α-type gliadins from wheat *(Triticum aestivum).* (From Kasarda, D.D. et al., *Proc. Natl. Acad. Sci. U.S.A.,* 81, 4712, 1984. With permission.)

The γ-type gliadins of wheat have been studied less extensively than the α-type. The structural organization of this type of gliadin is shown in Figure 12. As seen from the figure, all eight of the cysteine residues are located at the C-terminal domain and the characteristic repeats (PQQPFPQ) are at the N-terminal domain. All the cysteine residues are involved in formation of intramolecular disulfide bonds.

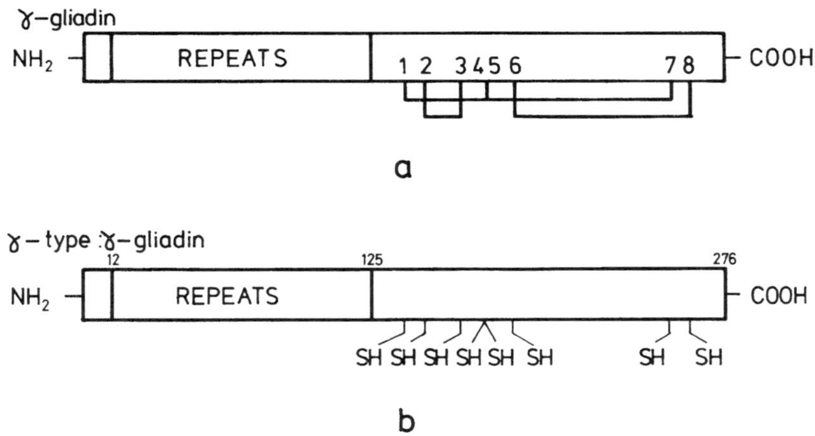

FIGURE 12 Structural organization of γ-type gliadins.[115] (a) Location of disulfide bonds; (b) location of SH groups.

Summarizing our knowledge concerning molecular structure of low molecular weight, S-rich gliadins (α-, β-, γ-gliadins), all appear to be compact, tightly folded molecules that are unusually stable to thermal treatment.[3] At least some of this stability derives from the presence of disulfide bonds which are intramolecular in the monomeric forms. CD spectroscopy and structure prediction both show that the members of this group of gliadins are remarkably similar in secondary structure, although some differences are also apparent. These differences would affect the overall dimensions of the polypeptides. This view is supported by studies of Popineau and Pineau,[118] who studied the conformation and surface hydrophobicity of α-, β-, and γ-gliadins under a range of conditions of pH and salt concentration by gel permeation chromatography and 2 p toluidinyl-naphtalene-6-sulfonate (TNS) binding, respectively. It was found that α- and β-gliadins (α-type gliadins) behaved as compact globular proteins; the γ-gliadin had a higher hydrodynamic value, suggesting a more extended structure.

The near- and far-UV CD spectra of ω-gliadins in 70% (v/v) aqueous ethanol and 0.1 *M* acetic acid and at temperatures ranging from 20°C to 80°C showed that these polypeptides are rich in β-turns.[119] These results together with observations of Popineau and Pineau[118] indicate that ω-gliadins are rod-shaped molecules with unusual secondary structures based predominantly on repetitive β-turns.

Despite the great progress in wheat gliadin chemistry, biochemistry, and genetics, we are far from having complete knowledge of all gliadins present in different wheat cultivars. To give an idea about the complexity of the problems to be solved some statements of a recent publication of Metakovski et al.[120] will be summarized here. Over several years 391 wheat cultivars from 7 countries were studied and 690 different gliadin electrophoretic patterns were found (Table 7). The number of patterns exceeded the number of cultivars because many cultivars have natural biotypes differing in gliadin allele composition. Differences in the electrophoretic patterns of wheat genotypes are a consequence of vast multiple allelism at the gliadin-coding loci. A recent catalogue describes more then ten alleles for each of the six main Gli loci (in total 111). This number of alleles is sufficient to distinguish (theoretically) more than 30 million different gliadin allele compositions.

TABLE 7
Number of Gliadin Genotypes in Different Countries and Breeding Centers[120]

Country	Number of Cultivars Studied	Number of Gliadin Genotypes Found
Australia	28	29
Canada	22	25
England	43	51
Italy	105	137
Bulgaria	36	72
Russia	106	298
Yugoslavia	51	82
Total	**391**	**694**

3. Gliadin-Lipid and Gliadin-Carbohydrate Interactions

It is well known that gliadin preparations always contain lipids. Bushuk et al.[121] and McMaster[122] reported that the ethanol-soluble fraction of gluten (mainly gliadin) contained about 10% nonprotein material, of which 0.6% was carbohydrate and the remaining 9.4% was presumed to be lipid. The lipid content of the preparations may vary according to the procedure used for the production of the gliadin preparation (preliminary defatting of the flour by different solvents, use of undefatted flour, extraction from flour or wet gluten, etc.). It is commonly known that the majority of protein-lipid complexes are detectable in doughs, being formed in the presence of phospholipids during the hydration of the proteins. On the other hand, various other lipoproteins may be obtained by extraction of flour with some organic solvents. Several different models have been proposed to explain the nature of protein-lipid interactions in the dough.[123]

The results of the investigation of some lipoproteins of wheat[124] support the assumption that the complex is formed by electrostatic interactions between the numerous polar side chains of protein and polar phospho- and/or glycolipids. The effect of hydrophobic interactions may not be excluded.

Most of the previous studies focused on the lipid components of the complexes and did not specifically address the nature of the protein component with special lipid-binding ability. Békés et al.[125,126] investigated the nature of the gliadin-lipid interaction. The compositions of gliadins prepared without defatting of the flour or with different defatting procedures are shown in Table 8. It can be stated that the gliadin obtained after extraction of the flour by water-saturated butanol does not contain lipids. After defatting with *N*-butanol and hexane or with hexane alone a portion of the lipids remains in the gliadin fraction. The lipid compositions of the gliadin samples are given in Table 9. Gliadin preparations were fractionated into five fractions by gel filtration chromatography on Sephadex G-200. Lipid was found in fractions I and III. Fraction I contained polar lipids and fraction III contained neutral lipids. For seven different gliadin preparations and fractions thereof the lipid and carbohydrate contents were directly related. Gliadin preparations from totally defatted flour contained no carbohydrate. Fraction I of the gliadin from defatted flour contained only high molecular weight components, whereas the analogous fraction of the gliadin from undefatted flour contained, in addition, low molecular weight components. The results indicate that, in the presence of lipids, low and high molecular weight subunits of gliadin can form aggregates of high apparent molecular weight. The lipid, mainly galactolipid, appears to play a key role in the formation of those aggregates, and this may be the main reason for the already demonstrated involvement of this lipid in the bread-making quality of bread flours. The reconstitution experiments with totally defatted gliadin fractions and the lipids originally present showed that the lipid-mediated aggregation of high and low molecular weight gliadins is reversible.

TABLE 8
Protein, Carbohydrate, and Lipid Contents of Gliadin Preparations[125,126]

Method of Defatting	Protein (%)	Carbohydrates (%)	Lipid (%)
Not defatted	72.00	1.80	8.95
	74.00	1.05	7.85
Hexane	76.25	1.28	5.63
Water-saturated butanol	86.00	0	0
n-Butanol-hexane	83.75	1.00	3.29

The important role of lipids in bread making has stimulated further investigation of lipid-gluten protein interactions. The majority of the more recent studies confirmed the presence of lipid-binding proteins in both of the major components (gliadin and glutenin) of gluten.[127-131] A specific lipid-binding protein was isolated by Frazier et al.[127] and named ligolin.

Another lipid-binding protein (S-protein) was isolated by Zawistowska et al.[132] from the gliadin fraction of flour. It also must be noted that according to the views of some authors the lipid-binding property of different wheat proteins is a general phenomenon and the lipid-binding property of ligolin-like proteins is not unique.[133] The possible mode of binding of lipids in the gluten complex is discussed by Lásztity et al.[129] (Figures 13 and 14).

TABLE 9
Lipid Compositions of Gliadin Preparations Obtained from Undefatted and Defatted (*n*-Hexane and *n*-Butanol) Flour (mg/100 g)[125,126]

Lipid Component	Undefatted	Defatted
Triglycerides and sterol esters	2041	142
Diglycerides	747	137
Free fatty acids	336	196
Monoglycerides	669	317
Acyl-stearyl glycerides	602	203
Monogalactosyl diglycerides	332	103
Monogalactosyl monoglycerides	583	113
Digalactosyl diglycerides	2175	1229
Digalactosyl monoglycerides	656	172
N-Acyl-phosphatidylethanolamines	166	57
Phosphatidylethanolamine + phosphatidylglycerol	347	185
Phosphatidylinositol + phosphatidylserine (and their lyso derivates)	72	21
Lysophosphatidylethanolamine + lysophosphatidylglycerol	56	30
Lysophosphatidylcholine	12	8

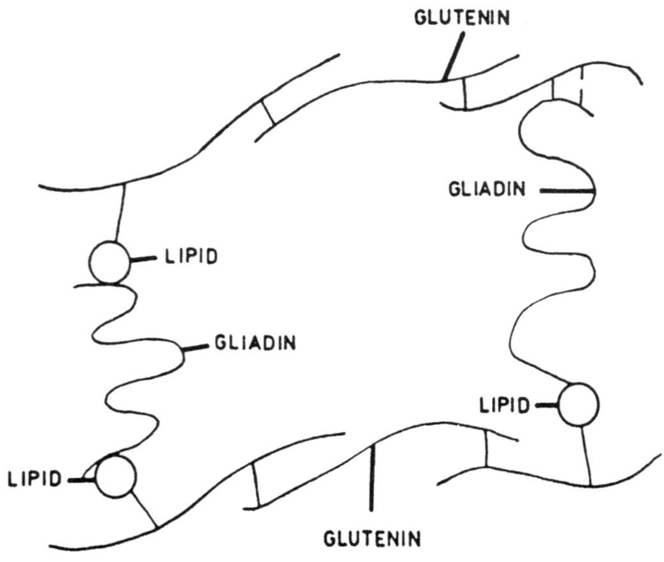

FIGURE 13 Possible location of lipids in the gluten network (Model A: lipids mediate the gliadin-glutenin interactions).[129]

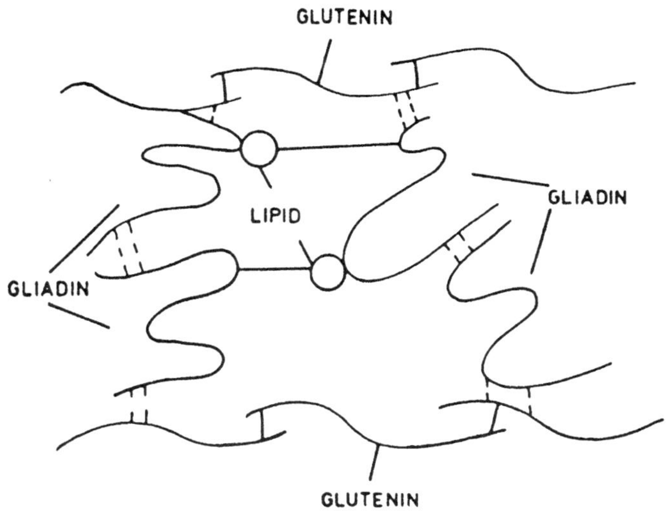

FIGURE 14 Possible location of lipids in the glutenin network (Model B: lipids mediate gliadin-gliadin interactions).[129]

More recent investigations concerning the carbohydrate content of gluten[134,135] showed that only a minor portion of carbohydrate is bound by gliadin components. The major components of the carbohydrate part are glucose, galactose, and mannose.

4. Other Proteins Found in Gliadin Preparations

Beckwith et al.[136] studied the gliadin fraction extracted from gluten with ethanol and found that it contained a high molecular weight fraction (100 kDa). This fraction was designated high molecular weight gliadin (HMWG). Later HMWG was exhaustively investigated by Bietz and Wall[137] and the results were compared with those obtained by the investigation of ethanol-soluble reduced glutenin (ESRG). PAGE of *S*-pyridyethyl (PE) derivatives of ESRG and reduced and *S*-pyridylethyl alkylated HMWG resulted in approximately 20 fairly sharp bands in each fraction. PE-ESRG and PE-HMWG were nearly identical, both quantitatively and qualitatively. Amino-terminal sequence analysis proved that many of the same polypeptides comprise HMWG and ESRG. On the basis of the obtained data a distribution of amino acids in the N-terminal sequences of the subunits common to HMWG and ESRG was proposed (see Figure 15). Heterogeneity of the fractions did not permit the determination of individual sequences. These data imply that many of these polypeptides are homologous and that the heterogeneity of HMWG and ESRG results from duplication and mutation of a common ancestral gene. During biosynthesis, kernel maturation, or drying these polypeptides can combine either with each other to form HMWG or with higher molecular weight, ethanol-insoluble polypeptides and with highly aggregating polypeptides to form glutenin.

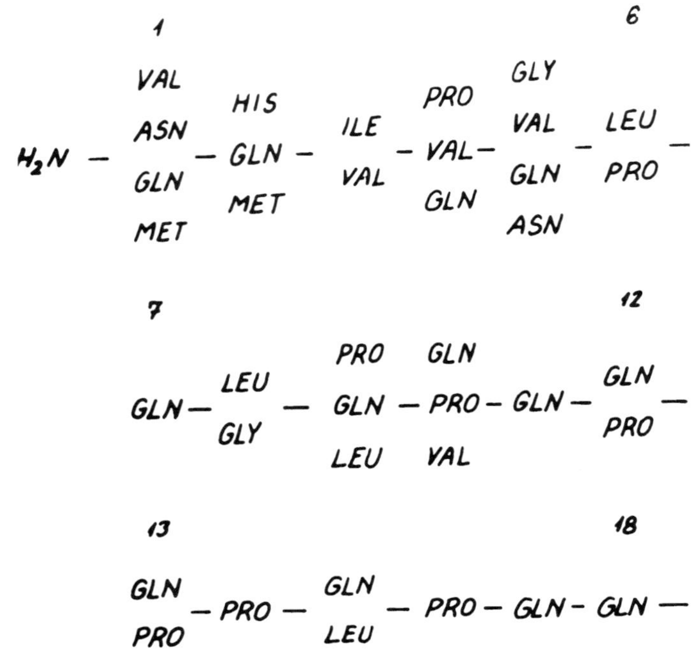

FIGURE 15 Distribution of major amino acids in the amino-terminal sequences of the major polypeptides common to high molecular weight gliadin and ethanol-soluble reduced glutenin.[118]

Taking into account the high ability of wheat proteins to interact with each other, it is understandable that the gliadin preparations always contain some other proteins in small quantity. These proteins may originate from the endoplasmic reticulum or from different biological membranes occurring in the wheat endosperm. In some cases enzymatic activity may be detected in electrophoretically separated components.

5. Nutritive Value of Gliadins

Due to their low lysine content (lowest among the wheat protein fractions) the gliadins belong to the less valuable protein fractions in wheat. In susceptible individuals a peptide (or peptides) derived from the digestion of gliadin proteins produces a specific immune response localized in the tissues of the small intestine. The resulting adverse changes in the intestinal mucosa diminish its ability to absorb nutrients. The resulting malabsorption syndrome is known as celiac disease. In the earlier studies the toxicity of α-gliadins and peptides derived from the α-gliadins has been demonstrated. Later Jos et al.[138] showed on the basis of the organ culture test results that β-gliadins are as noxious as α-gliadins and that the γ-gliadins are slightly noxious. Only ω-gliadins would be unnoxious. As the length of peptic-tryptic peptides has been shown to be a direct function of their proline content, the differences in toxicity between gliadins can be considered to be partially correlated with the differences between their proline contents since only peptides with molecular weights between 5,000 and 10,000 have been shown to be noxious.

B. High Molecular Weight Storage Proteins (Glutenins)

1. Separation, Nomenclature

As was discussed in Section II of this chapter, there are no internationally accepted good definitions for this group of proteins. It also can be stated that a standardized procedure for extraction and production of glutenin preparations does not exist. In this book the term high molecular weight storage proteins will be used. These proteins have two main characteristics: they are not soluble in dilute salt solutions and 70% ethanol, and the macromolecule is composed of more polypeptide chains bound by disulfide bonds. This definition also includes the HMWG described by Bietz and Wall.[137]

As reviewed by Kasarda et al.,[1] different procedures are used for obtaining the least soluble portion of the wheat endosperm storage proteins. Despite the lack of a uniform approach to the preparation of this group of proteins, and with the resultant difficulties in the definition of the term, the name "glutenin" is frequently used owing to the lack of a better terminology. Unfortunately, relatively little has been done to compare different preparations on a quantitative basis, but it seems likely that quantitative differences do occur and that they may be large for some preparations. Taking into consideration the differences in quality and quantity of the different preparations, the author would like to suggest the use of the term glutenin only for the preparations obtained by the traditional method of Osborne, which involves extraction of albumins and globulins from flour with dilute salt solution and extraction of gliadins with 70% ethanol, followed by solubilization with acid or alkali of the glutenin in the residue derived from the previous extractions. The products obtained by other procedures may be named in a way which gives information about the method of preparation. For example, a glutenin extracted by AUC may be noted as "glutenin prepared by the AUC method" or "AUC glutenin". As a suffix the name of the authors elaborating the method of preparation also may be used (e.g., "glutenin prepared by the method of Orth and Bushuk"). The extraction methods using reducing agents and splitting the disulfide bonds give products which cannot be named glutenin, since the term glutenin is reserved for the native molecule.[139]

The high molecular weight storage proteins may be separated by different techniques into fractions. One possibility for separation is based on solubility. Acetic acid is frequently used to solubilize glutenin. This method yields a soluble glutenin and residue protein. The ratio of these fractions may vary widely.[141,149]

Mecham et al.[142] found that exhaustive extraction of the flour with acetic acid resulted in the formation of a highly hydrated, gelatinous material containing about 30% of the total protein. This gel-forming protein was named "gel protein" by Mecham et al.[143] Gel protein was also prepared by other procedures. By dialysis against water the gel proteins were separated into a water-soluble gel (WSG) and a water-insoluble gel (WIG). WSG was separated into two fractions by gel filtration chromatography on Bio-Gel P60 or Sephacryl S-200. Two peaks were obtained.[28]

Huebner and Wall[144] separated the proteins of the AUC extracts of flour by gel filtration chromatography. Agarose gel columns (Sepharose 4B and 28B) were used. The first two peaks eluted from Sepharose 4B were considered to be two fractions of glutenin. Graveland et al.,[24] using a combined SDS-centrifugation separation procedure (see Figure 2), separated the high molecular weight proteins into glutenin I, II, and III, glycoprotein, and glutelin. The later fraction could be separated by gel filtration chromatography (Sepharose 4B columns) into four fractions (glutelin I, II, III, and IV). The name glutelin was proposed by Graveland et al.[23,24] because of the similarities between this fraction and the glutelins of other cereals. It seems that the name wheat glutelin may be more adequate. Because of their high molecular weight the glutenin fractions do not enter into the gel when using electrophoretic techniques for the separation. If they are reduced and alkylated the subunits obtained may be well separated by gel electrophoresis. The early investigations[145] showed that reduced glutenin contained about 20 subunits.

A major advance was made in characterizing glutenin subunits by using SDS-PAGE. These studies of reduced bread wheat glutenin have shown that this protein consists of approximately 17 to 20 polypeptide subunits. The molecular weights of these subunits, determined by the same technique, ranged from 12,000 to 134,000.[145]

Early reviews on the structure of glutenins were given by Bietz and Huebner[147] and Bushuk et al.[148] According to recent views of specialists, summarized in the reviews of Shewry and Miflin,[83] McRitchie et al.,[149] Ng and Bushuk,[150] and Shewry et al.,[151] the subunits of glutenin are divided into two groups: (1) high molecular weight glutenin subunits (HMW or HMW-GS) and (2) low molecular weight glutenin subunits (LMW or LMW-GS). Jackson et al.[152] classified glutenin subunits according to their mobility in SDS-PAGE and their relative acidity. The "A" group includes the entire group of HMW-GS, which have the slowest mobility. Low molecular weight glutenin subunits collectively form the "B", "C", and "D" groups. The "B" group is comprised of the greatest number of subunits, which are the most basic of the endosperm storage proteins and which are much slower in mobility than α-, β-, and γ-gliadins. The "D" subunits are the most acidic and are the slowest among LMW subunits: The "C" group presents a wide range of isoelectric points and overlaps with α-, β-, and γ-gliadins in SDS-PAGE.

The HMW-GS are identified according to electrophoretic mobility within the group and according to chromosome coding for the individual polypeptide. The HMW-GS designated 1A1 is a subunit coded by chromosome 1A having the lowest electrophoretic mobility. Genes coding for HMW subunits are located on the long arms of chromosomes 1A, 1B, and 1D. The coding loci are named Glu-A1, Glu-B1, and Glu-D1. A catalogue of genes coding for HMW subunits of wheat is given by Payne and Lawrence.[153] At this time more than 40 different HMW-GS have been found; they may be classified into two subgroups: X-type and Y-type subunits.

The LMW-GS are also coded by chromosomes 1A, 1B, and 1D, but on the short arms (Glu-3 loci) near the gliadin-coding loci. At this time no generally accepted nomenclature for LMW-GS is available. This fact is connected with the relatively fewer number of studies about this type of subunit and to the problems caused by overlapping of LMW-GS and gliadin electrophoretic spectra. It seems that a system similar to that used for HMW-GS must be developed.

2. Composition and Structure

The amino acid composition of high molecular weight storage proteins of wheat endosperm is in general similar to those of low molecular weight (gliadin) storage proteins. A slightly higher content of basic amino acids and lower amount of glutamic acid and proline may be observed. The average content of the amino acids having hydrophobic side chains is also smaller. Some differences may be observed also in the degree of amidation of the carboxyl groups of the glutamic and aspartic acids. The amidation degree is somewhat lower in glutenin. Generally, glutenin preparations have a more hydrophilic character. The different subfractions of high molecular weight storage proteins and some groups of subunits were also investigated by different research workers. Analyzing the compositional data published in the literature, Kasarda et al.[1] called attention first of all to the differences in glutamic acid (which is not differentiated from glutamine in most works) and proline content in various preparations and fractions. They stated that the compositions fall into two groups: the high group, with glutamic acid content from 250 to 350 residues per 10^5 g, and the low group, with glutamic acid content ranging from about 150 to 200 residues per 10^5 g. The low group is also notable for having higher levels of basic amino acids, particularly lysine, and a higher level of aspartic acid or asparagine. The low glutamic acid levels are relative, however, in that they are high in comparison with most other proteins. They amount to roughly 20 mol% in comparison with roughly 30 mol% in the high group. Some data-supporting views of Kasarda et al.[1] are summarized in Table 10.

The amino acid compositions of some high molecular weight storage protein groups were investigated by Graveland et al.[24] Some results of these investigations are shown in Table 11. As shown in this table, there are no big differences between the different fractions of glutenin prepared by the combined SDS-centrifugation method (see Figure 1). Also, the groups of subunits differ only slightly in glutamic acid and proline content. More expressed differences may be observed in the content of basic amino acids, first of all in the lysine content and also in the amount of cysteine. In Table 12 the amino acid compositions of glutenin fractions prepared by Ryadchikow et al.[30] using the Landry-Moureaux method[29] are demonstrated. Relatively great differences may be observed in the glutamic acid content and also in the proportion of basic amino acids. It was also stated that the amino acid compositions of the same fractions — prepared by the same method — show some differences between wheat varieties. However, the differences are mostly small and in many cases are not significant. On the other hand, significant differences were observed between the amino acid compositions of glutenin preparations — prepared by the same method — of tetra- and hexaploid wheat.[154]

Progress made in genetic and separation techniques resulted in separation of different individual polypeptides belonging to the HMW-GS and LMW-GS groups,

TABLE 10
Amino Acid Compositions of Glutein and Glutein Subfractions (Residues Per 10^5 g Protein)

Amino Acid	Gliadin[a]	Glutenin[a]	High Molecular Weight Gliadin	Glutenin I[c]	Glutenin II[c]	PE Glutenin[d]	PP Glutenin[e]	PH Glutenin[e]
Lysine	5	13	9	14	10	29	37	37
Histidine	15	13	12	13	13	18	19	17
Arginine	15	20	22	22	20	34	37	38
Aspartic acid	20	23	17	24	19	60	60	56
Threonine	18	26	22	27	25	36	36	37
Serine	38	50	60	60	60	62	52	58
Glutamic acid	317	278	324	281	297	185	174	196
Proline	148	114	130	105	108	82	69	74
Glycine	25	78	42	77	65	94	74	72
Alanine	25	34	23	34	40	58	60	55
Cystine	10	10	11	10	10	8	ND	ND
Valine	43	41	35	44	36	48	51	45
Methionine	12	12	11	16	14	15	19	7
Isoleucine	37	28	29	28	27	32	35	36
Leucine	62	57	64	58	57	34	72	69
Tyrosine	16	25	15	25	23	35	27	23
Phenylalanine	38	27	35	27	31	32	33	33
Tryptophan	5	8	ND	5	4	11	ND	ND

Note: ND, not determined.

[a] From Wu and Dimler.[155,156]
[b] From Bietz and Wall.[157]
[c] From Huebner and Wall.[158]
[d] From Huebner et al.[159]
[e] From Wasik and Bushuk.[154]

TABLE 11
Amino Acid Compositions of High Molecular Weight Storage Protein Fractions

Amino Acid	Glutenin I (Gel Proteins)[a]	A Component of Glutenin[a]	B and C Components of Glutenin I[a]	Glutenin II[a]	Glutenin III[a]	Glutelins[a]
Lysine	1.03	1.15	0.43	1.00	0.42	5.50
Histidine	1.60	1.30	1.65	1.62	1.60	2.90
Arginine	2.98	3.15	2.45	2.90	2.47	8.30
Aspartic acid + asparagine	2.48	2.60	1.75	2.50	1.75	7.90
Threonine	2.42	2.85	1.90	2.40	1.87	3.65
Serine	5.10	5.20	5.55	5.20	5.50	4.70
Glutamic acid + glutamine	38.12	39.45	38.60	38.10	38.70	39.95
Proline	11.20	10.50	11.60	11.10	11.55	12.65
Glycine	2.80	3.00	1.40	3.00	1.35	4.60
Alanine	2.05	2.30	1.45	2.05	1.45	5.10
Valine	3.25	2.40	3.25	3.25	3.25	5.35
Methionine	1.35	0.92	1.40	1.40	1.40	1.82
Leucine	5.56	4.95	6.20	5.56	6.24	6.85
Tyrosine	3.49	5.90	1.75	3.50	1.76	1.30
Phenylalanine	3.45	2.80	5.15	3.36	5.10	4.00
Tryptophan	0.70	1.10	0.35	0.80	0.40	0.90
Cysteine	2.00	1.10	2.30	2.10	2.18	1.55

[a] From Graveland et al. (g/100 g protein).[24]

TABLE 12
Amino Acid Compositions of Gliadin and Landry-Moureaux Glutenins (g/100 g Total Amino Acids)[30]

Amino Acid	Gliadin	Glutenin I	Glutenin II	Glutenin III
Lysine	0.85	0.97	4.8	4.3
Histidine	1.65	1.6	1.8	2.0
Arginine	1.7	1.9	3.8	4.1
Threonine	2.0	2.4	3.3	3.5
Aspartic acid	2.2	2.3	5.8	5.9
Serine	4.2	4.5	4.6	5.2
Glutamic acid	39.0	38.6	30.7	24.8
Proline	15.7	13.8	9.9	10.0
Glycine	2.7	2.6	7.9	5.5
Alanine	2.4	2.7	4.3	4.0
Cystine	3.1	3.6	2.1	3.2
Valine	3.7	4.2	4.1	4.6
Methionine	1.7	2.4	1.8	2.6
Isoleucine	4.0	4.2	2.6	3.5
Leucine	6.9	7.1	5.6	8.1
Tyrosine	2.8	1.9	4.2	3.8
Phenylalanine	5.5	5.2	3.0	4.2

respectively. Some data about the amino acid compositions of these polypeptides are shown in Table 13. As is seen from the data, although the high glutamic acid and proline content is characteristic for all polypeptides, there are some significant differences within the groups and also between the two type of polypeptides (e.g., glycine, valine, leucine content).

The most commonly held view of the structure of the high molecular weight storage proteins (glutenins) of wheat is that it consists of a mixture of polypeptide subunits cross-linked by intermolecular (intersubunit) disulfide bonds in such a way as to yield a broad spectrum of molecular weights ranging up to higher polymers with molecular weights in the millions.

A number of different models have been proposed for the structure of high molecular weight storage proteins (glutenins). The earliest ones were those proposed by Ewart[162] and Lásztity et al.[105,163] The latter is presented in Figure 16. As can be seen in this model, the polypeptide chains are bound by one disulfide bond. The molecules have linear character. This structure may be supported by the following experimental facts:

1. The splitting of disulfide bonds by reduction or oxidation results in a drastic change in the molecular weight.
2. The quantity of N-terminal groups calculated for 10^4g protein is practically the same in high (glutenin) as well as low molecular weight (gliadin) preparations.

TABLE 13
Amino Acid Compositions of Some Glutenin Subunits (in mol%-S)

	Subunit					
Amino Acid	**HMW 1A1[a]**	**HMW 1DX2[a]**	**HMW 1DX5[a]**	**HMW 1D12[a]**	**LMW 13 Variety REKTOR[b]**	**LMW 20 Variety REKTOR[b]**
Aspartic acid	1.0	0.6	0.6	1.4	2.5	5.2
Threonine	2.9	2.9	3.0	3.1	2.5	2.5
Serine	6.3	5.7	6.1	6.3	8.3	6.2
Glutamic acid	37.1	36.3	38.6	34.9	37.3	30.1
Proline	16.4	15.8	13.5	14.7	13.6	15.8
Glycine	14.7	20.0	17.9	13.9	4.7	5.7
Alanine	2.5	2.9	3.2	3.5	3.3	4.9
Cystine	0.8	0.6	0.6	1.3	ND	ND
Valine	2.4	1.6	1.8	2.9	4.6	5.6
Methionine	0.1	Trace	Trace	0.2	1.2	0.2
Isoleucine	1.4	0.6	0.6	2.0	4.0	4.5
Leucine	5.2	4.5	4.7	4.9	7.2	7.7
Tyrosine	4.7	5.7	6.0	3.9	2.0	0.1
Phenylalanine	1.1	0.5	0.4	1.8	3.9	4.8
Histidine	0.6	0.5	0.5	1.8	1.9	1.8
Lysine	0.6	0.9	0.9	1.2	0.8	2.2
Arginine	2.1	1.0	1.5	2.1	2.3	3.2

Note: ND, not determined.

[a] From Shewry et al.[160]
[b] From Belitz et al.[161]

3. The viscosity of the glutenin solutions decreases rapidly by splitting even a relatively small number of disulfide bonds.
4. High molecular weight fractions were consistently present and were demonstrated in the endosperm of the developing grain throughout the period of development.[164]

An alternative model for glutenin structure was proposed by Kasarda et al.[1] According to this model there are no interpolypeptide disulfide bonds in glutenin; all of the disulfide bonds are of the intramolecular type. The high molecular weight storage proteins of the endosperm aggregate strongly through secondary bonding forces such as hydrogen bonds, ionic bonds, and hydrophobic interactions. The authors mentioned above postulated that the intramolecular disulfide bonds constrain the glutenin subunits into a specific conformation which facilitates the interaction of specific secondary forces between adjacent polypeptides forming the functional aggregate. The subunits have a globular shape and the fibrils are formed by the interaction of the globular subunit molecules. This model is based on the observation

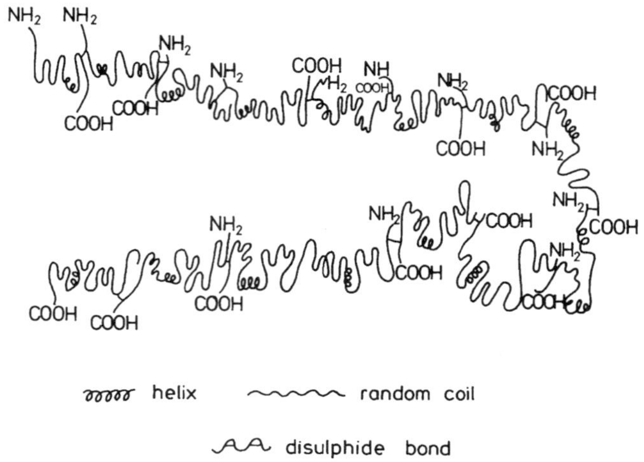

FIGURE 16 Structure of high molecular weight gluten protein.[105,169]

of the microfibrillar complexes formed by A-gliadin subunits, and it is supplemented by the observation of other fibrillar structures derived from endosperm proteins. For the elucidation of the fact that disruption of the disulfide bonds causes changes in structure, it was postulated that the secondary forces between globular subunits are so strong that they cannot be disrupted by any known solvent. Reduction of the intramolecular (intrasubunit) bonds changes the conformation of the subunit, which in turn leads to disruption of the specific interpolypeptide secondary forces, thereby releasing the glutenin subunits. A schematic drawing illustrating the ways in which different protein subunits (designated as A, B, and C) might aggregate into microfibrils is shown in Figure 17. The microfibrils may be formed from the same subunits; also, different subunits can interact to form a mixed subunit microfibril.

A third type of model was proposed by Bushuk et al.[121] The model of glutenin contains both inter- and intrasubunit disulfide bonds. Secondary forces (hydrogen bonds, ionic bonds, hydrophobic interactions) are also involved in the formation of the complex. A schematic representation of the model is shown in Figure 18. On the basis of the investigations of these authors it has been postulated that the complex contains two types of molecules: (1) subunits of 68,000 mol wt and lower named glutenin I and (2) glutenin II composed of subunits with higher than 68,000 mol wt that are joined to each other through at least one intersubunit disulfide bond. The glutenin I components are held in the complex through secondary forces through protein-protein interactions and protein-intermediate (carbohydrate, lipid)-protein interactions. These subunits provide a measure of the viscous flow in the model. On the other hand, the characteristic elastic properties of the glutenin are associated with glutenin II.

A recent review about newer glutenin models was published by Bushuk.[165] In the model of Graveland et al.[166] the backbone of the molecule is comprised of only HMW glutenin subunits (X and Y types) alternating in a head-to-tail arrangement.

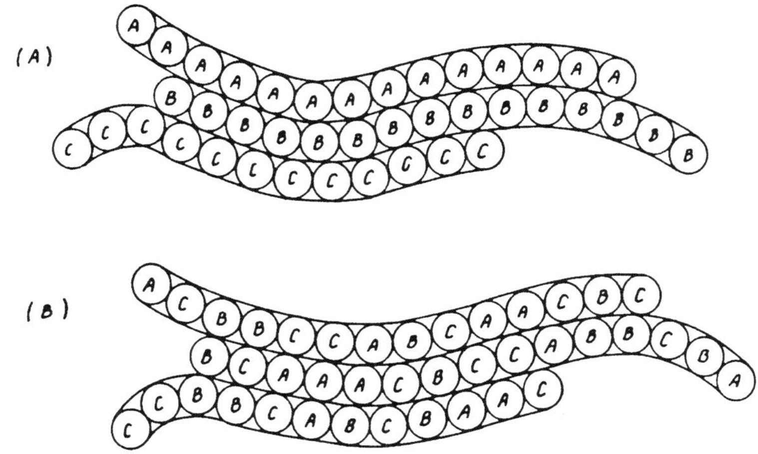

FIGURE 17 Schematic drawing illustrating ways in which different protein subunits, designated as A, B, and C, might aggregate into microfibrillar structures. (A) Specific aggregation in which only like subunits interact to form microfibrils; (B) random aggregation of subunits to form microfibrils. In either case lateral aggregation of microfibrils may occur. (From Kasarda, D.D., Bernardin, J.E., and Nimno, C.C., *Advances in Cereal Science and Technology,* Vol. 1, Pomeranz, Y., Ed., American Association of Cereal Chemists, St. Paul, MN, 1976, 158. With permission.)

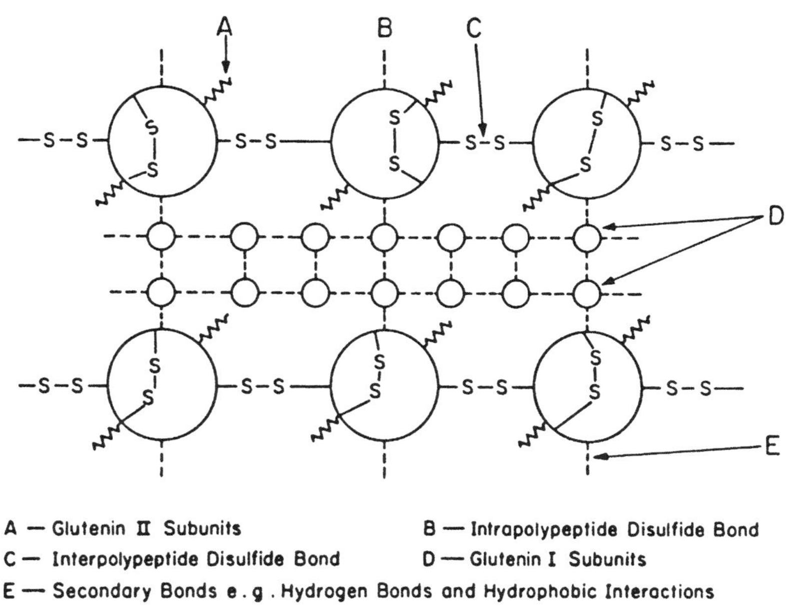

FIGURE 18 Schematic representation of the model of functional glutenin. (From Bushuk, W., Khan, K., and McMaster, G., *Ann. Technol. Agric.,* 29, 279, 1980. With permission.)

The LMW-GS are accommodated as short polymeric clusters linked by disulfide bonds to the Y-type subunits of the backbone. A somewhat different model was proposed by Kasarda.[167] In this model the LMW-GS are linked together by disulfide bonds in the C-terminal domains where most of the cysteine residues are located. Clusters of LMW subunits are interlinked by HMW subunits. Schematic representations of the two models are shown in Figure 19.

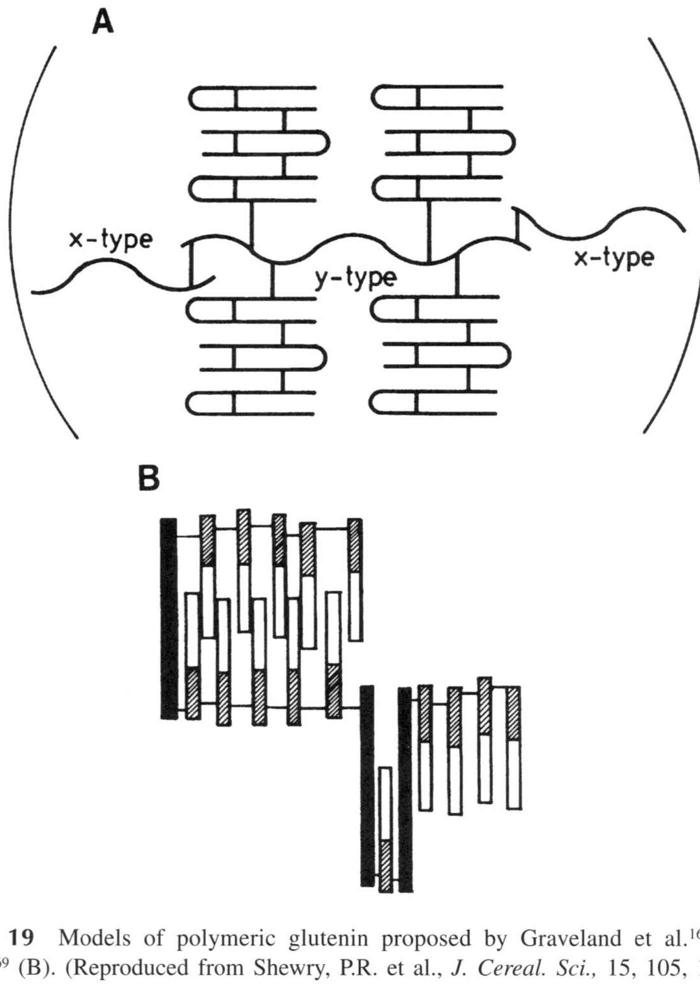

FIGURE 19 Models of polymeric glutenin proposed by Graveland et al.[166] (A) and Kasarda[169] (B). (Reproduced from Shewry, P.R. et al., *J. Cereal. Sci.,* 15, 105, 1992. With permission.)

Recently a model called the "block polymer model" was proposed for the structure of glutenin by Gao et al.[168] This model (Figure 20) is a substantial modification of the models of Graveland et al.[166] and Kasarda.[167] According to the block polymer model, submolecular blocks, comprising most or all of the subunits of glutenin, are interlinked by disulfide bonds. At least two different types of disulfide bonds are envisaged: those that link subunits together within the block and those

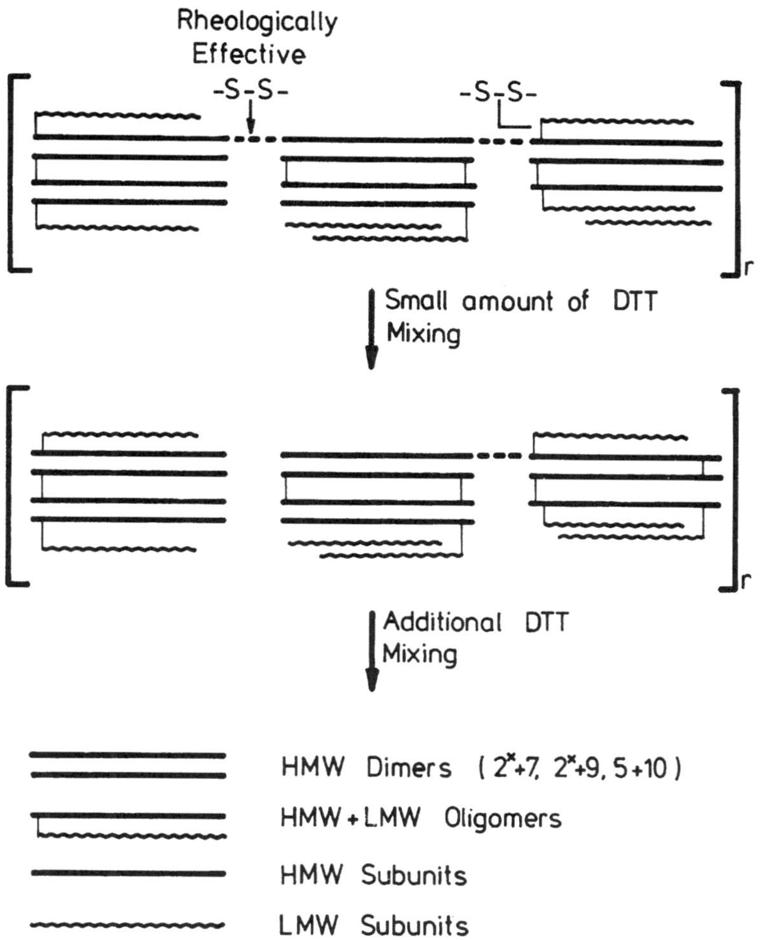

FIGURE 20 Block polymer model of glutenin and its breakdown by reduction with dithiothreitol (DTT). HMW = high molecular weight; LMW = low molecular weight. (From Gao, L. et al., *Cereal Chem.,* 69, 452, 1992. With permission.)

that interlink the blocks. Splitting of interblock disulfide bonds — under conditions of very mild reduction — results in free blocks which can be separated by gel filtration chromatography and analyzed by SDS-PAGE.[168] Further reduction produces dimers of HMW subunits only and of HMW and LMW subunits.

Summarizing knowledge accumulated to date about the structure of glutenin, it can be stated that it is formed from different subunits bound together by a network of disulfide bonds. Different subunits may differ in their tendency to polymerize and, once polymerized, may have different capacities for interaction with other constituents. The mechanism and control of disulfide bond formation are not yet clear; determination of the processes involved in formation of this network is a challenge for the future. The efforts to determine the structure of glutenin may be facilitated due to the significant progress in studies on individual glutenin subunits (for a review see Reference 149).

Genes encoding HMW subunits have been isolated.[169] The complete amino acid sequences have been deduced from the DNA sequences of the respective genes. The schematic representation of X-type and Y-type HMW subunits is shown in Figure 21. In general they consist of three structural domains. At the N-terminus is a nonrepetitive sequence of 80 to 100 residues containing three to five cysteine residues. At the C-terminus there is another nonrepetitive region of 42 residues including one cysteine, this region being identical for all subunits. The central region of the polypeptide (490 to 690 residues) consists of a number of repeated sequences. This region appears to contain repeated β-turns organized into a loose spiral. This spiral structure may be intrinsically elastic.

The intensive study of HMW-GS is continuing, including investigation of their amino acid sequences and interactions. As a result, newer allelic variants of HMW have been separated, and in many cases qualitative differences have been found in different cultivars between subunits with the same mobility.[170,171] From the point of view of glutenin structure the presence of HMW-GS dimers (containing one X-type and one Y-type subunit) is of interest.[172] Whether or not a chain of such dimers forms the backbone of glutenin, as proposed by Graveland et al.,[166] must be confirmed or rejected by further experiments.

It was found that D-subunits of glutenin from the Chinese Spring cultivar, coded by chromosome 1D, likely contain only one cysteine group. So it is possible that D-subunits would negatively influence quality characteristics because they would be able to form only intermolecular disulfide bonds, thereby acting as terminators of the growing glutenin polymer.[173]

Kazemie and Bushuk[174] reported the identification of a group of HMW proteins in some Canadian wheat varieties and referred to them as K-proteins. They were extractable with a solvent composed of acetic acid and urea, but not with solvents that contained detergents. In a more recent publication[175] it was reported that K-proteins were also present in developing grain; this confirms their genuine nature.

The LMW-GS were not studied as intensively as HMW-GS. Sequences derived from DNA clones have been reported by Okita et al.,[176] Colot et al.,[177] and Cassidy and Dvorák.[178] Ellen et al.[179] recently published a number of N-terminal sequences of LMW-GS isolated from reduced and pyridylethylated glutenin (see Table 14). Figure 22 models a typical LMW-glutenin subunit. All of the cysteine residues are found either in the C-terminal, nonrepetitive domain of the subunit or in the small N-terminal region in front of a repetitive domain.

3. Interactions of the High Molecular Weight Proteins with Lipids and Carbohydrates

The fact that glutenin components can interact with lipids is well known. It is also known that these interactions play an important role in the formation of the dough and that they influence dough properties. A good review concerning the

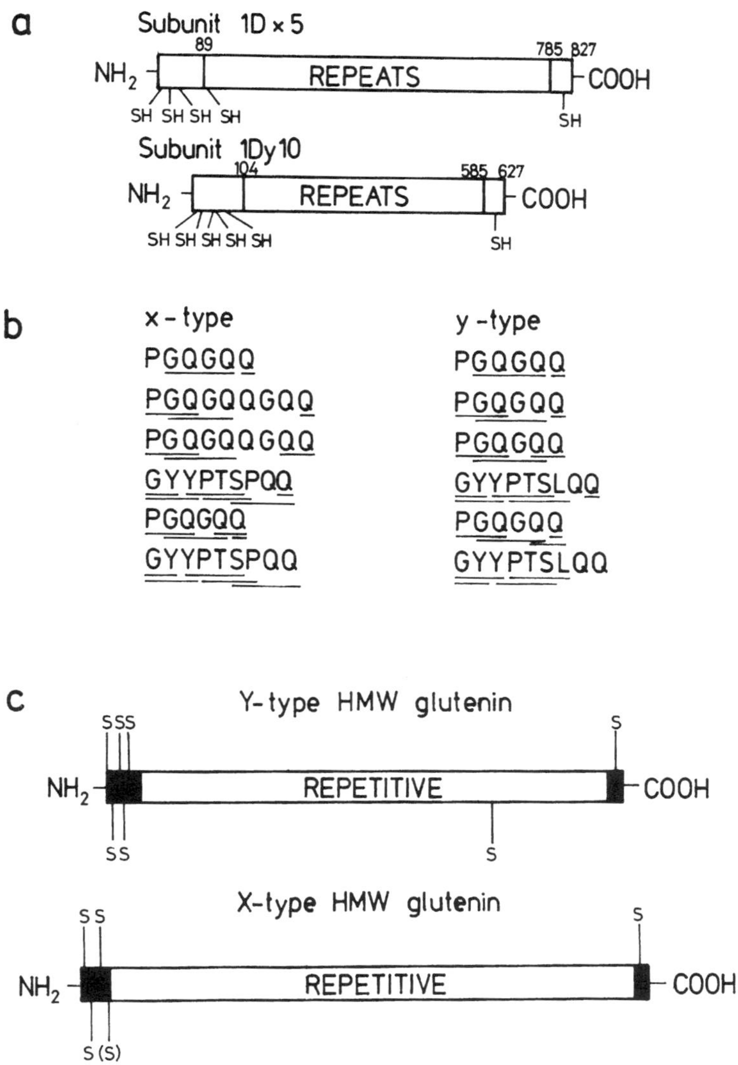

FIGURE 21 Schematic representation of x-type and y-type high molecular weight (HMW) glutenin subunits. (a) Structural organization of 1D × 5 and 1D × 10 subunits; (b) sequences of the central repetitive domains of x-type and y-type subunits (underlined tetrapeptides indicate predicted reverse turns); (c) general domain structure of 2 types of HMW subunits. (From Anderson, O.D. et al., in *Gluten Proteins,* Bushuk, W. and Tkachuk, R., Eds., American Association of Cereal Chemists, St. Paul, MN, 1990, 376. With permission.)

interactions of lipids and gluten proteins was published by Pomeranz.[181] Summarizing our knowledge at this time, it can be stated that free wheat-flour lipids interact with gluten proteins during dough mixing and gluten washing. In these processes the main role belongs to the phospho- and glycolipids which may be bound to the gluten proteins by ionic or hydrogen bonds. Hydrophobic interactions also play a role.

TABLE 14
N-Terminal Sequences of Reduced-Pyridylethylated Fractions[179]

Fraction Number	Sequence Type[a]	Percentage of Fraction	Sequence
	1	10	15
7Aa	α	54	V –R–V–P–V–P–Q–L–Q–P–Q –N–P–S– Q–
7Ab	γ	23	N–M–Q–V–D–P–S–G–Q–V–Q–W–P–Q–Q–
7Ac	LMW-s	16	S –X– I –P–G–L–E–R–P– S–Q–Q–Q–P– L–
7Ad	LMW-m	7	M–E–T–S–(C/H)–I–P–G–L–E–R–P–S–Q–Q–
7Ba	α	31	V–R–V–P–V–P–Q–L–Q–P–
7Bb	γ	28	N–M–Q–V–D–P–S–G–Q–V–
7Bc	LMW-s	25	S– H– I –P–G–L–E–R–P–S–
7Bd	LMW-m	15	M–E–T–S–H– I –P–G–L–E–
8A			Blocked? Hint of α type
8Ba	α	58	V–R–V–P–V–P–Q–L–Q–P–
8Bb	LMW-s	19	S–H–I–P–G–L–E–(R/K)–P–S–
8Bc	γ	15	N–M–Q–V–D–P–S–G–Q–V–
8Bd	LMW-m	8	M–E–T–S–H– I –P–G–L–E–
8Ca	LMW-s	48	S– H– I –P–G–L–E–X–P–S–
8Cb	LMW-m	25	M–E–T–S–H– I –P–G–L–E–
8Cc	α	15	V–X–V–P–V–P–Q–L–Q–P–
8Cd	γ	12	N–M–Q–V–D–P–S–G–Q–V–
9Aa	α	33	V–R –V–P–V–P–Q–L–Q–P–
9Ab	LMW-s	32	S–H–I–P–G–L–E–(R/K)–P–S–
9Ac	LMW-m	29	M–E–T–S–H– I –P–G–L–E–
9Ad	γ	6	N–M–Q–V–D–P–S–G–Q–V–
9Ba	LMW-s	81	S–H–I–P–G–L–E–(R/K)–P–S–

9Bb	LMW-m	19	M–E–T–S–H– I –P–G–L–E–
10	LMW-s	100	S–H–I–P–G–L–E–(R/K)–P–S–Q–Q–Q–P–L–P–P–Q–Q–$\overset{20}{\text{T}}$–L–X–X–X–(Q/P)–X–Q–Q–P–$\overset{30}{\text{(I/P)}}$–
11Aa	a	81	V–R–V–P–V–P–Q–L–Q–P–Q–N–P–S–Q–Q–Q–P–Q–(K/E)–Q–V–
11Ab	LMW-s	15	S–H–I–P–G–L–E–(R/K)–P–S–Q–Q–Q–P–L–
11Ac	LMW-m	4	M–E–T–S–(R/K)–I–P–G–L–E–
11Ba	LMW-s	80	S–H–I–P–G–L–E–(R/K)–P–S–Q–Q–Q–P–L–P–L–X–Q–X–L–
11Bb	LMW-m	20	M–E–T–S–H–I–P–G–L–E–K–P–(L/S)–Q–Q–Q–P–X–P–X–Q–
11Ca	LMW-s	62	S–H–I–P–G–L–E–(R/K)–P–
11Cb	LMW-m	38	M–E–T–S–C– I –P–G–L–
12Aa	LMW-s	64	S–H–I–P–G–L–E–(K/R)–P–S–
12Ab	LMW-m	36	M–E–T–S–H– I –P–G–L–E–
12B	LMW-m	100	M–E–T–S–(H/R)–(I/V)–P–G–L–E–
13Aa	LMW-m	55	M–E–T–S–H–(I/V)–P–G–L–E–
13Ab	LMW-s	45	S–X–I–P–G–L–E–R–P–S–
13B	LMW-m	100	M–E–T–S–R–V–P–G–L–E–K–P–S–Q–Q–
14	LMW-m	100	M–E–T–R–C–I–P–G–L–E–R–P–X–Q–Q–Q–P–L–X–(P/Q)–
15A+B	γ	100	N–M–Q–V–D–P–S–G–Q–V–Q–V–P–Q–Q–Q–P–F–P–Q–P–Q–Q–P–F–C–$\overset{26}{\text{Q}}$–Q–P–Q–R–T–I–
16a	γ	74	N–M–Q–V–D–P–S–G–Q–V–Q–V–P–Q–Q–Q–P–F–P–Q–P–Q–Q–P–F–C–Q–Q–
16b	HMW-1	14	G–G–S–F–Y–P–G–Q–T–T–P–P–Q–Q–L–Q–Q–
16c	HMW-2	12	G–Q–Q–P–G–Q–G–Q–Q–P–G–Q–G–Q–Q–G–Q–Q–P–G–Q–G–Q–Q–G–Q–Q–P–

[a] LMW-m, the sequence type described by Okita et al.,[176], Colot et al.,[177] and Cassidy and Dvorák[178] (m represents methionine, the first amino acid of the sequence); LMW-s, the sequence type described by Shewry et al.,[379] Kasarda et al.,[380] and Tao and Kasarda[381] (s represents serine, the first amino acid of the sequence); α, the α-type sequence; γ, the γ-type sequence (see Kasarda[167] for α- and γ-type gliadin nomenclature).

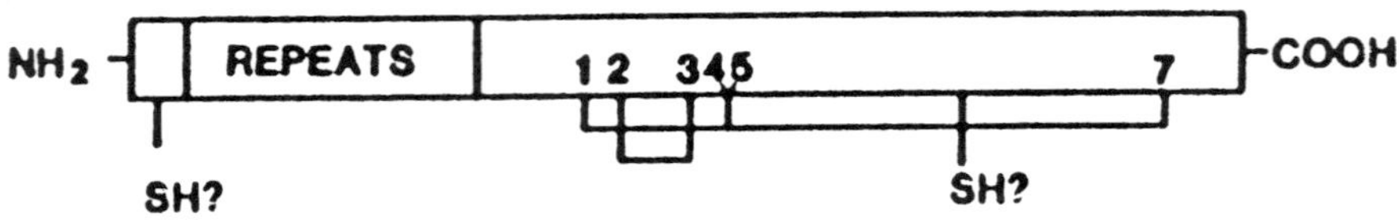

FIGURE 22 Low molecular weight (LMW) glutenin subunit structure. The signal peptide is cleaved during processing. S = cysteine residues. (From Anderson, O.D. et al., *Gluten Proteins,* Bushuk, W. and Tkachuk, R., Eds., American Association of Cereal Chemists, St. Paul, MN, 1990, 376. With permission.)

Some experimental data have confirmed that lipid-protein (lipid-carbohydrate-protein) complexes also may be present in the dry endosperm. They are extractable from the flour using organic solvents. Lásztity et al.[124] extracted the flour with a chloroform-methanol mixture (2:1) after defatting the flour using petroleum ether. A glycolipoprotein was isolated and investigated. The protein content of the complex was found to be 85.3%. The following lipid components were separated: phosphatidylcholine, phosphatidylethanolamine, phosphatidic acid, digalactosyl diglyceride, polyglycerol phosphatide, monogalactosyl diglyceride, sterol glycosides, and neutral lipids. Of the carbohydrate constituents, arabinose and galactose were identified unambiguously in the hydrolysate.

N-terminal amino acid analysis and PAGE both indicated the presence of four fractions. The amino acid composition of the lipoglycoprotein is given in Table 15. Most of the glutenin preparations contain small amounts of carbohydrates. This fact was observed by many research workers; e.g., Bushuk et al.[182] observed that a relatively significant amount of carbohydrates was present in the high molecular weight fraction of gluten. The carbohydrate portion is comprised of 97% glucose and trace amounts of arabinose, xylose, galactose, and mannose.

TABLE 15
The Amino Acid Composition of the Lipoglycoprotein Complex

Amino Acid	g/100 g Protein	Amino Acid	g/100 g Protein
Aspartic acid	1.17	Methionine	0.45
Threonine	2.76	Isoleucine	5.31
Serine	1.22	Leucine	4.60
Glutamic acid	23.40	Tyrosine	1.60
Proline	22.20	Phenylalanine	4.71
Glycine	1.55	Arginine	2.20
Alanine	1.65	Lysine	2.35
Cystine	8.20	Histidine	1.22
Valine	2.14	Ammonia	1.46

Recently Chen et al.[183,184] reported about the isolation of carb
proteins from wheat gluten and about isolation of a glycopepti
containing fraction, possibly a glycopeptide, was isolated from a p
gluten. The glycopeptide contained three sugar components — xylose, a
and galactose — and had a highly branched structure. Occurrence of glycosyla
HMW glutenin subunits was confirmed recently by Tilley et al.[185]

IV. THE GLUTEN COMPLEX AND FACTORS INFLUENCING ITS RHEOLOGICAL PROPERTIES

It is generally accepted that the properties of the storage proteins of wheat govern its suitability for processing into bread. Among cereals only bread wheats — and to a lesser extent triticale — possess storage proteins, which interact with water to yield doughs having the necessary cohesiveness and elasticity for making leavened bread. The reason for this and the structure of gluten and its protein constituents have intrigued cereal chemists since the days of Osborne. It is evident that the factors playing a role in defining the rheological properties of gluten are of complex character. Based on theoretical considerations, and also on all the studies which have been carried out, it would appear that the following two groups of factors are the most important:

1. The quantity and quality (solubility, amino acid composition, molecular weight distribution, structure, etc.) of the protein components of the gluten complex
2. The interactions (disulfide bonds, hydrogen bonds, electrostatic and hydrophobic interactions) between the protein fractions present in the gluten complex

A. The Quantity and Quality of the Components of the Gluten Complex

It is clear that an insoluble protein matrix is an essential prerequisite for the formation of a cohesive dough. Not only must the protein be insoluble, but there must be a sufficient amount of it to form a continuous protein phase in the presence of starch and water. In early investigations the ratio of the readily dispersible proteins (using dilute organic acids such as lactic or acetic acid) was measured. The results indicate that the amount of readily dispersible components correlates negatively with the rheological quality of gluten and dough. An increase in the nondispersible fractions has an improving effect. These observations are in good agreement with the practical work, and some methods for the determination of baking value of wheats (swelling test of gluten, sedimentation test of Zeleny, etc.) are based on these observations.

The proportion of acetic acid-soluble and acetic acid-insoluble proteins (residue protein, gel protein) of gluten and glutenin was investigated by many authors. A review of this work was given by Feillet.[186] Orth and Bushuk[187] have shown that bread-making quality is correlated negatively with the proportion of acetic acid-soluble glutenin and positively with the proportion of the residue protein (acetic acid-insoluble glutenin). Kobrehel and Bushuk[17,18] and, more recently, Kobrehel[21] investigated the solubilization of glutenins in distilled water containing soaps. On the basis of the investigation of different French wheat varieties, a correlation was found between the quantity and characteristics of the solubilized proteins.

In the early investigations concerning correlations between the composition and rheological properties of gluten, the effect of amino acid composition was also studied. The results of these and some newer investigations are summarized by Lásztity.[188]

The amino acid compositions of the glutens prepared from different wheats show slight differences which may, in many cases, be statistically significant. Nevertheless, the amino acid composition of gluten is relatively stable and may be characterized as follows:

1. High glutamic acid content
2. Relatively high proline content
3. Low amount of basic amino acids (lysine, arginine, histidine)
4. High degree of amidation nearly equivalent to the aspartic and glutamic acid content
5. Remarkable cysteine and cystine content

The mathematical-statistical evaluation of the overall amino acid composition results and the rheological characteristics do not exhibit a significant correlation in most cases. The total disulfide bond (cystine) content shows a significant correlation with the rheological properties. This is characterized by a linear correlation coefficient varying from 0.3 to 0.6. The lower degree of correlation may be explained by the assumption that not only the absolute number of disulfide bonds but also their distribution is important from the perspective of rheological properties. The problem of the disulfide bonds will be discussed later.

The correlation between the degree of amidation (calculated on the basis of aspartic and glutamic acid content and ammonia content, respectively) and the rheological characteristics is shown in Figure 23. The results indicate that an optimum degree of amidation exists. The observation may be explained partly by the work of Holme and Briggs,[189] Cunningham et al.,[190] and Beckwith et al.[192] They postulated that an increase in the number of amino groups would increase the possibility of formation of secondary bonds in the gluten structure, thereby improving the rheological properties of the gluten. However, this hypothesis does not explain the negative effect of the highest degrees of amidation.

An interesting correlation was found between the amount of amino acids with hydrophobic side chains (leucine, isoleucine, proline) and relaxation time. The correlation can be described by a second-order equation.

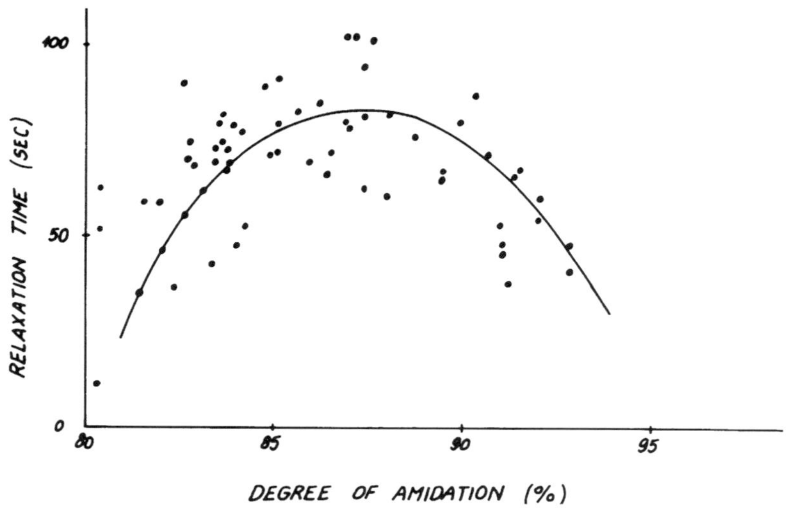

FIGURE 23 Correlation between the degree of amidation and the relaxation time of gluten.[188]

Based on the results mentioned above a new "quality index" was proposed, serving as a preliminary evaluation of the baking value of wheat, from the data of the amino acid composition of the gluten:

$$QN = 10\ C + 0.15\ A - K_A + 0.4\ H - K_H \qquad (1)$$

where C = cystine content (%); A = degree of amidation (%); H = proline, leucine, and isoleucine content; K_A = (87 – A) (absolute value); and K_H = (22.5 – H) (absolute value).

It is generally accepted that the proportion of different fractions comprising the gluten complex may influence the rheological properties of gluten and dough. In early studies the ratio of low (gliadins) and high molecular weight (glutenins) storage proteins was investigated in relation to the baking properties of wheat and flour. The ratio of gliadin and glutenin fractions appeared to be a most important factor controlling the rheological properties of wheat gluten and dough. The permissible range over which this ratio may vary appears to be quite small. The first investigators used the classical technique of Osborne for the separation. The most commonly held view concerning the role of the two main fractions of gluten was that a ratio near 1:1 was optimal from the point of view of baking quality.

More recent studies have suggested that the solubility and molecular weight distribution of the gluten proteins are major factors in determining gluten quality. Using reconstitution techniques McRitchie[192,193] has shown that dough strength appears to be a function of the molecular weight distribution of the gluten proteins. The more insoluble high molecular weight protein fractions were found to increase farinograph dough development time and extensigraph height and area and to reduce farinograph dough breakdown. Reconstitution studies by the same author[194] have also suggested that differences in baking quality of bread wheat flours varying in quality may be closely related to the properties of the more insoluble high molecular weight glutenin proteins.

Investigating a large number of Hungarian wheats by gel filtration chromatography, Lásztity[188] found that the correlation between the relaxation time and the amount of high molecular weight gluten fractions can be expressed by a second-order equation and a corresponding curve having a maximum value. This means that over a given optimal concentration the addition of high molecular weight fractions may have the opposite effect. These findings are in good agreement with the studies of Preston and Tipples.[195] They investigated the effects of adding increasing levels of acid-soluble and acid-insoluble gluten protein fractions on the rheological and baking properties of wheat flours. It was observed that the acid-insoluble (high molecular weight) gluten proteins at higher levels had a slight dough-weakening effect. The loaf volumes were also significantly reduced. The results of these studies also suggest that the acid-insoluble (glutenin) flour proteins that disaggregate during mixing (or gluten preparation), rather than more insoluble gluten proteins which are resistant to mechanical disaggregation, are of major importance in determining bread-making quality.

Hamada et al.[196] reported on the investigation of the relationship of protein fractions of spring wheat flour to baking quality. Flour proteins of wheat cultivars with a broad spectrum of dough-mixing requirements and baking characteristics were fractionated into glutenin, gliadin, albumin, and nonprotein nitrogen using gel filtration chromatography on Sephadex G-150 columns. A positive relationship was found between the amount of glutenin in wheat flour protein and mixing strength. A negative relationship appeared to exist between gliadin in flour protein and mixing strength. The glutenin fraction was additionally separated into a high (glutenin I) and a low (glutenin II) molecular weight fraction using gel filtration chromatography on Sepharose CL-2B columns. The mixing strength and the loaf volume correlated positively with the glutenin I content. Residue protein (insoluble in 0.5 *M* acetic acid) also had an increasing effect on loaf volume. Residue protein may be predominantly a high molecular weight glutenin similar to glutenin I. Doekes and Wennekes[197] and Lásztity et al.[198] investigated the changes of the glutenin, gliadin, albumin, and globulin fractions at different levels of nitrogen fertilization. An increase in the total protein content was observed. The analysis of the distribution of fractions showed changes in distribution of high and low molecular weight fractions and also in technological quality.

Some characteristic elution diagrams of AUC extracts on Sephadex G-100 columns are shown in Figure 24. The results showed significant changes in both high and low molecular weight protein fractions. Recently the important role of gel protein (according to Graveland[24]) was stressed by Pritchard and Brock.[375]

The development of gel electrophoresis and the growing knowledge of the genetics of wheat opened up new possibilities in the investigation of the correlation between the protein fractions and baking value of wheat and wheat flours. Early

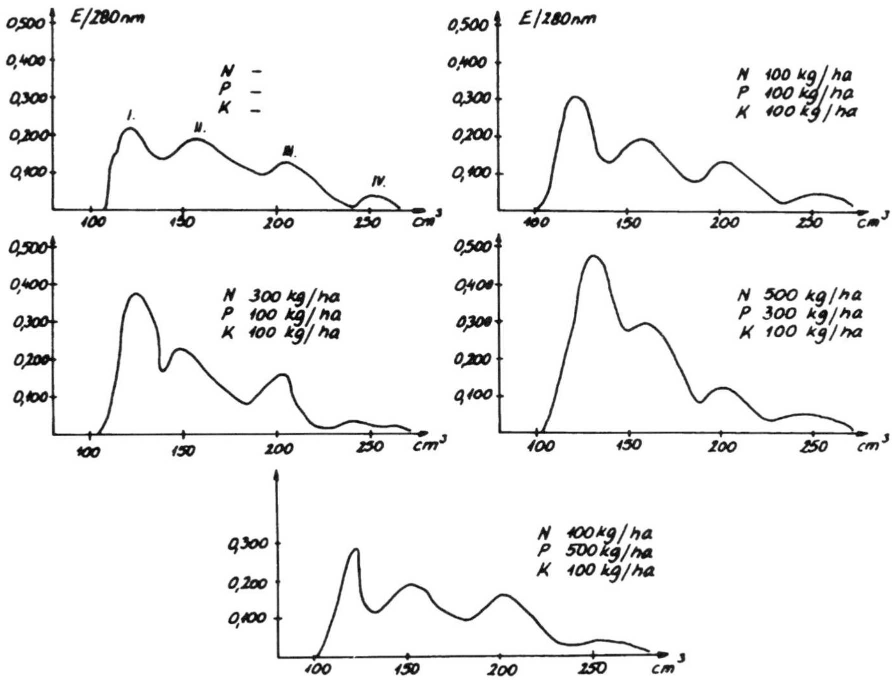

FIGURE 24 Characteristic elution diagrams of acetic acid-urea-cetyltrimethylammonium bromide (AUC) extracts of wheat grown under different levels of fertilization with N, P, and K fertilizers. (From Ragasits, Z. and Varga, J., *Növénytermelés,* 27, 131, 1978. With permission.)

studies were connected with gliadin components because their extraction was relatively easy and the separation of gliadin components was successfully solved by gel electrophoresis. In a pioneering work Doekes[200] claimed that α-, β-, and ω-gliadins occur in only a few different configurations. Based on this finding, the wheat varieties were characterized with the aid of a simple code, e.g., 1423 for a combination α1, β4, γ2, and ω3. The author hypothesized that this configuration is correlated with the baking quality of wheat varieties. In the late 1970s and early 1980s a lot of research was done in different countries, and correlations were found between the varietal intrinsic quality of wheats and the occurrence of some specific gliadin bands in electrophoretic patterns (for a review see Reference 149).

As a typical example of these results, studies by Damidaux et al.[201] may be mentioned. They have found a consistent relationship between the "gliadin 45" band and strong dough properties in durum wheats, whereas poorer quality was associated with band 42. Of the 117 samples investigated, 66 belonged to group 45 and 47 varieties to group 42; 4 varieties could not be classified into one or the other of these two groups.

Russian workers (Sozinov and Poperelya[202]) proposed a system which took into account genetic relationships between the gliadins. As mentioned earlier, gliadins are inherited in blocks associated with six loci on chromosomes 1A, 1B, 1D, 6A, 6B, and 6D. The gliadin composition of any wheat could be defined by giving the numbers for these six blocks. For example, the Russian wheat Bezostaya-1 has the gliadin composition 1A4, 1B1, 1D1, 6A1, 6B1. Based on an investigation of 50,000 samples, Sozinov[203] ranked the blocks according to their beneficial effect on grain quality (Table 16). Application of the Sozinov system in former Czechoslovakia and in Hungary has led to general agreement with the Sozinov quality ranking.[204,205]

TABLE 16
Gliadin Blocks Arranged According to the Degree of Influence on the Grain Quality

GLD 1A7 > GLD 1A4 > GLD 1A2 > GLD 1A5 > GLD 1A3 > GLD 1A1 > GLD 1A6
GLD 1B1 > GLD 1B2 > GLD 1B7 > GLD 1B5 > GLD 1B4 > GLD 1B3 > GLD 1B6
GLD 1D4 > GLD 1D6 > GLD 1D1 > GLD 1D2 > GLD 1D3
GLD 6A3 > GLD 6A1
GLD 6B2 > GLD 6B1
GLD 6D2 > GLD 6D1 > GLD 6D3

The study of the correlations between gliadin spectra and wheat quality is continuing, as shown by recent publications.[120,206,207] This could be explained by the fact that although many publications have reported the existence of significant associations between the presence of specific gliadin components and aspects of grain quality, there is no generally accepted relationship. Newer observations relating to the role of glutenin subunits in determination of baking quality suggest that the gliadins play a secondary role due to genetic linkage to another protein that more directly influences functional properties. In addition, we may be faced with the difficulty that gliadin proteins of similar electrophoretic mobility are not necessarily identical. The use of more effective separation techniques (two-dimensional gel electrophoresis, RP-HPLC, capillary electrophoresis) will help to overcome such problems.

In the 1970s the first studies[208-210] were published showing that the HMW-GS varied between wheat genotypes of different quality. Correlation studies on HMW subunits and quality characteristics were performed throughout the 1980s on a large number of wheats grown in many countries. A review of the results of these studies is given by McRitchie et al.[149] Based on worldwide observations relating to correlation between HMW-GS patterns and wheat quality, Payne[211] proposed the use of the so-called "Glu-1 quality score" for evaluation of baking quality of wheat varieties. The system proposed by this author is widely used in many countries. The contribution of different HMW-GS to quality (expressed in scores) is shown in Table 17. Although it seems that according to more recent investigations the quality score system should be modified, the Glu-1 quality score system is widely used[375-377] and has a good predictive value. In Table 18, Glu-1 quality scores of wheat cultivars grown in Hungary are shown.

TABLE 17
Glu-1 Quality Scores Assigned to High Molecular Weight Glutein Subunits[211]

Chromosome	Subunit	Score 1	2	3	4
1A	1			+	
	2*			+	
1B	17+18			+	
	7+8			+	
	13+16			+	
	7+9		+		
	7	+			
	6+8	+			
	20	+			
1D	5+10				+
	2+12		+		
	3+12		+		
	4+12	+			

There is accumulating evidence that, in addition to the qualitative effect, the quantity of subunits also contributes to the functionality of glutenin.[212,213]

The LMW subunits of glutenin, of which there are about 15 varieties, have received less attention than the HMW subunits. However, recent evidence[207,214,215] suggests that they too contribute to the intergenotype variation in bread-making quality. Whether or not the observed relationship between subunit composition and baking quality is a direct effect or an indirect effect through the structure of polymeric glutenin, which itself would depend on subunit composition, remains to be determined. In future studies the fact that there exists the possibility of producing relatively high amounts of individual subunits using expression of these polypeptides by yeast, insect cells, tissue cultures, and transgenic plants will open up new pathways in research.

The experiments of Békés and Gras,[216] using 2 g of mixograph and a direct addition of isolated HMW glutenin subunits to dough are very promising.

B. Interactions Between Protein Components

1. Disulfide Bonds

Although the idea that dough structure is based on an extensive three-dimensional network of protein subunits joined together by disulfide cross-links seems to

TABLE 18
High Molecular Weight (HMW) Glutenin Subunit Compositions of Hungarian-Grown Wheats

Variety	HMW Glutenin Subunits			Glu-1 Score
	1A	1B	1D	
Adriana	N	6+8	2+12	4
Alfold	2*	7+9	5+10	9
BLC 2125	N	7+9	5+10	7
Bucsanyi 20	N	7+9	5+10	7
Danka	1	20+9	5+10	8
Derzsanka	1	7+9	5+10	8
FD-5	N	7+8+9	5+10	8
GK Abel	N	7+9	5+10	7
GK Aron	N	7+9	2+12	5
GK Barna	1	7	2+12	6
GK Bence	1	7+9	5+10	9
GK Csanad	N	7+9	5+10	7
GK Csuros	N	7	2+12	4
GK Gergo	1	7+8	4+12	7
GK Ilma	2*	7+9	5+10	9
GK Istvan	N	7+9	5+10	7
GK Kalaka	N	7+9	5+10	7
GK Kalangya	N	7+9	5+10	7
GK Kincso	1	7	2+12	6
GK Orseg	N	7	2+12	4
GK Orzse	1	6+8	2+12	6
GK Othalom	2	7+9	5+10	9
GK Pusztaszer	1	7	2+12	6
GK Szoke	N	7+9	5+10	7
GK Zombor	N	7	2+12	4
GK 1035	1	7	2+12	6
GK 32-82	1	7	2+12	6
GK 45-87	N	20	2+12	4
Jubilejnaja 50	2*	7+9	5+10	9
Korona	2*	6+8	5+10	8
Lonja	1	20	2+12	6
MV 3	1	7+9	5+10	9
MV 9	2*	7+9	5+10	9
MV 12	2*	7+9	5+10	9
MV 14	1	7	2+12	6
MV 15	2*	7+9	5+10	9
MV 16	2*	7+9	5+10	9

TABLE 18 (continued)
High Molecular Weight (HMW) Glutenin Subunit Compositions of Hungarian-Grown Wheats

Variety	HMW Glutenin Subunits 1A	1B	1D	Glu-1 Score
MV 17	2*	7	2+12	6
MV 75-84	2*	7+9	5+10	9
MV 08-85	N	7+9	5+10	7
MV 21-85	2*	6+8	2+12	6
MV 03-86	N	7+9	2+12	5
MV 06-83	2*	7+9	5+10	9
MV 15-86	1	7+9	5+10	9
MV 107-86	N	20+9	5+10	6
MV 04-87	2*	7+9	5+10	9
MV 32-87	2*	7+9	5+10	9
MV 37-87	2*	7+9	5+10	9
MV 10-88	2*	7+9	5+10	9
MV 12-88	1	7+9	5+10	9
MV 23-88	N	7	3+12	4
MV 109-88	2*	7+9	5+10	9
MV 119-88	2*	7	2+12	6
MV 130-88	1	7+9	5+10	9
MV 213-88	2*	7+9	5+10	9
MV 218-88	N	7	2+12	4
MVHB 26-87	2*	7	5+10; 2+12	8
MVHB 47-87	N	7+9+20	5+10	8
MVHB 48-87	N	7+9	5+10	7
MVHB 69-87	2*	7+9	5+10	9
SZ 26-88	N	7	2+12	4
SZ 146-88	1	7+9	5+10	9
Skopjanka	N	7	2+12	4
Zagrebcsanka	1	6+8	2+12	6
ZG 52-10	2*	7+9	5+10	9
ZG 7057/79	N	6+8	2+12	4
ZG 163/82	N	6+8	2+12	4
ZG 213/83	2*	6+8	4+12	5
ZG 2008/85	1	6+8	2+12	6
ZG 167/86	2*	6+8	4+12	5
ZG 291/86	N	7	2+12	4
Vitka	N	7+8+9	5+10	7

be phasing out[217,218] and the role of the other, noncovalent binding is being stressed,[1] there is no doubt that thiol groups and disulfide bonds play an important role in determining gluten and dough properties. The gluten proteins contain relatively small quantities of cystine and cysteine (average 2 to 3%). Their importance was observed primarily in relation to problems of flour improvers. As a consequence, very extensive research work was started in this domain. Nevertheless, there are still many unsolved problems. To clarify the role of disulfide bonds, further comprehensive investigations are needed. Some useful data may be obtained by studying the changes occurring in the rheological properties due to the decomposition of the disulfide bonds.

Earlier tests of Beckwith et al.[219,220] on wheat gliadin and glutenin showed that reduction (breakdown) of the S–S bonds of gliadin involves no perceptible change in molecular mass. Though ferograms obtained by gel electrophoresis show minor deviations in mobility, these can be explained by changes in conformation.

In the case of reoxidation in a diluted solution, investigations by the above-mentioned authors show that the native gliadin is practically recovered. Their finding has been confirmed by ultracentrifugal, electrophoresis, and rotatory dispersion tests. No data have been published about the rheological properties of the reoxidized product. Their observation that solution (5%) yields products with higher molecular masses and less solubility than the original gliadin is very interesting. Presumably, intermolecular disulfide bonds are being formed in this case.

The decomposition of the disulfide bonds in glutenin by reduction results in the disintegration of the large gluten component molecules. In the case of reoxidation in solutions of higher concentration, a product with properties very close to those of native glutenin may be obtained. According to the cited authors, the physical properties of the product formed in the course of reoxidation are highly influenced by the reoxidation conditions, primarily by pH and urea concentration. No numerical data on the rheological properties of the glutenins produced under different conditions have been reported; probably no such measurements have been carried out.

In the author's laboratory, studies were conducted on the conditions of reoxidation following gluten reduction and on the rheological properties of the products obtained in order to provide the necessary information. To reduce and reoxidize the gluten samples the author adopted the method applied by Beckwith et al.,[219,220] its rough outline being as follows: 5% solutions of the gluten samples in a 6 mol/dm^3 urea solution were prepared. The reduction was subsequently carried out with β-mercaptoethanol under nitrogen circulation for 12 h. Part of the reduced gluten was alkylated with acrylonitrile, yielding after dialysis and lyophilization the *S*-cyanoethyl gluten derivative. Reoxidation was carried out in different urea concentrations (solutions of 1 to 8 mol/dm^3) and at different pH values (3.5 to 5.5 to 8.5). The gluten content of the solution ranged from 1 to 10% since preliminary tests showed this concentration range to be the most favorable for producing a product similar to native gluten.

Reoxidation was performed by oxygen circulation for 168 h. By the end of the reoxidizing process the product was purified by dialysis and compacted in a centrifugal apparatus, and finally free water was removed from the agglomerating mass by hand kneading in a polyethylene bag. The samples were tested for stress relaxation by the method of Lásztity.[372,373] Table 19 summarizes the rheological properties of reoxidized glutens produced under different conditions. Data in Table 19 show that the rheological properties of the products obtained are highly influenced by the reoxidation conditions. Products best demonstrating the properties of native gluten are produced with a 3 mol/dm^3 urea solution at pH 5.5 and with a 6 mol/dm^3 urea solution at pH 3.5. In general, with low urea concentrations, cohesive products lacking elasticity are obtained, whereas in the case of 8 mol/dm^3 urea concentration the reoxidized gluten is tougher but has no appropriate elasticity. In alkaline media (pH 8.5) no product with properties similar to native gluten could be obtained at any urea concentration. It should be noted that reoxidation was essentially more rapid in alkaline media, and in general the reoxidized product yielded a practically inelastic, cohesive mass when mixed with water. Its properties were largely similar to those of gluten which has been extensively denaturated by heat. On the basis of the results it is apparent that the absolute number of disulfide bonds alone does not unambiguously define these properties. In this respect the site of the disulfide bonds is also important.

TABLE 19
Rheological Properties of Reoxidized Glutens

Sample No.	Urea Concentration (mol/dm^3)	pH	τ h (N/m^2)	t_r (s)	Remarks
1	1	3.5	15	Not measurable	—
2	1	5.5	22	—	—
3	1	8.5	35	—	—
4	2	3.5	24	30	—
5	2	5.5	28	42	—
6	2	8.5	120	Not measurable	—
7	4	3.5	54	68	Elastic
8	4	5.5	77	92	—
9	4	8.5	180	150	—
10	6	3.5	30	42	Slightly
11	6	5.5	27	29	Elastic
12	6	8.5	190	180	—
13	8	3.5	32	35	—
14	8	5.5	270	Not measurable	Nonelastic
15	8	8.5	280	Not measurable	Nonelastic
16	Native gluten (control sample)		59	83	Gluten of average elasticity and extensibility

The influence of pH and urea concentration on the properties of the reoxidized products can be explained as follows: depending on pH and urea concentration, changes may occur in the conformation of the peptide chains, the steric position of the individual groups, their dissociation conditions, and their reactivity, defining the type and site of the disulfide bonds formed. The effect of urea, pH, and ion concentration on protein conformation are generally known.

The disulfide bonds formed might be either intra- or intermolecular bonds. The ratio of inter- and intramolecular disulfide bonds is presumably very important in the development of rheological properties. To check this assumption, changes in the viscosity of the solution during decomposition by performic acid of reoxidized glutens obtained in different ways have been followed. Characteristic curves are presented in Figures 24 to 26.

It can be seen distinctly that the viscosity vs. time graphs are different for reoxidized gluten products having different rheological properties. The simplest curve was obtained for a gluten reoxidized in alkaline medium at a high urea concentration (Figure 24). After a relatively rapid decrease in viscosity it remains at an approximately constant value during further oxidation with performic acid. The reoxidized product, with properties approximating those of the native gluten, follows a different course (Figure 25). After a rapid decrease in viscosity a minimum is reached. Viscosity then rises to reach a limit value. The solution of a reoxidized gluten product prepared at a low urea concentration at acid pH (Figure 26) is subject to a smaller decrease in viscosity during performic acid oxidation, the viscosity graph shows a sharp minimum, and the subsequent increase in viscosity is higher than in Figure 26.

The results clearly show the differences between the disulfide bond systems of the reoxidized glutens with different rheological properties. The decrease in viscosity occurring in all cases at the beginning of the disintegration of the disulfide bridges indicates that, owing to the rupture of intermolecular disulfide bonds, larger protein molecules will break down to smaller units. The subsequent course of the viscosity curve will depend on whether or not the smaller units formed contain intramolecular disulfide bonds at all — and if they do, to what extent — since the disintegration of these intramolecular disulfide bonds will result in a change in the conformation of the molecule, and the molecule, "opening" to a certain extent, will increase in viscosity. When disintegration of the intramolecular disulfide bonds comes to an end, both the conformation of the molecule and the viscosity will attain constant values. Studying the curves from this point of view, it may be seen that the reoxidized gluten prepared in an alkaline medium at a high urea concentration practically contains intermolecular disulfide bonds only. In the product close to native gluten the number of intramolecular disulfide bonds is high, and the same applies also to reoxidized gluten obtained at acid pH and a low urea concentration.

In principle the viscosity recovery after a minimum could also be ascribed to new aggregates forming secondary bonds after the breakdown of the primary disulfide bonds. This assumption is, however, improbable because no such increase is recorded for the reoxidized gluten prepared at alkaline pH and a high urea concentration.

Reduction and reoxidation studies of gluten indicate the importance of the disulfide bonds in the structure of gluten molecules and also in their rheological properties. According to these studies, high molecular mass gluten protein fractions consist of polypeptide chains connected by disulfide bridges. In addition, the number

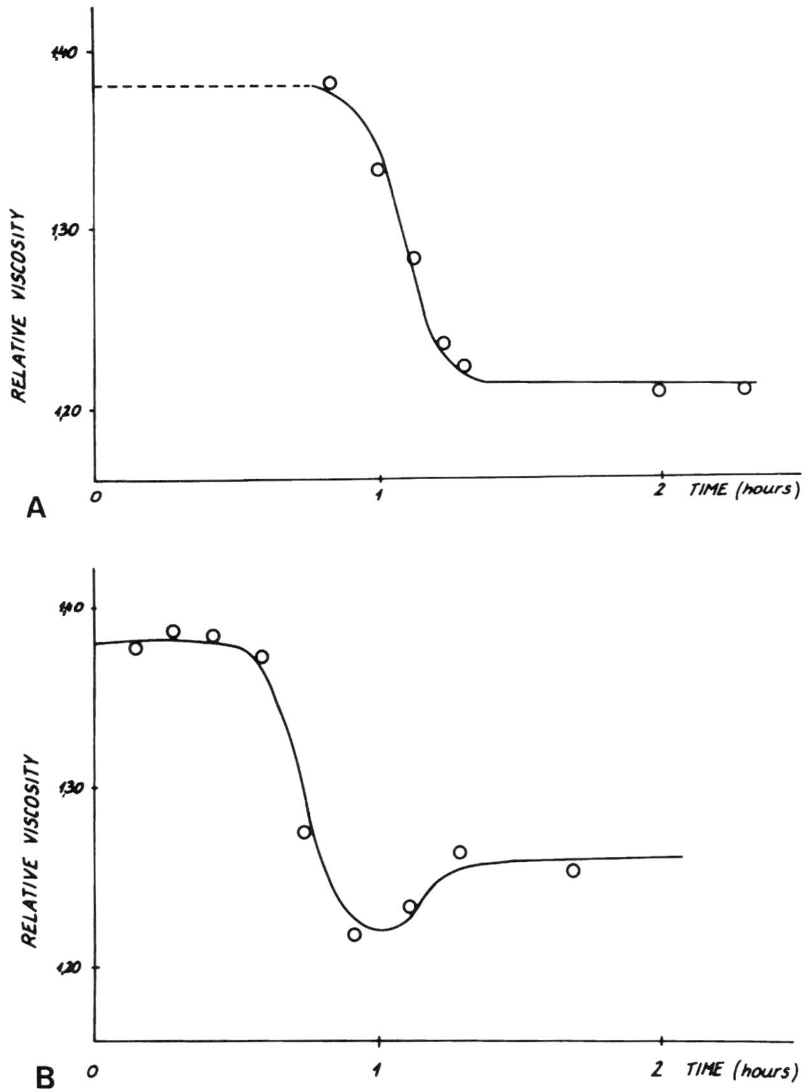

FIGURE 25 Changes in the viscosity of reoxidized gluten solution during splitting of the S–S bonds with performic acids. (A) Product B: reoxidized in 3 mol/dm^3 urea at pH 5.5; (B) product C: reoxidized in 8 mol/dm^3 urea.

of disulfide bonds within the molecule is also of importance. During the reduction of the gluten all disulfide bonds will break down, and the product obtained lacks the rheological properties of the original gluten. When reoxidized, the reversion is practically quantitative. However, the site of newly formed bonds and the ratio between inter- and intramolecular disulfide bonds will depend on reoxidizing conditions. This fact is reflected in the rheological properties of the reoxidized product.

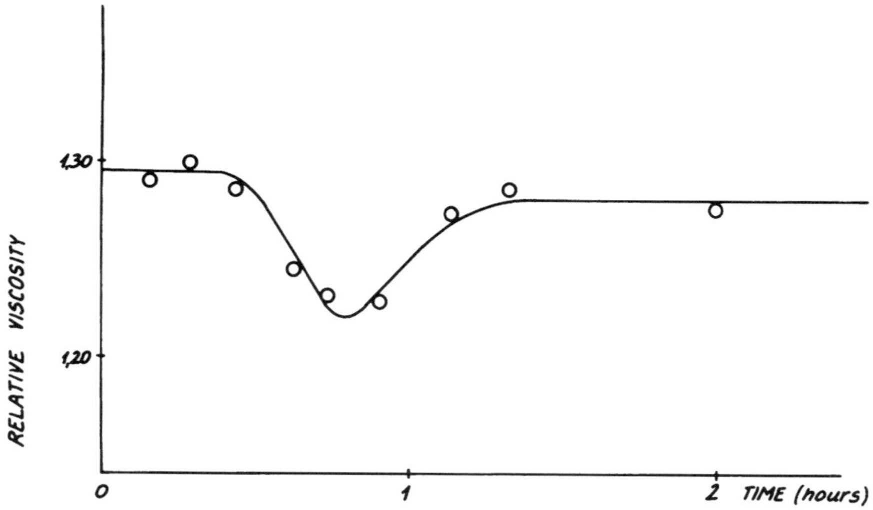

FIGURE 26 Changes in the viscosity of reoxidized gluten solution during splitting of the S–S bonds with performic acid (product A: reoxidized in 1 mol/dm^3 urea at pH 3.5).[188]

It follows from the above that the absolute number of disulfide bonds alone does not unambiguously define the structure and the rheological properties. It becomes clear why, in general, no closer correlation could be established between the disulfide bond content and the rheological properties. It also explains why the correlation is stronger in gluten of the same wheat variety: it may be assumed that in a given wheat variety the protein biosynthesis proceeds similarly, and hence the distribution of the disulfide bonds will also be similar. The looseness of the correlation is likely to be attributed to the many other factors involved in the development of the rheological properties.

The finding that products with differing rheological properties can be obtained, depending on the conditions of reoxidation after reduction of a given gluten, could be of paramount importance in practice. It implies the possibility of developing an economically feasible method of reduction and reoxidation for breaking down the native glutens into units consisting of the fundamental polypeptide chains, and subsequently, by selecting the appropriate conditions for reoxidation, to produce glutens with rheological properties as required by the particular grain-processing technology in question. The underlying concept of this gluten-processing method is presented in Figure 27.

The disulfide bonds of the gluten and dough form a dynamically changing system. The changes are related to both the quantity and the distribution of the S–S linkages: the conclusions mentioned above are based on numerous investigations concerning changes in disulfide bonds and thiol group quantity during mixing or resting of the doughs. The thiol groups may affect the disulfide bonds in two ways: by oxidation new disulfide bonds may be formed; and interchange reaction may occur between S–S bonds and thiol groups, causing a dynamic change in the distribution

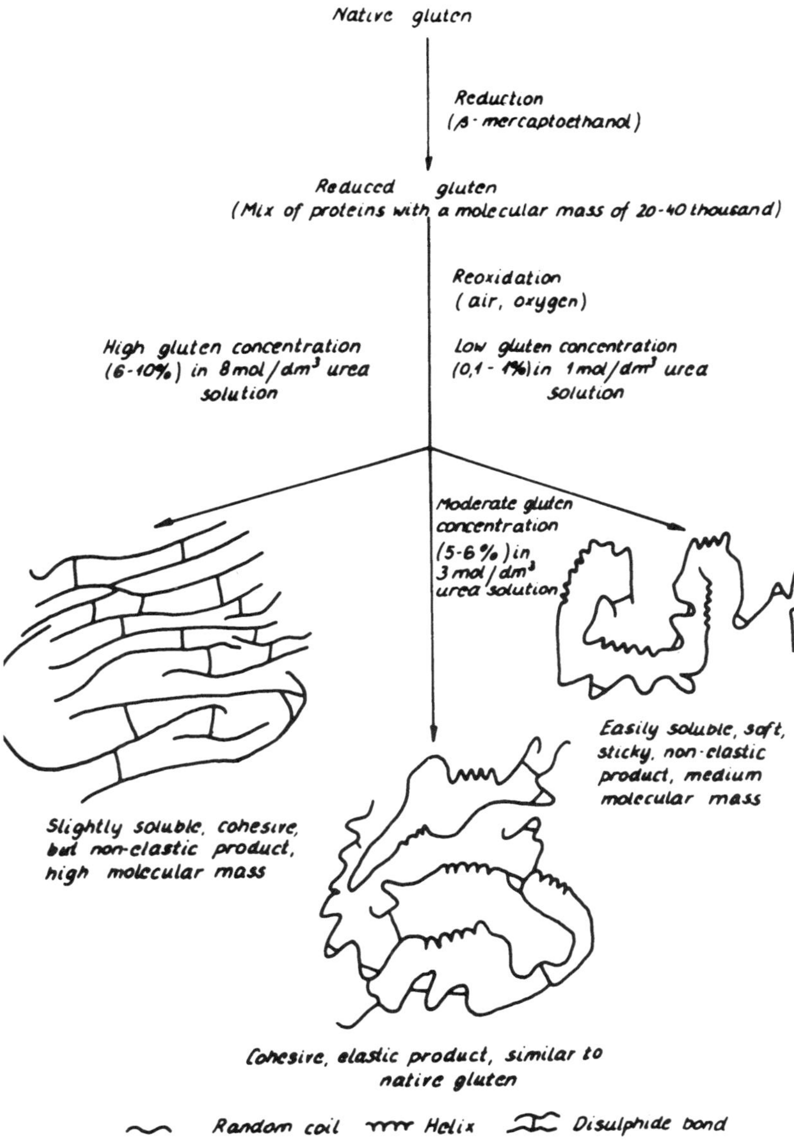

FIGURE 27 Scheme of the process producing gluten with modified rheological properties.

of disulfide linkages.[217,221,222] Conversely, a reduction of disulfide bonds causes an increase of SH groups. Oxidation strongly affects the rheological properties of doughs. A widely accepted explanation is that oxidation removes thiol groups and forms new disulfide bonds. Some authors[223] are of the opinion that this explanation is too simplified and that the process is more complex. The experimental facts supporting this view may be summarized as follows:

1. The quantity of oxidizing agents used for improving the rheological properties of dough is very small, and the precondition for the formation of new disulfide bonds is the sterically favorable positioning of two thiol groups. Under such conditions the quantity of the newly formed S–S bonds may be extraordinarily small.
2. Although the decrease in thiol content has been well established experimentally, the increase in disulfide bond content has not been confirmed.
3. The thiol content of protein groups having the most important role in gluten formation is relatively smaller than in albumin and globulin fractions.
4. Addition of thiol group blocking agents has the same effect as the use of oxidizing improvers.
5. In many cases the change in the rheological properties is much slower than the oxidation process.

The problems mentioned above are partly solved by the fact that disulfide-thiol interchange may occur, which causes a change in the distribution of S–S linkages. The latter may be connected with rheological changes. By blocking the thiol groups the interchange or oxidation of these groups is not possible. An improvement of the theory concerning the role of SH and S–S groups was elaborated by Bloksma[221,222] and introduced the term "rheologically effective" SH groups and S–S bonds. It was supposed that the rheologically effective groups are only fractions of the total content of thiol and disulfide groups. In the author's laboratory the effect of *N*-ethylmaleimide on the thiol groups of gluten and on its rheological properties was investigated.[224] The rheological features of *N*-ethylmaleimide derivatives of gluten are listed in Table 20. Data in Table 20 suggest that no significant change occurs in the viscoelastic behavior of gluten when its free thiol groups are blocked.

The viscosity of the gluten derivative suspended in 0.1 *N* acetic acid was also studied; results are collected in Figure 28. The diagram indicates a small but clearly observable decrease in the viscosity of gluten solutions blocked with *N*-ethylmaleimide, referred to as controls.

These two series of experiments allow us to draw the conclusion that free thiol groups have no significant effect on the rheological properties of glutens. The thiol-disulfide interaction observed in pasta or dough does not play any practical role in gluten. It is probable that thiol groups participate in intra- or intermolecular bonding; however, no noticeable effect due to this is exerted upon rheological behavior.

This refers also to eventual hydrogen bonds, as well as to supposed thiol-carbonyl interactions. Theoretically, in the latter case, due to an addition reaction, a thiol ester is formed.

The breaking of the disulfide bonds during mixing was experimentally confirmed by many research workers. Also, a reconstitution of S–S linkages was observed during resting. From the point of view of the explanation of the mechanism changes, the observation of Dronzek and Bushuk[225] was important. They obtained evidence that free radicals are produced in dough during mixing. An increase in thiol group content on mixing under nitrogen was also noted.[226,227]

Recent investigations concerning the occurrence and distribution of disulfide bonds and thiol groups revealed the important role of some redox systems present in dough. Grosch and Sarwin[228] found free reduced glutathione (GSH), oxidized

TABLE 20
Viscoelastic Properties of the N-Ethylmaleimide Derivative of Gluten

Sample No.	Blocking (%)	Relaxation Time (s)	I (g)
1	0	57	69
	57	64	75
	100	59	60
2	0	39	60
	57	41	65
	100	38	58
3	0	80	106
	57	89	125
	100	93	98
4	0	68	75
	57	75	80
	100	69	82
5	0	43	68
	57	39	59
	100	59	69
6	0	68	85
	57	70	80
	100	73	78
7	0	46	92
	57	50	97
	100	50	91
8	0	58	106
	57	54	120
	100	49	122
9	0	104	140
	57	121	130
	100	98	119
10	0	82	98
	57	78	96
	100	91	107

glutathione (GSSG), and protein-glutathione mixed disulfides (G-S-S-Prot) in flours and their doughs. A decrease in GSH and an increase in cysteine was observed. Experiments involving addition of l-threonine-ascorbic acid (L-TAA) confirmed the hypothesis that the improver action of L-TAA is caused by a rapid oxidation of GSH to its rheologically inactive disulfide. Kobrehel et al.[229] studied the role of a thioredoxin-linked redox system in selective reduction of wheat storage proteins. It was suggested that this system could be applied as an improver.

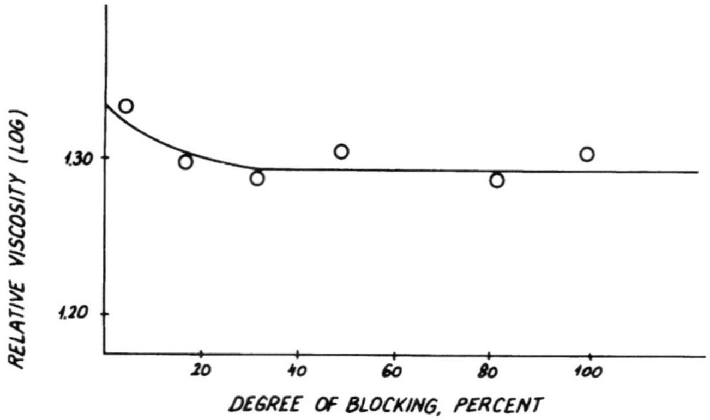

FIGURE 28 Change of viscosity of solutions of the *N*-ethylmaleimide derivative of gluten as a function of the degree of blocking.[180]

The deeper knowledge of polypeptides occurring in the gluten complex combined with new, more effective separation techniques provides new possibilities for studying the localization and nature of disulfide bonds in gluten. Some recent results were published by Tao et al.,[230] Köhler et al.,[231] and Weegels et al.,[232] among others. Cystine peptides isolated from tryptic and thermolytic digests of glutenin were analyzed for their amino acid sequences and assigned to known sequences of gluten proteins. The peptides exhibited inter- and intramolecular disulfide bonds within the group of HMW subunits, LMW subunits, and γ-gliadins.[231]

Weegels et al.[232] studied the subunit composition of the glutenin macropolymer (GMP) during dough mixing. During mixing GMP partly depolymerized and became partially extractable in SDS, resulting in a changed subunit composition for the remaining GMP. For flours with glutenin subunit composition 7 + 9 and 2 + 12, 10% (Camp Remy) or 25% (Obelisk) of subunit 9 remained in the GMP. For the variety Rektor (7 + 9, 5 + 10), 11% of subunit 5 remained in the GMP. For all other subunits less was left after mixing. During resting, repolymerization occurred and subunits were incorporated to different levels and at different rates. Y-type subunits 9, 10, and 12 were incorporated at a higher rate and to a larger relative level than X-type subunits $1/2^x$, 2, 5, and 7. Although it is tempting to explain these results by the varying cysteine content of the N-termini of X-(4 SH) and Y-type (5 SH) subunits, the repolymerization of individual subunits could be almost completely (91%) explained by the amount of a subunit in flour GMP and the resting time. This shows that the composition of GMP during processing can be predicted on the basis of flour and processing parameters only and that differences in the amounts are more important than quality differences.

2. Hydrogen Bonds

Although the important role of the disulfide bond system in the determination of rheological properties of gluten has been confirmed by many experimental facts, the investigations of the last few decades have shown that the explanation of rheological properties of gluten is not possible without taking into account the other possible interactions in the gluten network. A purely theoretical approach to the problem indicates that the gluten proteins contain a great number of side chain groups forming hydrogen bonds. In Table 21 the average number of functional groups in gluten proteins is shown.[233] This fact supports the hypothesis that hydrogen bonds also contribute to the rheological properties of gluten. Many experimental facts confirm the possible role of noncovalent bonds. Most insoluble glutens can be dispersed in strong urea solutions or in other hydrogen bond-disrupting agents.

TABLE 21
Functional Groups in the Gluten Proteins (mmol/100 g Protein)[233]

Group	Amino Acids	Gliadin	Glutenin
Acidic	Glutamic acid	27	36
	Aspartic acid		
Basic	Lysine	39	52
	Arginine		
	Histidine		
	Tryptophan		
Amide	Glutamine	309	266
	Asparagine		
Thiol and disulfide	Cysteine	12	12
	Cystine		
Total ionic	Acidic + basic	66	87
Total polar	Hydroxy + amide	381	365
Total nonpolar		390	301

The contributions of hydrogen bonds and reactive sulfur-containing groups of proteins to the rheological properties of dough were studied by Jankiewicz and Pomeranz[234] by addition of urea and *N*-ethylmaleic imide. Vakar et al.[235] have reported that freshly washed gluten becomes stronger and more elastic after it is dipped into D_2O. These facts also indicate that hydrogen bonds play an important role in gluten structure. The known role of amido groups, the more recent hypotheses for the proposed structure of glutenin, and the investigations of SDS-soluble and soap-dispersible proteins also confirmed the importance of hydrogen bonds in the formation of the gluten complex. In the author's laboratory an extended research program was established with the purpose of explaining the role of different groups in the formation of hydrogen bonds and rheological properties of gluten. The role of amide groups, the effect of esterification of carboxyl groups, and the acylation of primary amino groups were investigated. Some results of these investigations are summarized in the next part of this chapter.

a. Influence of Deamidation

A great number of amidated carboxyl groups are present in gluten proteins. In view of this number, high in comparison with other polar groups, the role of amino groups in the formation of secondary bonds might be important. Therefore, penetration indexes of glutens deamidated to various degrees were determined, and the viscosities of deamidated gluten dissolved in acetic acid and in 8 mol/dm^3 urea solutions were measured. Results are listed in Tables 22 to 24. The data demonstrate that, compared to control samples, deamidated glutens are of softer consistency; i.e., their rheological properties are inferior. The differences, in terms of relative percent penetration, increase with the degree of deamidation, substantially at the start and then tending toward a limit value.

TABLE 22
Rheological Properties of Deamidated Glutens

Sample	Degree of Deamidation (%)					
No.	10	30	50	70	90	100
1	15	24	31	39	39	42
2	12	23	35	46	47	50
3	17	29	39	51	55	57
4	10	21	31	35	34	39
5	8	17	29	37	42	42
6	7	23	29	35	37	39
7	13	21	34	45	49	53
8	15	21	29	42	47	48
9	11	19	33	42	47	48
10	14	23	32	44	43	43

Note: Values are differences in penetration (%) vs. control sample.

As far as solubilities are concerned, deamidated gluten is more difficult to dissolve in strongly acidic media (below pH 3), but is easily dissolved — in contrast to controls — in pH 8 phosphate buffer. Considering the substantial increase of free carboxyl groups and the acidic character of the protein formed, this fact seems to be understandable.

Based on the results of viscosity measurements it can be stated that deamidation primarily affects the viscosity of solutions in acetic acid. According to the data in Table 23, modification leads to an increase in intrinsic viscosity, demonstrating that a change has occurred in the conformation of the molecules, which results in higher

TABLE 23
Intrinsic Viscosity of Deamidated Gluten Solutions in Acetic Acid

Series	Degree of Deamidation (%)						Acetic Acid Concentration
No.	10	30	50	70	90	100	(mol/dm³)
1	0.425	0.445	0.462	0.480	0.505	0.510	0.05
	0.430	0.435	0.440	0.437	0.435	0.420	1.0
2	0.480	0.485	0.492	0.507	0.580	0.510	0.05
	0.475	0.480	0.481	0.475	0.470	0.469	1.0
3	0.460	0.475	0.490	0.502	0.500	0.499	0.05
	0.462	0.467	0.470	0.465	0.459	0.458	1.0
4	0.502	0.520	0.530	0.536	0.535	0.537	0.05
	0.490	0.501	0.506	0.508	0.506	0.501	1.0
5	0.397	0.412	0.431	0.432	0.430	0.429	0.05
	0.400	0.405	0.405	0.402	0.400	0.390	1.0

Note: Values are η (dl/g).

TABLE 24
Intrinsic Viscosity of Solutions of Deamidated Gluten in 8 mol/dm³ Urea

Series	Degree of Deamidation (%)					
No.	10	30	50	70	90	100
1	0.480	0.475	0.475	0.478	0.468	0.450
2	0.550	0.552	0.545	0.547	0.530	0.527
3	0.501	0.497	0.502	0.504	0.486	0.479
4	0.560	0.550	0.552	0.540	0.531	0.535
5	0.480	0.482	0.480	0.470	0.447	0.450

Note: Values are η (dl/g).

asymmetry of the structure. For an explanation, one might suggest that the removal of the amido groups involves the elimination of secondary (e.g., hydrogen) bonds, resulting in a looser structure. Presumably, due to the dissociation of carboxyl groups liberated within a molecule, repulsive forces will be operative between groups with identical charge. This assumption is supported by the experimental finding that an increase in viscosity is substantially less in 1.0 mol/dm^3 acetic acid at higher pH and lower dissociation or that under these conditions no increase in viscosity is found in some cases. Probably on the one hand electrostatic repulsion is weaker, and on the other hand new hydrogen bonds are formed between groups at sterically favorable sites.

Similar conclusions can be drawn from viscosity data relating to glutens and to deamidated glutens dissolved in 8 mol/dm^3 urea. A comparison of viscosity data from solutions in 0.05 mol/dm^3 acetic acid and in 8 mol/dm^3 urea reveals that as compared to the acetic acid solution the increase in viscosity of nondeamidated control samples is significantly higher than that of partially deamidated samples. The differences can be explained on the basis that in amidated glutens there are substantially more hydrogen bonds present and that these are disrupted by the urea added, and thus the conformations are altered.

At lower pH (1 mol/dm^3 acetic acid) deamidated gluten samples also show viscosity data widely differing from those of solutions with urea. In some cases these values are very nearly the same as those for the control samples. This finding supports the idea of new hydrogen bonds being formed, as mentioned in the discussion of the data shown in Table 23.

b. Effect of Esterification

Esterification is one of the possible ways to transform the free carboxyl groups. Partial conversion of amido groups into esters is also feasible. In the author's experiment the rheological properties of glutens esterified with methanol or ethanol were studied together with the viscosities of the solutions prepared from the derivative with 0.05 mol/dm^3 acetic acid. Results are listed in Tables 25 and 26.

TABLE 25
Relaxation of Gluten Esterified with Methanol

Series	Extent of Methylation (mmol/g)						
No.	0	0.30	0.50	1.0	1.5	2.0	3.0
1	82	79	60	54	48	45	46
2	45	44	36	30	28	25	26
3	73	70	60	52	45	40	41
4	55	56	51	41	35	32	34
5	69	65	54	48	40	36	30

Note: Values are relaxation time (s).

The data in Table 25 show that with increasing degrees of esterification the rheological properties of gluten deteriorate, and relaxation time becomes significantly shorter. In the first stage, corresponding to the esterification of the free carboxyl groups

TABLE 26
Intrinsic Viscosity of Solutions of Gluten Esterified with Methanol

Series	Extent of Methylation (mmol/g)						
No.	0	0.30	0.50	1.0	1.5	2.0	3.0
1	0.442	0.439	0.384	0.350	0.321	0.295	0.280
2	0.495	0.480	0.401	0.362	0.318	0.288	0.275
3	0.480	0.469	0.360	0.331	0.297	0.291	0.302
4	0.530	0.529	0.460	0.431	0.390	0.321	0.305
5	0.420	0.415	0.340	0.291	0.270	0.258	0.261

Note: Values are [η] dl/g.

present, no essential change occurs; this suggests that the role of free carboxyl groups in the formation of secondary bonds is insignificant.

The viscosity data indicating a substantial decrease in intrinsic viscosity implicate more compact and less asymmetric molecules, possibly due to the fact that alkylated protein is highly hydrophobic, and hence its hydration degree will be lower.

c. *Effect of Acylation*

In order to study the rheological properties of acylated gluten, the penetration values of the hydrated gluten derivatives and the viscosities of their solutions in 0.1 mol/dm^3 acetic acid were measured. Results are summarized in Tables 27 and 28.

TABLE 27
Penetration Values (0.1 mm) of Acylated Gluten

Series	Acylation (%)			
No.	0	40	80	100
1	72	142	152	160
2	58	108	112	135
3	85	120	135	142
4	700	105	121	143
5	994	143	162	180
6	45	92	108	125
7	48	89	102	117
8	73	104	130	135

TABLE 28
Intrinsic Viscosity of the Solutions of Acylated Gluten

Series	Acylation (%)			
No.	0	40	80	100
1	0.425	0.396	0.392	0.388
2	0.480	0.428	0.420	0.422
3	0.460	0.432	0.417	0.418
4	0.502	0.477	0.472	0.465
5	0.397	0.368	0.362	0.365
6	0.485	0.444	0.427	0.430
7	0.510	0.482	0.469	0.461
8	0.447	0.417	0.405	0.396

Note: Values are $[\eta]$ dl/g.

The data reveal that the rheological properties of acylated gluten are very much inferior to those of native gluten. The decrease in cohesiveness suggests that primary amino groups play a substantial role in the formation of intermolecular noncovalent bonds.

Experimental results show that no major alteration in viscosity takes place; after an initial small decrease the viscosity values remain practically constant. Thus, it can be concluded that no important change in molecular conformation occur or that primary amino groups participate principally in the formation of intermolecular bonds. Nierle and El Baya[236] reported that alkylation of ε-amino groups does not significantly influence gluten functionality.

The rheological properties of chemically modified gluten were investigated by Batey.[237,238] The reaction of gluten with sodium hydroxide produced some very interesting results. The alkali treatment caused a destruction of disulfide bonds, but affected practically no amino groups. At 40°C and a relatively long time of action only 6% of the amide groups were hydrolyzed. The molecular weight distribution of the alkali-treated gluten remained practically unchanged — being controlled by gel filtration chromatography on Sephadex G-150 columns. Small differences were observed, probably as an effect of the exocleavage of short oligopeptides. If gluten consisted of relatively small subunits held together by disulfide bonds, the molecular weight of the gluten should be drastically reduced by this treatment. That no such reduction in molecular weight range is observed is evidence that disulfide groups are not the major force holding small subunits together in large aggregates. Hydrogen bonding, hydrophobic interactions, and electrostatic attractions together must contribute the major forces determining the quaternary structure of the protein complex. The views of Batey concerning the role of noncovalent bonds in formation of gluten structure are in agreement with the newer results published in the literature. Nevertheless, it has not been explained why a drastic deterioration of dough and gluten rheological properties occurs without changes in molecular weight distribution.

The charged residues (lysine and arginine) can be modified extensively with relative ease, thus indicating that they are in accessible positions on the surface of the molecule. The glutens so modified show a marked deterioration in their mixing properties. Tyrosine residues react slowly with *N*-acetylimidazole under nondenaturating conditions, but more rapidly in strong urea solutions. These results suggest a gluten conformation characterized by charged residues on the surface of the modified molecule and by the hydrophobic side chains in the interior.

Flow properties of aqueous gluten and gluten methyl ester dispersions were studied by Mita and Matsumoto.[239] Characteristic flow curves of the gluten dispersion are shown in Figure 29. Gluten dispersion exhibited Newtonian flow behavior at concentrations below 4%, but non-Newtonian flow behavior became pronounced with increasing concentrations. With higher concentrations a hysteresis loop was observed. The gluten methyl ester dispersions differ considerably from those of gluten. The differences are clearly shown in Figure 30. The differences in the flow properties of gluten and gluten methyl ester dispersions are explained by the author as being due to the hydrogen bond interactions between molecules. This effect becomes more pronounced at higher concentrations. In the gluten methyl ester dispersion the number of side chains participating in the formation of hydrogen bonds is much lower. It was supposed that hydrogen bond interactions between glutamine (asparagine) side chains might occur more rapidly in a dough system because the water content of dough is much lower than that of the gluten dispersions investigated.

3. Hydrophobic Interactions

As was shown in Table 21, gluten proteins contain several amino acids with hydrophobic side chains (alanine, leucine, phenylalanine, isoleucine, valine, proline). Moreover, taking into consideration that the hydrophobic parts of longer polar side chains (e.g., in the case of lysine and glutamic acid) may also interact, there can be no doubt concerning the potential for hydrophobic bond formation.

Dough and gluten formation proceeds in aqueous media. Owing to the fact that an interaction of the nonpolar groups with water is "unfavorable" from the thermodynamic viewpoint, the thermodynamic tendency points toward a linkage of the nonpolar groups with each other (with a consequent weakening of the interaction between these groups and water). In general, the formation of hydrophobic bonds is an endothermic process; i.e., the change in thermodynamic potential is negative since the effect of the change in entropy ($T\Delta S$) exceeds that of the change in enthalpy (ΔH). Up to a certain temperature limit the strength of hydrophobic bonds increases with increasing temperature, so that hydrophobic bonds are of particular importance from the viewpoint of thermal stability of proteins.

The solubility of gliadin in nonpolar solvents and the influence of the latter on solubility are also indicative of the possible importance of the role of hydrophobic bonds. All this shows convincingly that a study of the hydrophobic bonds is unavoidably

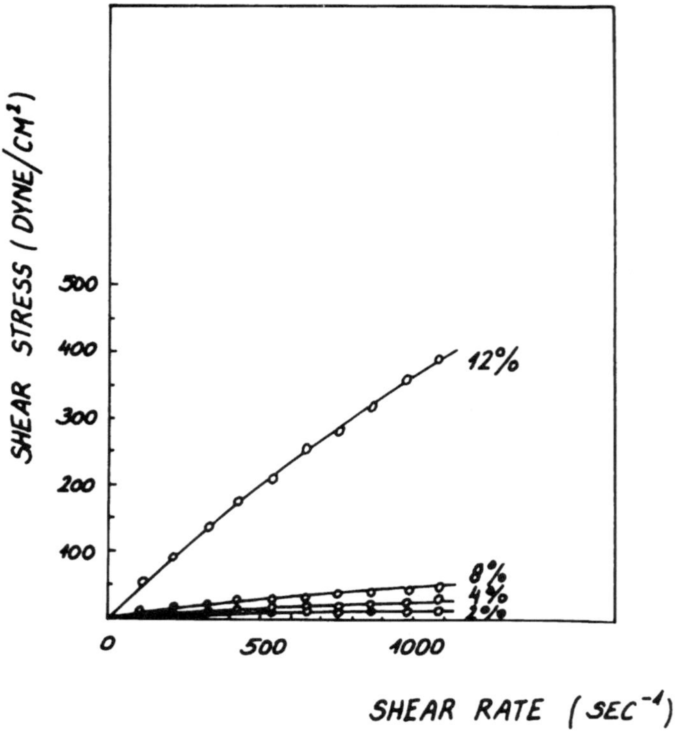

FIGURE 29 Characteristic flow curves of aqueous solutions of gluten methyl ester. (From Mita, T. and Matsumoto, H., *Cereal Chem.,* 58, 57, 1981. With permission.)

necessary for the understanding of factors which influence the structure and rheological properties of gluten proteins.

From earlier research the observation might be mentioned that the rheological properties of doughs are already changed by small quantities of certain aliphatic hydrocarbons.[240,243]

In the author's laboratory the effect of compounds able to react with the hydrophobic groups of the gluten complex has been studied; they were able, through these groups, to interfere with the hydrophobic bonds existing earlier. Some results of this work will be summarized in the next part of this chapter.

a. *Effect of Hydrocarbons on the Rheological Properties of Gluten*

These tests were carried out as follows. Dehydrated gluten was brought into contact with water containing a known amount of hydrocarbons. After hydration and swelling, the hydrated mass was subjected to mechanical working until a coherent, homogeneous material was obtained. The excess solution was removed and relaxation was measured. Some experimental results are presented in Table 29.

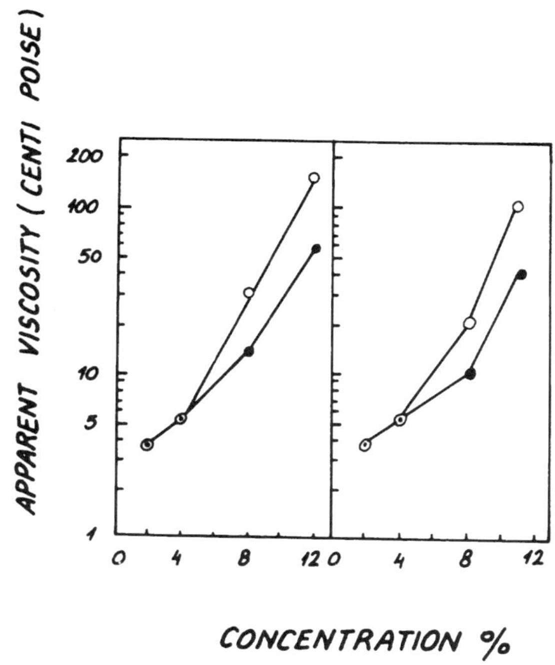

FIGURE 30 Plots of apparent viscosity vs. concentration at $\gamma = 110\ s^{-1}$ (left) and $\gamma = 1.076\ s^{-1}$ (right); -●-gluten, -○-gluten methyl ester. (From Mita, T. and Matsumoto, H., *Cereal Chem.*, 58, 57, 1981. With permission.)

These data show that the rheological properties of gluten are affected unfavorably by the presence of higher aliphatic hydrocarbons. When tested organoleptically, gluten becomes less stretchable and more crumbly. In the case of pentane and hexane an increase in the relaxation time and in the force necessary to cause a deformation of identical degree can be observed, particularly with glutens of poorer quality.

The pronounced changes which can be detected even at the relatively low concentrations used definitely indicate an interaction between the hydrocarbons and the proteins of gluten. Concerning the character of this interaction, on the basis of thermodynamic considerations one can assume that a linkage is formed between the hydrocarbons and the hydrophobic side chains of proteins. In the case of pentane and hexane a weaker bond is formed, extending or rather protecting those hydrophobic nuclei which — in the course of hydration, osmotic uptake and swelling, and peptization — prevent the aggregates from unlimited swelling and disintegration. When higher hydrocarbons are added, the interaction may become stronger due to the higher affinity, so that existing interactions between side chains may cease; i.e., existing hydrophobic bonds may be ruptured and replaced by bonds between added hydrocarbon and the side chains. This situation is analogous to that assumed for the hydrogen bonds by urea. The two analogous processes are illustrated by the scheme shown in Figure 31.

TABLE 29
Effect of Hydrocarbons on the Rheological Properties of Gluten

Series No.	0.03 mol/100 g Gluten					
	Control	Pentane	Hexane	Heptane	Octane	Undecane
1	102	106	101	94	82	65
2	95	95	96	82	76	72
3	88	91	82	71	66	50
4	73	72	70	72	68	53
5	69	65	63	58	55	48
6	62	65	60	55	54	45
7	58	60	62	59	51	45
8	53	48	49	44	40	37
9	43	44	40	38	37	35
10	38	45	40	38	40	41

Note: Values are relaxation time (s).

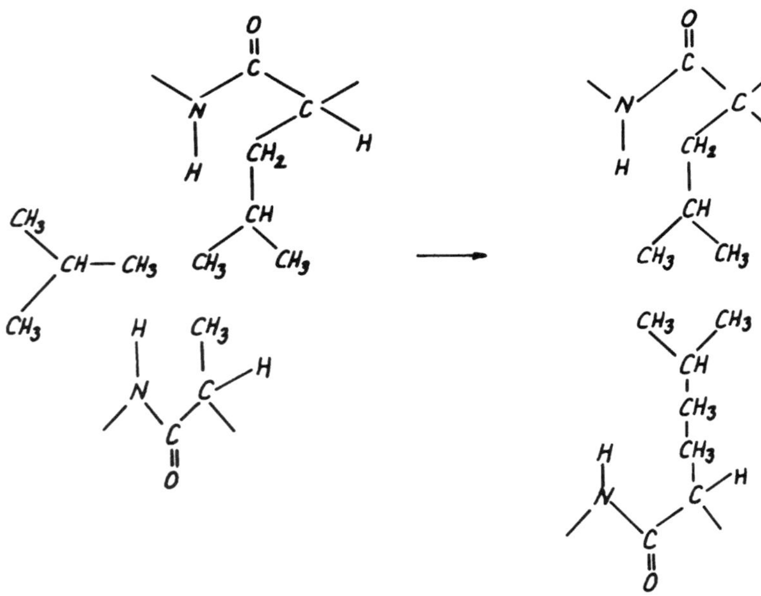

FIGURE 31 Proposed scheme of the rupture of hydrophobic bonds by hydrocarbon molecules.[188]

b. *Effect of Fatty Acids on the Rheological Properties of Gluten*

The procedure was the same as in the preceding series of experiments; some of the fatty acids were dissolved, and others were emulsified in the aqueous medium. The rheological properties of the glutens treated under these conditions are summarized in Table 30.

TABLE 30
Effect of Fatty Acids on the Rheological Properties of Gluten

Series	Acid Added: 0.01 mol/dm^3 Solution (Emulsion)								
No.	Control	Formic	Acetic	Propionic	Butyric	Valeric	Palmitic	Oleic	Stearic
1	102	39	40	56	72	85	80	—[b]	75
2	95	47	30	50	68	80	82	—[b]	71
3	88	39	28	52	59	69	79	—[b]	80
4	73	48	—[a]	41	48	53	63	—[b]	65
5	69	41	—[a]	44	50	60	62	—[b]	58
6	62	42	—[a]	48	47	50	52	—[b]	47
7	58	29	—[a]	32	39	40	52	—[b]	49
8	52	—[a]	—[a]	30	30	42	48	—[b]	41
9	43	—[a]	—[a]	27	30	40	42	46	30
10	38	—[a]	—[a]	25	28	32	32	57	28

Note: Values are relaxation time (s).

[a] Not measurable (sticky, spreading mass).
[b] Not measurable (crumbling, disintegrating mass).

The data in this table show an interesting pattern. The changes in rheological properties differ depending on the acid and the gluten. In the case of formic and acetic acid the peptizing effect predominates, which brings about rapid deterioration of the rheological properties. Acids with increasing numbers of carbon atoms up to and including valeric acid cause an increase in relaxation time, while palmitic and stearic acid lead to a slight deterioration of the rheological properties.

To explain the observed changes it may be assumed that, as with pentane and hexane, fatty acids with three to five carbon atoms bring about hydrophobicity. On the other hand, the decreasing relaxation time observed with higher fatty acids indicates that the interaction of more strongly hydrophobic compounds with proteins may result in the rupture of existing hydrophobic bonds.

Unsaturated oleic acid does not fit at all into the series. Oleic acid causes a change similar in character to a very high degree of normal denaturation. Presumably this is caused by the interaction of oleic acid with a preferred side chain.

c. *Effect of Hydrocarbons on the Formation of Gluten in the Presence of Urea*

In earlier work concerned with the role of hydrogen bonds, the effect of the addition of increasing amounts of urea on the rehydration of dry gluten and on gluten formation was studied. These experiments were repeated with the variation that various hydrocarbons were added to the urea solution (0.03 mol/1 g of gluten). The experimental results obtained under these conditions indicate the absence of gluten formation or a considerable decrease in the amount of gluten formed already at a lower urea concentration. The results are plotted in Figures 32 and 33.

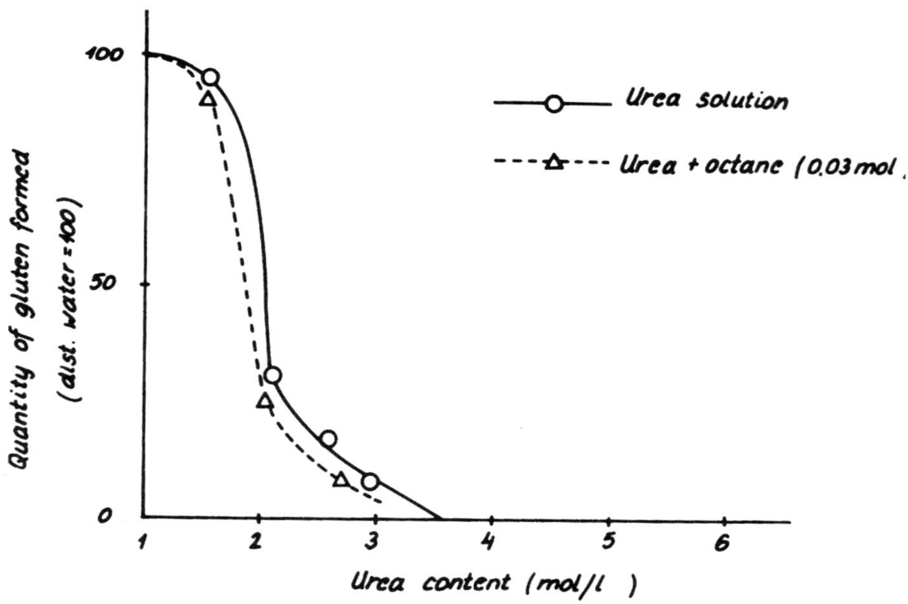

FIGURE 32 Effect of octane on the formation of gluten in the presence of urea.[188]

The observed behavior can be explained by assuming that a combined addition of urea and hydrocarbon hinders not only the formation of intermolecular hydrogen bonds, but also the formation of the corresponding hydrophobic bonds as a result of the interaction between hydrocarbon and nonpolar side chains of the protein.

Recently the surface hydrophobicity of the gliadins was investigated by Kaczkowski et al.[244] and Popineau.[245] It was shown that differences in hydrophobicity exist between gliadins from wheats of poor and good baking quality. It was also hypothesized that a hydrophobic interaction might occur between gliadin and glutenin components of gluten.

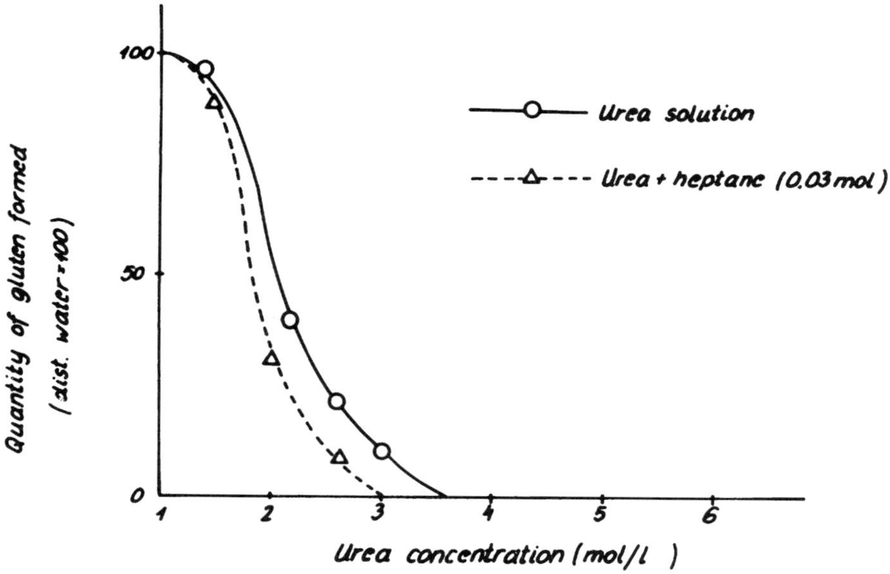

FIGURE 33 Effect on heptane on formation of gluten in the presence of urea.[188]

C. The Structure of the Gluten Complex

It is generally accepted that the gluten complex consists of a mixture of more than 100 types of polypeptides aggregated by covalent and noncovalent systems of bonds and interacting ions. A scheme of the major polypeptide types taking part in gluten complex formation according to Shewry and Miflin[83] is given in Figure 34.

An early model of the possible structure of the gluten protein complex is shown in Figure 35. Another model, proposed by Wall,[246] is presented in Figure 36.

The gluten is formed from three types of proteins (gliadin, glutenin, and residue protein) packed together by covalent and noncovalent linkages.

A third, more complex interpretation of the origin and interaction of wheat proteins taking part in the formation of gluten has been proposed by Bietz and Wall[137] (see Figure 37). Further studies are needed to determine the exact position of the interacting nonprotein components (especially lipids and carbohydrates) of the gluten complex. A model proposed by Lásztity et al.[129] was shown earlier in Figures 13 and 14.

Two major groups of storage proteins, the gliadins and the glutenins, are found in wheat endosperm. Recently another class of storage proteins with legumin-like properties was identified in wheat endosperm.[247,248] The proteins, originally called triplet proteins and now referred to as tricicin, are coded on the short arm of chromosomes 1A and 1D. They are synthesized between 8 and 21 days postanthesis and are concentrated in the protein bodies as inclusions.[248,249] The possible role of these proteins in gluten formation needs further studies.

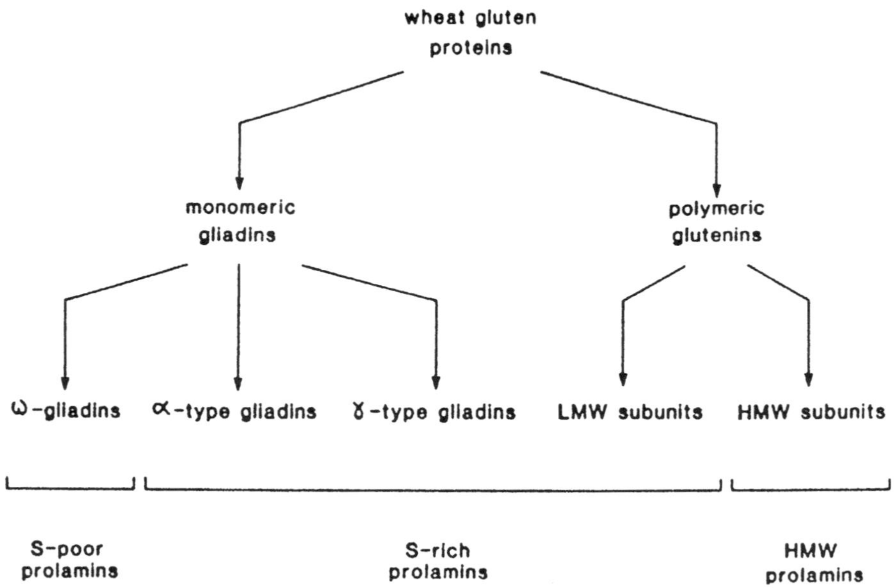

FIGURE 34 Major polypeptide types taking part in gluten formation. LMW = low molecular weight; HMW = high molecular weight. (From Shewry, P. R. and Miflin, B. J., in *Advances in Cereal Science and Technology,* Vol. 7, American Association of Cereal Chemists, St. Paul, MN, 1985, 1. With permission.)

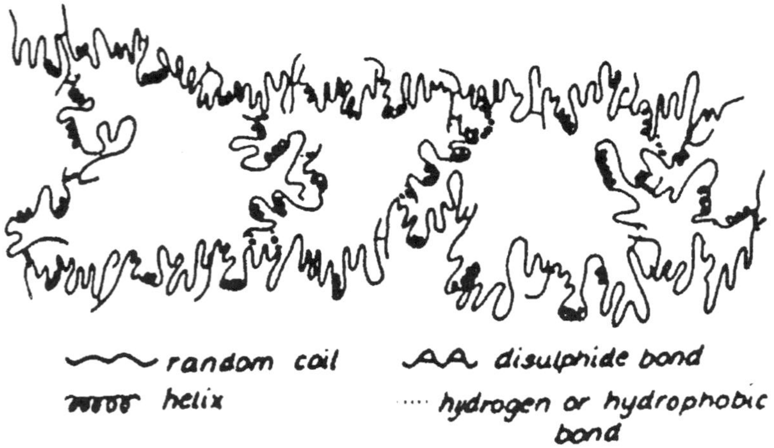

FIGURE 35 Proposed structure of the gluten complex.[105]

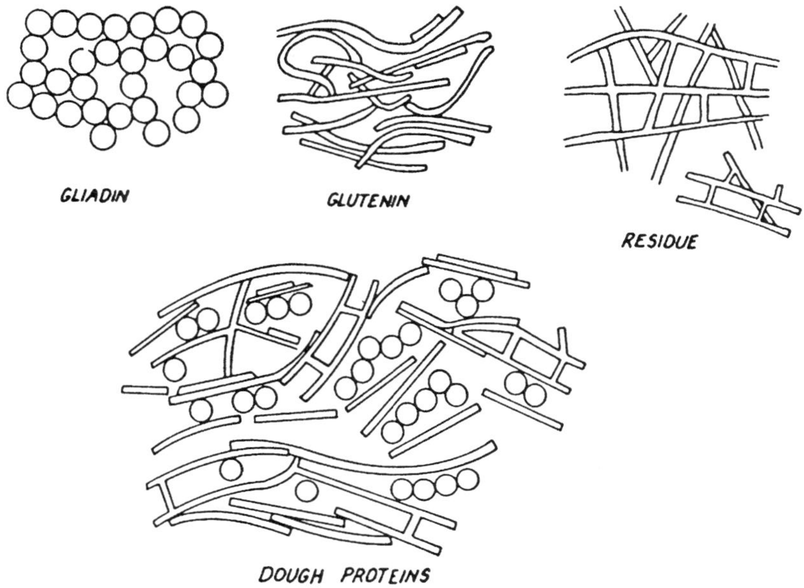

FIGURE 36 Model of interactions of wheat proteins in dough.[246]

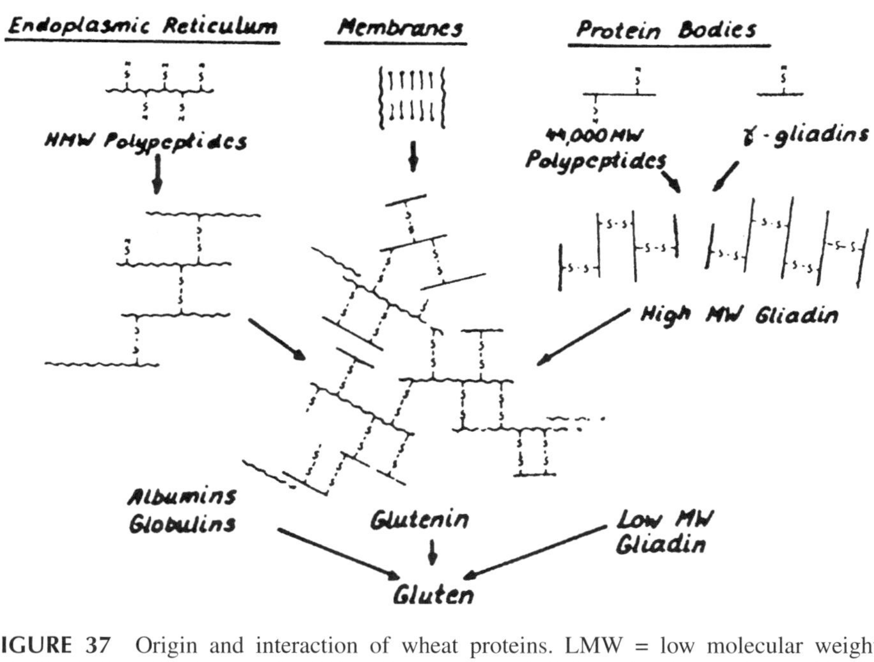

FIGURE 37 Origin and interaction of wheat proteins. LMW = low molecular weight; HMW = high molecular weight. (After Bietz, J. A. and Wall, J. S., *Cereal Chem.*, 57, 415, 1980. With permission.)

V. METABOLICALLY ACTIVE (CYTOPLASMIC) PROTEINS

The group consisting of cytoplasmic proteins is very inhomogeneous and not so intensively studied as the storage protein group. In comparison with the classification of Osborne, the cytoplasmic proteins are somewhat identical with the group of albumins and globulins. Due to good solubility the problems of extraction do not play as important a role in these investigations as in the case of the storage proteins. Nevertheless, the ionic strength of the extracting media and also the qualitative composition of the aqueous salt solution may affect the quantity of extracted proteins. The greatest quantity of proteins can be extracted using sodium chloride solutions, but the extract also may contain low molecular weight storage proteins. The lowest proportion of prolamin-type proteins may be assured using phosphate and magnesium sulfate buffers. For further separation of the components the techniques commonly used in protein investigation (gel filtration chromatography, gel electrophoresis, HPLC, etc.) are used. Of the proteins belonging to this group, the enzyme proteins (and inhibitors) and some special low molecular weight proteins (e.g., purothionins) have been investigated.

A. Enzymes of Wheat

The wheat grain, as a living entity in a dormant state, contains all the enzymes (in active or inactive form) which catalyze the biochemical reactions characteristic for the grains. It is well known that biochemical processes connected with respiration also continue in the postharvest period during the storage of grain. This means that all enzymes taking part in the decomposition of starch are present in the grain until it is oxidized to CO_2 and water. The wheat grain contains a lot of other enzymes. Some of them have technological importance; others have been considered interesting — until now — only from the scientific point of view.

The presence of several enzyme inhibitors, especially in germ but also in the endosperm, was observed in all cereal grains. These compounds, together with some other antinutritive components, have some importance with regard to the nutritive (feeding) value of the cereals.

Relatively little is known about the localization of different enzymes. Some observations are summarized in the review by Simmonds and O'Brien.[250] In aleurone protein bodies the association of certain degradative enzymes (protease, α-amylase) with the outer membrane has been established with some certainty. Acid phosphatases surround the inclusions of phytin. The presence of hydrolytic enzymes was also observed in close association with protein bodies of the endosperm and starch granules.

The isolation of enzymes is generally a difficult task because of the small quantity of enzyme proteins and the interference of other types of proteins present in greater amounts. After extraction and preliminary purification by precipitation and gel filtration chromatography, preparative gel electrophoresis, ion exchange, and affinity chromatography may be used.

Early work concerning the enzymes of wheat and their significance in baking technology was reviewed by Anderson.[251] More recent results were later summarized by Rohrlich[252] and Reed and Thorn.[253] Recently an excellent review was published by Fox and Mulvihill.[6]

1. Amylases and Proteases

Amylases are technologically the most important enzymes of wheat and wheat flours. In the production of yeast-leavened bakery products, optimal yeast growth and adequate CO_2 production must be achieved in order to obtain a good-sized, well-aerated bread. The normal level of fermentable sugar in flour is not sufficient, and during dough fermentation further fermentable sugar must be produced from starch by the amylases. Therefore, the level of amylase activity in wheat flours is an important quality factor. Ungerminated wheat contains an abundance of β-amylases and a low, variable level of α-amylases. In the germinating wheat grains an increase of α-amylase activity may be observed due to synthesis in the aleurone cells. The α-amylase activity of flour milled from germinated grains is too high; the excessive α-amylase activity in the flour leads to bread with sticky crumbs. The α-amylases of the developing wheat grain are located mainly in the pericarp, and they decrease in activity throughout kernel development, becoming largely undetectable at maturity. Investigating amylases of ungerminated wheat, Kruger[254] found three isoenzymes of α-amylase in the developing wheat grain. Later three isoenzymes were also resolved by Marchylo et al.[255] using acetone fractionation, ion exchange, and affinity chromatography. More recently, using isoelectric focusing and rocket immunoelectrophoresis, Sargeant[256] found that the developing wheat grain contains two groups of α-amylase isoenzymes. Group II, composed of three isoenzymes with isoelectric points of 4.5 to 4.8, was observed 10 days after anthesis. Later the concentration of this group decreased and diminished 35 days after anthesis. Group I contained four isoenzymes with peaks of 6.0 to 6.5 which appeared 35 days after anthesis and increased in intensity until maturity. Group I isoenzymes may result from the modification of those in group II.

Marchylo et al.,[255] using isoelectric focusing, separated from nongerminated seeds three groups of isoenzymes (G I, G II, G III) with a total of 22 components. The isoenzymes of the G I group were similar to isoenzymes described by Kruger[254] and those in group II of Sargeant.[256] The G II isoenzymes had weak activity and were absent from many tissues at many stages of ripening. The G III isoenzymes had components similar to those of the isoenzymes obtained from malted wheat. These results suggest that small amounts of malt α-amylase are also present in the ungerminated grains.

The properties and actions of amylases in sprouted grain are summarized in a review by Meredith and Pomeranz.[257]

Different amylases may be found in sprouting grains, immature grains, moldy grains, and even in situations where grain development has been cut short by frost or disease. Each of these kinds of α-amylase comprises a group of similar, but not identical, enzymes that differ slightly in what they do to starch. The genetic control of isozymes and a preferred nomenclature were discussed by Gale.[258]

Recently Zawistowska et al.,[276] using immobilized metal affinity chromatography and isoelectric focusing, achieved a more effective separation of wheat α-amylases.

The β-amylases of wheat are located in the endosperm. Much of the β-amylase in the endosperm of the maturing grain is inactive and can be activated by reducing agents. Rowsell and Goad[259] concluded that latent β-amylase is bound to glutenin via disulfide linkage and that proteinases release the enzyme still bound to glutenin polypeptides. Kasarda et al.[1] expressed the view that the inactive β-amylase is probably associated with membranes which can be included in glutenin preparations. Granulated glutenin is capable of binding added soluble β-amylase.

In an earlier work Tipples and Tkachuk[260] reported on the separation of five β-amylase isoenzymes (A, B, C, D, E) from NaCl extracts of wheat flour using DEAE-cellulose chromatography. The three principal components (A, B, and E β-amylases) were homogeneous on gel electrophoresis, contained thiol groups, and had very similar amino acid composition profiles. Small differences were observed in isoelectric point and pH optimum (4.6 to 6.2).[261] In a series of investigations Kruger[262-264] separated different β-amylase isoenzymes by diethyl-amino-ethyl (DEAE)-cellulose chromatography and isoelectric focusing. Two β-amylase isoenzymes, β-2 and β-3, occur early during the development of hard wheats. Four additional isoenzymes appear during the later stages of development; they represent only a small proportion of the total activity. The seventh isoenzyme, β-4, is present during early development and disappears as ripening progresses. An eighth isoenzyme, β-1, occurs in some varieties, especially in soft wheat.

During germination the principal isoenzymes, β-2 and β-3, disappear and are replaced by a new β-amylase with slower electrophoretic mobility. The proteolytic nature of these changes was confirmed by Kruger.[264] It was shown that papain and wheat malt proteinase converted β-1, β-2, β-3, and β-4 isoenzymes to the slower, more alkaline forms (β-5 to β-9) plus some additional minor forms.

Although the significance of the proteolytic enzymes in bread-making technology is not as great as that of amylases, the investigation of these groups of enzymes gives valuable additional data for a more detailed information on wheats. The proteases play only a minor role in the changes of gluten proteins and the rheological properties of dough (except the case of germinated wheat which is milled into flour), but their activities contribute via Maillard reaction to the formation of crust color and some specific components of bread aroma.

The proteolytic activity of ungerminated wheat is located in the outer layer (aleurone, germ, pericarp) of the wheat kernel. The proteolytic activity found in the endosperm is very low. The greatest portion of proteolytic activity may be extracted using a 10% sodium chloride solution. Further purification could be achieved by gel filtration chromatography, ion exchange, and gel electrophoresis. The best results may be obtained with affinity chromatography. Different groups of proteinases and peptidases occur in wheat grain. Because of difficulties associated with separation and purification most of them are not characterized in detail, and therefore their classification has not yet been achieved. Kaminski and Bushuk[265] separated the proteolytically active components using starch gel electrophoresis. Four groups of proteases were found, each of which showed microheterogeneity. Most of the proteolytic activity was observed in the alcohol-soluble fraction.

The proteases of unmalted wheat were exhaustively studied by Skupin and Warchalewski.[266] The 10% sodium chloride extract prepurified by fractionation with ammonium sulfate was studied using column chromatography on SE-Sephadex G-50. Two active fractions were obtained (A and B). Component A, representing the greatest part of the activity, was separated by rechromatography on SE-Sephadex G-50 into two components. On the basis of the investigation of the amino acid composition, they stated that proteinase A contains both disulfide and thiol groups. Enzymatic activity was destroyed by various thiol blocking agents. Skupin and Warchalewski concluded that these proteases resembled a papain-like thiol enzyme.

Salgó and Lásztity[267] reported on the proteases of Hungarian wheats. Salt solution extraction, gel filtration chromatography, ion exchange, and affinity chromatography were used for the separation of proteolytically active components. Three groups of proteases were separated and characterized. The pH optima of the enzymes were in the acidic region (pH 3.8 to 4.4). Studies of the possible active sites of the enzymes showed that most of them belong to the serine proteinase group (inhibition by diisopropyl fluorophosphate [DFP]). A slight inhibitory effect of complexing agents was also observed, which suggests the presence of metallic proteinases, too. No inhibitory effect of thiol group blocking agents was observed.

The changes in proteolytic activity during the development and ripening of the wheat grain were also studied. A comprehensive study by Kruger[268] showed that the proteolytic activity of maturing wheat increased to a maximum 16 to 18 days after flowering and then declined to less than 50% at maturity. The proteinase was concentrated in the pericarp, seed coat, and aleurone layers.

The proteolytic activity of germinated grains was also investigated. Protease production in early germination was reviewed by Kruger and Preston.[269] The presence of peptidases is characteristic for germinated wheat grains, but peptidases also may be observed in ungerminated wheat. Ungerminated wheat contains no PHB activity,[270] and acid-stable acidic BAEEase is also absent.[271] Two carboxypeptidases (A and B) were observed by Preston and Kruger[272,273] in germinating wheat kernels. Isoelectric focusing demonstrated two main aminopeptidases in both immature and germinated wheat.[274] They were concentrated in the endosperm.

In more recent work Salgó,[275] using separation by affinity chromatography on a hemoglobin-Sepharose column, isolated a relatively pure fraction characterized by high proteolytic activity. With isoelectric focusing nine proteolytically active components were separated. Five bands were obtained in the region pH 4.2 to 4.6, two bands were found in the region pH 5.3 to 5.6, and there was an intensive discrete band with isoelectric point at pH 7.4. The enzymes were inhibited by phenylmethylsulfonyl fluoride (PMSF) and ethylenediamine tetraacetic acid (EDTA). No inhibitory effect of *p*-chloro-mercury-benzoate (PCMB) was observed. The proteases are stable in the pH range 2.5 to 5, and their heat stability is slightly high (see Figures 38 and 39). The activity of proteases was investigated using hemoglobin, wheat albumin, globulin, gliadin, and glutenin as substrate. The rate of hydrolysis was the same for hemoglobin and wheat gliadin, but other wheat protein fractions were hydrolyzed faster than hemoglobin.

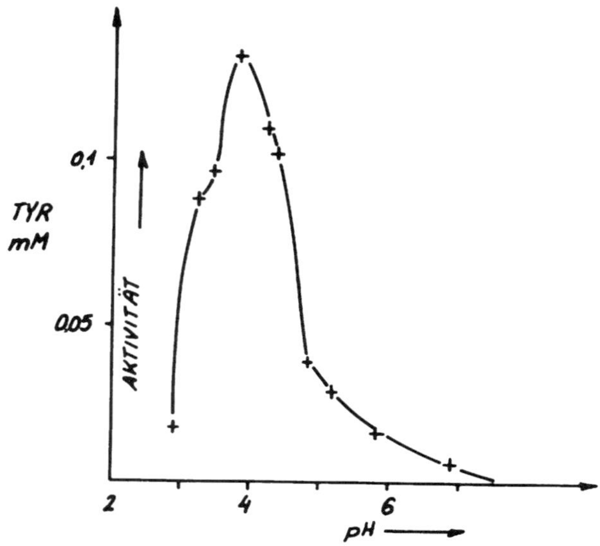

FIGURE 38 The effect of pH on the activity of wheat protease.[275]

It was found first by Kneen and Sandstedt[277] that the albumin fraction contains α-amylase inhibitor proteins. Petrucci et al.,[278] using gel filtration chromatography, separated three groups (families) of albumin components having an α-amylase inhibitory effect. The molecular weights of the families are 12,000, 24,000, and 60,000. The principal inhibitors of the 12,000 and 24,000 families have relative electrophoretic mobilities of 0.28 and 0.19, respectively, and are frequently referred to by these codes. Reviews covering the molecular properties, biology (including genetics), and possible nutritional significance of wheat α-amylase inhibitors were published by Buonocore et al.[279] and Belitz and Weder.[280]

The α-amylase inhibitors from wheat do not inhibit the α- and β-amylases from wheat or other cereals, but do inhibit in various degrees the α-amylases from various animal species, insects, and bacteria. It may be supposed that the protein α-amylase inhibitors evolved in wheat to provide the plant with protection against insect predators.[281] Such inhibitors may be important in controlling α-amylase activity in wheat kernels. The low α-amylase activity of mature kernels may be caused by an inhibitor-enzyme complex which dissociates upon germination.

It is probable that these inhibitors may be used in the control of α-amylase activity in flour and dough prepared from germinated wheat.

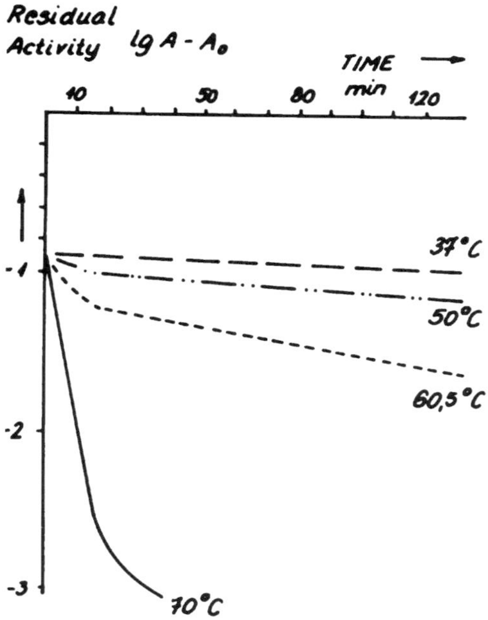

FIGURE 39 Heat stability of wheat proteases.[275]

The inhibitors are relatively thermostable, but the greatest portion of these compounds is inactivated during baking or boiling of macaroni products.[282] Although they are inactivated by pepsin, some of the α-amylase inhibitors survive passage through the stomach if large amounts are ingested. These facts suggest the necessity of the inactivation of α-amylase inhibitors in foods and feeds. The problem may be interesting in high-cereal diets and breakfast cereals.

Protease inhibitors were first found in wheat germ by Hochstrasser and Werle.[283] They separated two trypsin inhibitors having molecular weights of about 12 and 17 kDa. Later other research workers found protease inhibitors in wheat germ and endosperm, too.[284] A review of protease inhibitors found in cereals is given by Shewry and Miflin.[83]

Two extracts of whole wheat kernel and flour were investigated by Petrucci et al.[278] The trypsin inhibitors separated by gel filtration chromatography are basic proteins with a molecular weight between 10 and 24 kDa; they could be separated into more components by gel electrophoresis. Mitsunaga[285] isolated two major trypsin inhibitors (I and II) and two minor inhibitors from wheat germ by chromatography on DEAE-Sephadex, CM-Sephadex, Bio-Gel, and Sephadex. Inhibitors I and II had molecular weights of 16,000 and 10,000.

Trypsin inhibitors extracted from the whole grain of hard red winter wheat, durum wheat, rye, and triticale were investigated by Chang and Tsen.[286,287] Affinity chromatography, CM-cellulose ion-exchange chromatography, and gel filtration chromatography were used for the separation. Products of highly specific activity were isolated. Each cereal sample with the exception of triticale had three different trypsin inhibitors. The molecular weights of wheat trypsin inhibitors were as follows: hard red winter wheat, 36,800, 21,000, and 5,000; and durum wheat, 38,500; 22,500, and not determined.

Disc gel electrophoresis of these cereals showed them to be heterogeneous. All of the isolated trypsin inhibitors contained carbohydrates except trypsin inhibitor II isolated from durum wheat. No free thiol was detected in any of the inhibitors. The amino acid compositions of the inhibitors were similar. All inhibitors were heat stable; only heating at 125°C resulted in full inactivation. Boisen and Djurtoft[288] isolated an electrophoretically homogeneous trypsin inhibitor from wheat with a molecular weight of about 12,000. The inhibitor was very stable to pepsin and heat at 100°C.

Reviews relating to protease inhibitors were published also by Laskowski and Kato[290] and Belitz and Weder.[280]

2. Other Enzymes

In addition to α- and β-amylases, wheat kernels contain some other enzymes which hydrolyze carbohydrates. Low levels of α(1,6)-D-glucosidases (pullulanases) were found by Kruger and Marchylo.[291] They are present only in the endosperm and are not inhibited by thiol blocking agents or EDTA. Isoamylases have also been recognized.[292] The presence of enzymes hydrolyzing pentosans of wheat was demonstrated by Lee and Ronalds.[293]

Lipases of wheat may cause an increase in fatty acid levels if wheat is stored under adverse conditions of temperature or humidity. The fatty acids lower the acceptance of the cereal products by the consumer and may affect the gluten properties. Early work concerning lipases was reviewed by Sullivan.[294] A summary of the more recent results was given in the review by Fox and Mulvihill.[6] In spite of the considerable literature on wheat lipases, the enzyme has not been isolated to homogeneity from either sound or germinated wheat. A more comprehensive study is needed. It was reported by different authors that wheat also contains a range of phospholipases (for review see Reference 295).

Among the phosphatases found in wheat the phytase is widely known. After early research work the investigations have continued since the 1970s using modern separation techniques. A review about the role of phytase in cereals and cereal proteins is given by Lásztity and Lásztity.[296]

Lipoxygenase — an enzyme which catalyzes the peroxidation of unsaturated fatty acids — also occurs in wheat, where it is located mainly in the scutellum and embryo. The endosperm contains very low quantities of this enzyme. Lipoxygenase may take part in the oxidative destruction of unsaturated fatty acids and some biologically important fat-soluble compounds such as carotenoids, tocopherols, and others. Lipoxidase activity apparently improves the rheological properties of dough. Four lipoxygenase isoenzymes were found in wheat extracts by Guss et al.[297] and Hale et al.[298] The four isoenzymes were purified using gel filtration and DEAE chromatography. The fractions were not homogeneous. Further research is needed for the isolation and characterization of these groups of enzymes. The biochemistry and role of lipoxygenases in bread making were recently reviewed by Faubion and Hoseney.[299]

Polyphenoloxidases (PPO) may cause darkening of the wheat dough; therefore a screening of new wheat varieties for PPO activity is desirable. The more recent investigations involving PPO have concentrated on the isolation, separation, and characterization of different types of polyphenoloxidases and isoenzymes. The intervarietal differences were also studied.

The PPO activities of hard red winter, soft red winter, hard red spring, white common, club, and durum wheats were studied by Lamkin et al.[300] The PPO activities of some wheats are shown in Table 31. A very significant difference was observed between the activities of common and durum wheats. The lower PPO activity of durum wheat makes the identification of these wheats possible. Several differences were observed between bread wheats. This fact also may be useful as a secondary characteristic in variety identification. The distribution of PPO activity in flour millstreams was studied more recently by Marsh and Galliard,[301] McCallum and Walker,[302] and Hatcher and Kruger.[303] Less than 10% of total activity was present in flour streams corresponding to a 70% extraction rate. PPO activity was linearly correlated with ash content. PPO activities of Australian and U.S. wheat cultivars were recently studied by Baik et al.[384]

Peroxidases and catalases are among the most important oxidoreductases in plants. Both enzymes have been found in wheat. The most extensive research was realized by Kruger and La Berge.[304,305] They found 12 isoenzymes in immature kernels, and varietal and anatomical differences were observed. The isoenzyme patterns changed considerably during ripening. In the framework of intervarietal studies 32 cultivars were examined. It was found that the principal isoenzymes were present in all varieties. Differences were observed in minor components. Wheat peroxidases were found to be relatively heat stable.

The catalases of wheat were recently studied intensively by Kruger.[306] During early ripening catalase was located mainly in the endosperm. At the end of ripening the scutellum was the only tissue with significant catalase activity. The activity of this enzyme increased approximately fivefold during germination. Electrophoretically only one major isoenzyme was detectable that was present in both hard and durum wheats. High-resolution catalase zymograms from different anatomic locations revealed the presence of several different isoenzymes, but no significant intervarietal differences were observed in isoenzyme patterns. Concerning the significance of peroxidases and catalases, it is interesting to note the observation of Kobrehel et al.[307] that a positive high correlation exists between brownness of macaroni and the peroxidase activity of durum wheat semolinas, indicating that wheat cultivars with low peroxidase activity should be selected for macaroni and spaghetti production.

From the point of view of explanation of the gluten formation process a better knowledge of disulfide reductases and thiol oxidases may have importance.[289,374]

TABLE 31
Polyphenol Oxidase Activities of Wheat Cultivars[300]

Class and Cultivar	l-Tyrosine	Catechol	l-Dopa	Dopamine	Gallic Acid	Pyrogallol
Hard red winter						
Eagle (1978)	26.7 ± 1.3	28.9 ± 1.3	13.7 ± 0.7	26.9 ± 1.8	3.4 ± 0.5	24.1 ± 0.7
Bucksin (1978)	26.0	28.2	14.1	24.8	3.1	23
Scout (1978)	27.7	25.3	13.2	21.5	3.7	23.7
Centurk (1978)	27.2	25.7	15.6	27.5	3.0	21.6
Parker (1977)	25.9	26.4	14.9	24.0	3.0	20.0
Soft red winter						
Abe (1978)	26.4	28.5	15.6	25.4	3.1	26.6
Arthur (1977)	27.7	21.4	9.2	17.4	4.2	23.8
Monon (1977)	53.9	18.1	19.3	15.7	3.6	23.2
Arthur 71 (1977)	30.2	26.7	14.8	26.1	3.3	25.0
Arthur 71 (1977)	27.6	25.0	16.6	26.2	3.5	24.2
Logan (1978)	40.1	15.3	14.6	13.7	3.1	24.2
Hard red spring						
Coteau (1978)	56.9	23.7	19.6	25.2	3.4	24.6
Olaf (1978)	16.7	17.5	7.4	16.4	3.5	24.5
Waldron (1977)	23.5	26.7	15.0	23.7	4.0	25.0
Era (1978)	15.7	15.4	7.4	15.6	2.4	22.1
Thacher (1978)	20.2	20.4	10.0	19.0	3.4	25.3
Kitt (1978)	21.8	21.0	9.2	19.7	3.7	22.2
White common						
Luke (1977)	8.6	12.2	7.4	13.4	3.6	23.8
Nugaines (1977)	19.0	22.0	13.7	22.7	1.9	20.4
Ionia (1977)	23.0	21.1	10.9	20.1	5.4	21.9
Genesee (1977)	5.2	6.8	4.3	4.0	7.8	3.8
Hyslop (1977)	44.0	16.1	18.5	13.4	3.3	28.3
Club						
Paha (1977)	5.3	7.5	3.9	9.2	2.8	14.6
Moro (1977)	5.1	8.3	4.4	9.0	2.9	18.0
Omar (1975)	6.0	8.3	4.0	8.8	3.6	17.5
Barbee (1977)	10.8	15.7	7.7	15.9	3.6	17.1
Durum						
Roletta (1978)	3.6	4.5	2.6	3.8	0.4	7.5
Rugby (1978)	5.2	2.8	2.1	3.8	0.6	12.5
Ward (1978)	4.3	3.4	1.4	3.7	1.1	9.9
Calvin (1978)	5.0	3.8	1.6	3.5	1.4	12.2
Cando (1978)	6.0	4.1	1.4	4.2	0.7	8.4

Note: Values are $\mu l\ ml^{-1}\ min^{-1}$.

The mechanism of action of flour improvers generally involves some oxidoreductases. Ascorbic acid-oxidizing and dehydroascorbic acid-reducing enzymes were studied by Elkassabany et al.[308] and Walther and Grosch.[309]

Glutamic acid decarboxylase (GAD) was first detected by Rohrlich.[310] GAD activity may be a useful index of grain quality and storage conditions, especially if the moisture content of the grain increases to over 15%.

The stability of glucose-6-phosphate dehydrogenase in wheat was studied by Salgó and Feller.[311]

B. Purothionins

About 40 years ago a low molecular weight protein rich in sulfur-containing amino acids and lysine was isolated from wheat by Balls and Hale.[312] The protein, called purothionin, was extracted by petroleum ether, the lipid-protein complex obtained was cleaved by hydrochloric acid, and finally the apoprotein was isolated. Later other methods of isolation were elaborated using salt solution[313] and dilute sulfuric acid.[314] A review concerning the work on purothionin and including a complete bibliography was published by Békés and Smied.[313] Gel electrophoresis in aluminum lactate buffer showed two closely spaced bands which have been designated α- and β-purothionin according to their relative mobility.[314] The amino acid sequence of purothionins was reported by two independent research teams.[315-317] The sequences are shown in Figures 40, 41, and 42.

Purothionins differ markedly from most flour proteins because they contain about 20% cystine and about 20% lysine + arginine. On the other hand, the amount of glutamic acid (glutamine) and proline is low. All three purothionins have very similar amino acid sequences, and each consists of 45 amino acid residues. Later purothionin-like proteins (purothionin analogs) were isolated from barley,[318-321] rye,[322] and oat.[323]

The genetic control of purothionins has also been studied exhaustively in recent years. The work in this field was reviewed by Garcia-Olmedo et al.,[324] and a scheme was proposed for the evolution of the purothionins in wheat (see Figure 43). According to this proposition a primitive plant acquired a gene that coded for a protein similar to purothionin, presumably before the monocotyledonous and dicotyledonous plant lines separated because several dicotyledonous mistletoe species contain proteins (viscotoxins) that are remarkably homologous with purothionins.[325,326] The gene was carried down to an ancestor common to the different Triticineae species. This ancestral plant evolved into several species, and via mutations and hybridization were formed the purothionin genes of common wheat.

The genes coding for purothionins appear to be relatively stable. Based on these observations and the comparative study of amino acid composition[321] a general formula for the structure of thionins was proposed by Békés and Lásztity[321] (see Figure 44).

The functions of purothionin in plant physiology are practically unknown. A significant change in the quantity of this protein fraction could not be proved during

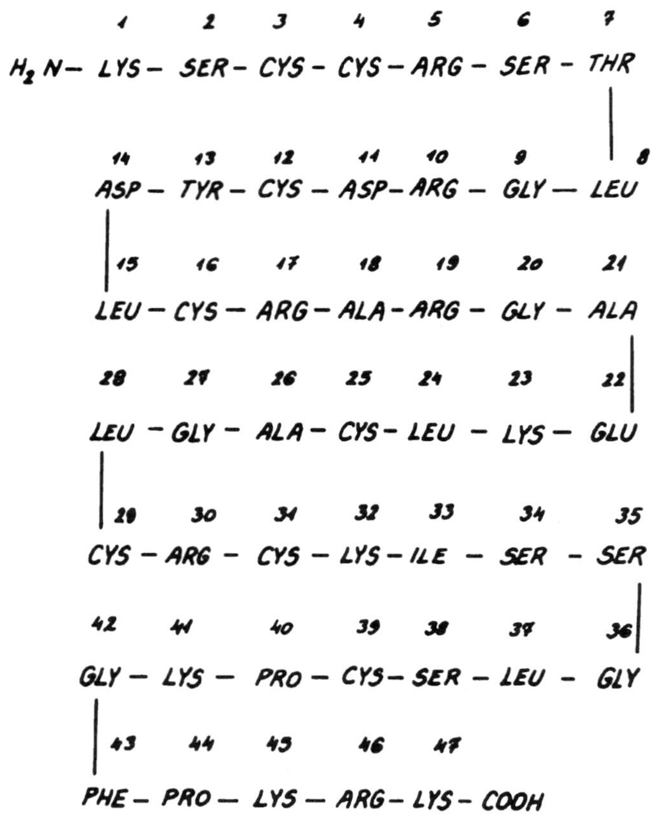

FIGURE 40 Amino acid sequences of α_1-purothionin.[315-317]

ripening or germination.[327] The purothionins seem to be associated with the endoplasmic reticulum and are potent inhibitors of an *in vitro* wheat translation system.[328] The few data found in the literature[1,324] on the enzyme inhibitory character of purothionin are not convincing: the trypsin and chymotrypsin functions have been disproven and papain inhibition has not been confirmed.[1,329] On the other hand, it has been known for some time[330-332] and confirmed by several authors[322,332-335] that purothionin and hordothionin are active against yeasts (see Figure 45) and have a toxic effect on some bacteria. It has been reported that they affect membrane permeability[320,336] and inhibit protein, RNA, and DNA synthesis[337] in mammalian cells.

Jones and Meredith[338] reported on the inactivation of α-amylase by purothionins. The amounts of purothionin used in these experiments were greater than those normally extractable from flour used as an amylase source. However, they postulated that if the purothionins were compartmentalized in the seeds the effective concentration of purothionin in this small area might be comparable to that used in experiments.

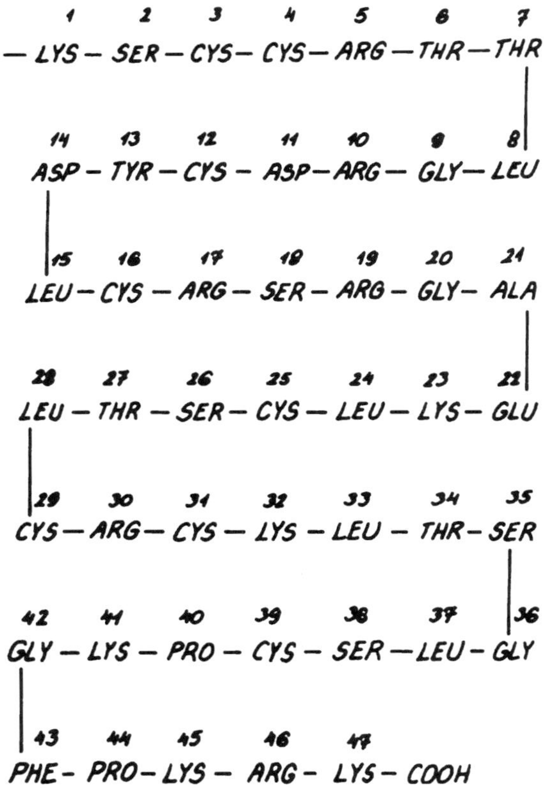

FIGURE 41 Amino acid sequence of α_2-purothionin.[315-317]

More recent investigations by Johnson et al.[339] revealed reduction of purothionin by the thioredoxin system. It was suggested that purothionin might be a secondary thiol messenger in redox control.

In contrast to the extensive work and literature on the apoprotein (purothionin), relatively little is known about the lipid complex of this protein, called lipopurothionin. An isolation method, based on precipitation from methyl acetate solution, was developed by Redman and Ewart.[346] They also separated the crude purothionin on Sephadex LH-20 columns with an ethanol-chloroform mixture and investigated lipid components of the complex. It was stated that the main lipid components of the complex are phosphatidylcholine and other polar lipids. Hoseney and Pomeranz[340] reported that the major lipid components of lipid-protein complexes are mono- and digalactosyl glycerides, phosphatidylethanolamine, and phosphatidylcholine. Later lipopurothionin and some of its lipid components were studied by Hernandez-Lucas et al.[341] They found that the lipids of lipopurothionin, in addition to the sterol ester present in trace amounts, are polar in the majority of phospholipids (phosphatidylcholine, phosphatidylethanolamine), and there are two glycolipids (digalactosyl diglyceride, monogalactosyl diglyceride).

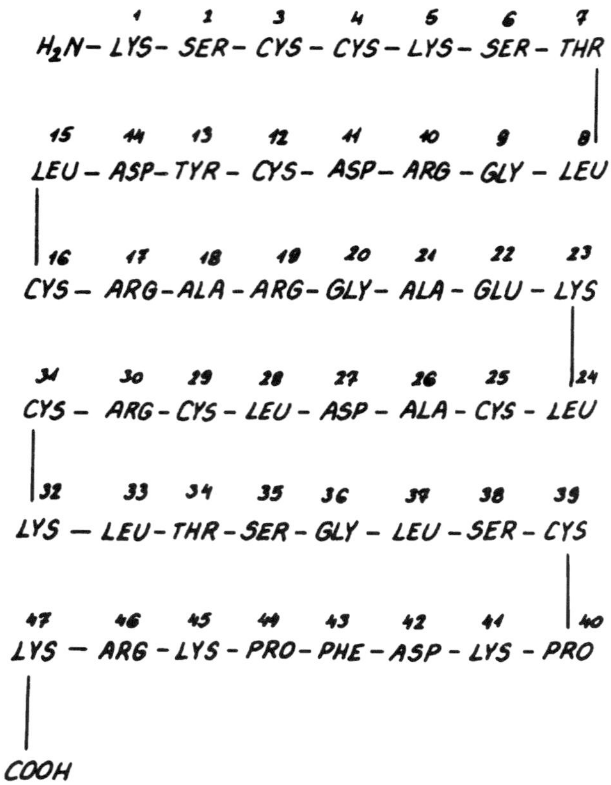

FIGURE 42 Amino acid sequence of β-purothionin.[315-317]

More recently Békés and Smied[313] reported the results of an exhaustive investigation of these lipoproteins realized in the author's laboratory. Four kinds of lipopurothionin were obtained from the petroleum ether extract of wheat flour and were fractionated on Sephadex LH-20 columns. Apoproteins were prepared, and the lipids bound in the complexes were separated and investigated (see Figure 46). The gross composition of lipopurothionin obtained by a methyl acetate precipitation procedure and its components separated on Sephadex LH-20 columns are given in Table 32. Table 33 summarizes the data concerning the composition of lipids bound in the complex prepared by the methyl acetate precipitation procedure (see Figure 46).

Differences were found in the composition of the lipids if lipopurothionins prepared by different procedures were compared. Some preparations contained a considerable amount of neutral triglyceride.

They also investigated the interactions occurring in model solutions containing pure purothionin fractions and different lipids (egg lecithin, L-α-dipalmitoyl lecithin, phosphatidylethanolamine, phosphatidylcholine, phosphatidylserine, phosphatidylinositol, cholesterol, ergosterol palmitate, monogalactosyl diglyceride, digalactosyl

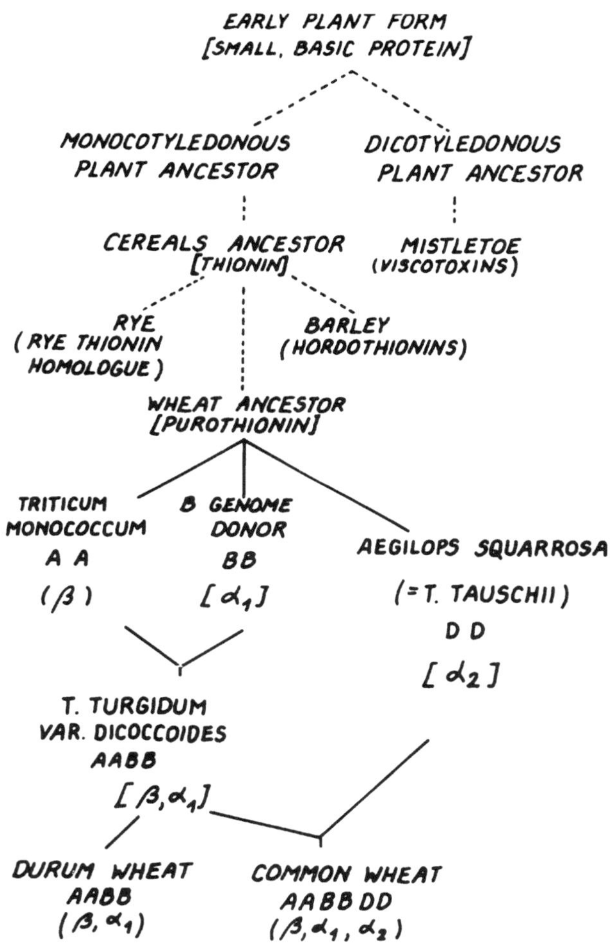

FIGURE 43 Scheme of the evolution of ancestral genes controlling purothionin biosynthesis. (After Garcia-Olmedo, F., Carbonero, P., and Jones, B. L., *Advances in Cereal Science and Technology,* Vol. 5, Pomeranz, Y., Ed., American Association of Cereal Chemists, St. Paul, MN, 1982, 1. With permission.)

diglyceride). The bound lipid content and the lipid-protein complexes were studied. Modified purothionins (basic side chains were masked using maleic acid or cyclohexanedione) were also used in model experiments. The authors stated that the interaction between purothionin and polar phospholipids was the strongest. If the basic side chains were blocked the binding of phospholipids decreased rapidly. From this fact it can be concluded that the phospholipids are bound by side chains of arginine and lysine. Model experiments have shown that glycolipids may be integrated in the complex only if the protein-phospholipid is preliminarily formed. Data on the quantity of glycolipids suggest the formation of phospholipid-glycolipid bonds rather than protein-glycolipid bonds. The occurrence of neutral lipids in some

Amino acid sequence in thionins

NH_2-LYS-SER-CYS-CYS-X_1-X_2-THR-X_3-GLY-ARG-ASP-X_4-TIR-ASP-LEU-CYS-ARG-X_5-X_6-GLY-ALA-X_7-LYS-LEU-

CYS-X_8-X_9-X_{10}-CYS-ARG-CYS-LYS-X_{11}-X_{12}-SER-GLY-LEU-SER-CYS-PRO-X_{13}-X_{14}-PHE-PRO-LYS-ARG-LYS-COOH

Serial number		Purothionin			Hordothionin			Secale-thionin	Avenothionin		Viscotoxin
		α_1	α_2	β	α_1	α_2	β		α	β	
X_1	5	ARG	ARG	LYS	ARG	ARG	LYS	LYS	ARG	LYS	PRO
X_2	6	SER	THR	SER	SER	THR	SER	SER	ASP	ASP	ASP
X_3	8	LEU	LEU	LEU	LEU	LEU	LEU	LEU	LEU	LEU	THR
X_4	12	CYS	CYS	CYS	CYS	CYS	CYS	CYS	CYS	CYS	ILE
X_5	18	ALA	SER	ALA	ALA	ALA	SER	GLY	SER	ALA	LEU
X_6	19	ARG	ARG	ARG	ARG	ARG	ARG	ARG	ARG	ARG	THR
X_7	22	GLU	GLU	GLU	GLU	GLU	GLU	GLU	PRO	PRO	PRO-THR
X_8	26	ALA	SER	ALA	ALA	SER	ALA	ALA	ALA	SER	ALA
X_9	27	GLY	THR	ASP	GLY	THR	ASP	GLU	THR	THR	LYS
X_{10}	28	LEU	LEU	LEU	LEU	LEU	LEU	LEU	LEU	LEU	VAL
X_{11}	33	ILE	LEU	LEU	VAL	LEU	LEU	ILE	ILE	LEU	LEU
X_{12}	34	SER	THR	THR	SER	THR	THR	THR	SER	THR	ILE
X_{13}	41	LYS	LYS	LYS	LYS	LYS	LYS	LYS	LYS	LYS	—
X_{14}	42	GLY	GLY	ASP	GLY	GLY	ASP	ASP	ASP	ASP	SER

FIGURE 44 General sequence formula of thionins. (From Békés, F. and Lásztity, R., *Acta Aliment.,* 10, 357, 1981. With permission.)

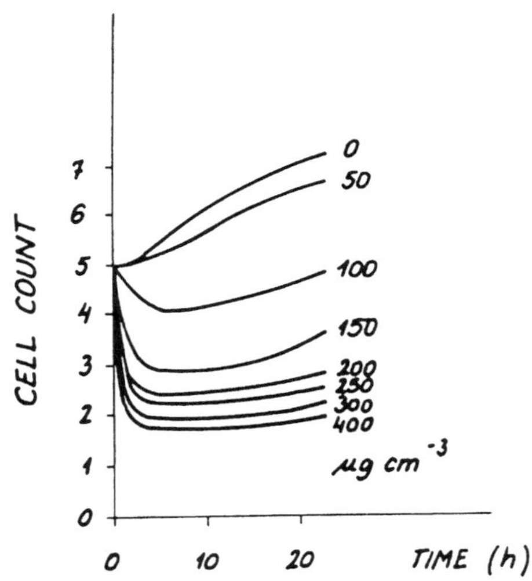

FIGURE 45 Growth of *Saccharomyces uvarum* in a medium containing yeast broth and varying amounts of purothionin. (From Békés, F., *Acta Aliment.,* 10, 343, 1981. With permission.)

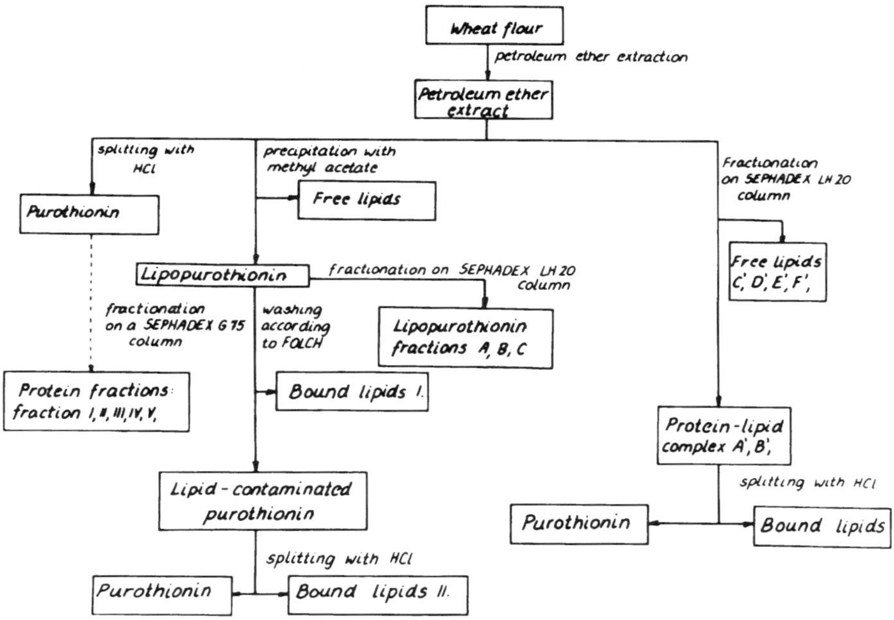

FIGURE 46 Scheme of the protein complexes isolated from the petroleum ether extract of wheat flour and the isolation of apoproteins and bound lipids. The isolated substances and their fractions are shown as noted in the text. (From Békés, F. and Smied, I., *Acta Aliment.*, 1, 229, 1981. With permission.)

preparations was interpreted as phospholipid (or glycolipid)-neutral lipid interaction (not excluding the hydrophobic protein-lipid interactions occurring between hydrophobic side chains of amino acid residues and neutral lipids). The hypothetical structure of lipopurothionin as proposed by Békés and Smied[313] is shown in Figure 47. The conformational structure shown in Figure 47 originates from the work of Mak and Jones.[342]

The extractability of some wheat endosperm proteins by chloroform-methanol mixtures was first reported by Meredith et al.[349] Later work showed that one portion of the lipoproteins extracted by a methanol-chloroform mixture had protein components identical to some α-, β-, γ-, and ω-gliadins. The other portion (lower molecular weight fraction) was composed almost entirely of two clearly defined groups of hydrophobic proteins: CM proteins[344-348] and the low molecular weight gliadins (LMWG).[349-351] Five components, designated CM1, CM2, CM3, 16, and 17, were found in *Triticum aestivum* cultivars.[348] In tetraploid wheat an infrequent allelic variant of CM3 exists, designated CM3.[347-352] Proteins CM1, CM2, CM3, CM3′, and 16 from *T. turgidum* have been purified and partially characterized.[345,346] These proteins have a molecular weight of about 12,000 to 13,000 and they contain a high proportion of hydrophobic amino acids (49 to 59% of the total amino acid residues, excluding cysteine and tryptophan). They also contain lower amounts of glutamic

TABLE 32
Gross Composition of Lipopurothionin Prepared by Methyl Acetate Precipitation Procedure (See Figure 46) and Its Fractions Separated on Sephadex LH-20 Columns[337]

		Fraction		
Characteristic	**Lipopurothionin**	**A**	**B**	**C**
Distribution of fractions (%)	100.0	41.2	32.2	26.5
Protein content (%)	27.4	30.4	26.4	25.7
Lipid content (%)	72.6	69.6	73.6	74.3
Phosphorus content (μg/mg)	20.0	21.3	18.4	19.2

TABLE 33
Lipid Composition of Lipopurothionin and Its Fractions as Percentage of Total Lipid Content (Bound Lipids I; See Figure 46)[313]

		Main Fractions		
Lipid Fraction	**Lipopurothionin**	**A**	**B**	**C**
Sterol ester	1.64	1.68	1.74	1.49
Sterol glycoside	1.84	1.86	1.90	1.77
Phosphatidylethanolamine	36.88	39.73	41.72	28.23
Phosphatidylcholine	30.49	24.83	31.94	36.60
Phosphatidylinositol	5.23	3.42	4.90	8.80
Phosphatidylserine	ND	ND	ND	ND
Lysophosphatidylethanolamine	0.80	0.39	0.78	1.30
Monogalactosyl diglyceride	7.86	9.20	6.54	7.41
Digalactosyl diglyceride	14.42	15.90	12.48	14.40
Monogalactosyl monoglyceride	0.84	3.02	4.10	Traces

Note: ND = not determined.

acid (glutamine) and proline and have a higher lysine content than do typical gliadins. The high proportion of hydrophobic side chains may explain the solubility of LMWG in organic solvents. They can be made water soluble by dialysis against an acid buffer containing urea without losing their solubility in organic solvents.[347] The genetics of CM proteins were recently reviewed by Garcia-Olmedo et al.[324]

Molchanova et al.[353] reported that these proteins originate in the plastids of the endosperm cells. Based on their primary structure[354] it has been suggested that wheat CM proteins are a subgroup of a large plant protein family related to some cereal α-amylases and trypsin inhibitors and to the 2S storage proteins of legumes. Shewry

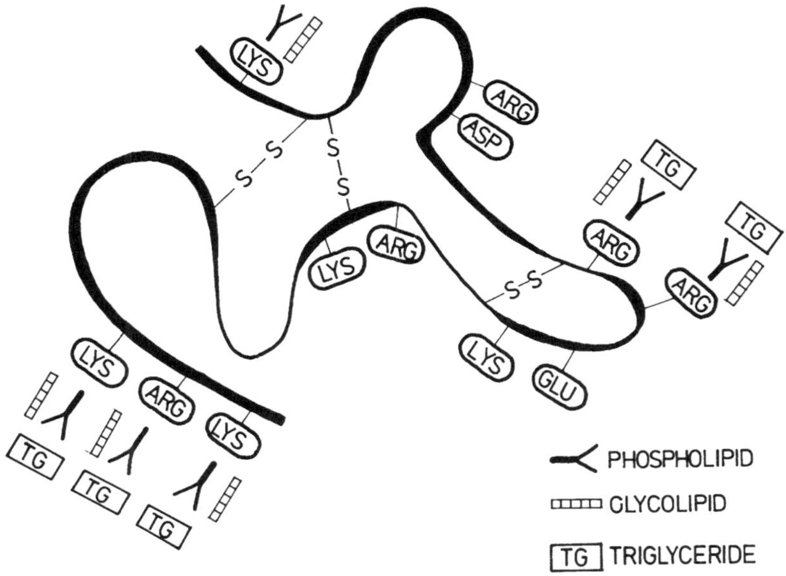

FIGURE 47 Hypothethical structure of purothionin lipid complex. (After Békés, F. and Smied, I., *Acta Aliment.,* 1, 229, 1981. With permission.)

and Miflin[83] defined the CM proteins according to their lipid-binding capacity, their size (mol wt 11,300 to 13,000), and their particular amino acid composition (low glutamine and glutamic acid content and higher cysteine content).

Gautier et al.[355] isolated and characterized a cDNA clone encoding DSG protein (durum wheat sulfur-rich glutenin fraction) and found that the main DSG proteins were identical to CM proteins.

C. Other Cytoplasmic Proteins

The albumin-globulin fraction, which represents 15 to 25% of the total protein in wheat, includes not only the enzymes and some well-defined protein groups discussed previously, but a lot of other proteins. These are important from the point of view of their biological functions, but they may play a role in the formation of the technological properties of wheat. In the early stages of investigation these proteins were studied as a group and data were collected about gross amino acid composition and molecular weight distribution.

Introducing the gel electrophoresis techniques in cereal protein research stimulated more intensive investigation of wheat albumins and globulins. The earliest results of investigations of these proteins by gel electrophoresis[356,357] suggested that they differ little among varieties.

According to many research workers, the albumin and globulin fractions of wheat are poorly suited to variety identification. On the other hand, this varietal uniformity makes the water-soluble wheat proteins suitable for comparisons between species because of the obvious differences in composition at this taxonomic level. Electrophoretic analysis of this group of proteins has thus proven valuable in determining the presence of *Triticum aestivum* in durum wheat products. Electrophoretic patterns of reduced albumin and globulin fractions of wheat cultivars grown in the former West Germany were studied by Ohms.[358] The baking value of flours and the protein patterns of the corresponding wheats were analyzed to detect possible correlations. Cultivar-specific protein patterns were observed after disc electrophoresis of wheat proteins soluble in buffer. Reduction of protein extracts by 2-mercaptoethanol induced the formation of six additional bands. Two of these 2-mercaptoethanol-dependent protein components occur preferentially in cultivars of good baking quality. Three specific protein bands are found in the majority of wheats of good baking value, and practically none are present in wheats of poor baking value. It was also stated the agrotechnical and climatic conditions did not influence the electrophoretic patterns.

Recent studies of Figueron and Khan[359] showed that many of the components of water-soluble wheat proteins are associated with carbohydrates. The nature of the binding and the amino acid residues involved are not yet clear.

Salt-soluble proteins of soft wheats were studied by Clements using PAGE.[360] Choice of extraction medium had little effect on patterns, and good results were obtained with both meals and single kernels. Genotypical differences in patterns were noted, but major differences were quantitative rather than qualitative. Patterns of high- and low-protein specimens of selected cultivars showed only minor differences.

The water-soluble wheat proteins were studied by Pogna et al.[361] using biochemical and immunological methods. Numerous protein components were separated by SDS-PAGE fractionation. The major proteins in this fraction occurred in two different size groups: the HMW albumins (about 60 kDa in size) and the LMW albumins (14 to 16 kDa). Only a few major proteins were found in basic PAGE separation, and these were named A, B, and C. Band A was found to be encoded by the short arm of chromosome 3D.

The analysis by SDS-PAGE of homozygous single chromosome recombinant lines of Cappelle-Desprez (Bezostaya 5A) realized by Krattiger et al.[362] allowed the identification and provisional mapping of a nonprolamin endosperm protein, a HMW albumin of 68 kDa, the presence of which reduced dough strength. The locus, designated Alb-Al, is located on the long arm of chromosome 5A (as are other HMW albumins).

Greenwell and Schofield[363] reported the existence of friabilin, a starch granule protein with a molecular weight of 15 kDa which controls wheat endosperm hardness. Friabilin (softness protein) was prominent in SDS extracts of starch granules of washed soft, but not hard, wheats in a survey of many wheat varieties. Based on these observations Greenwell and Schofield[363] suggested that this softness protein (friabilin) serves the function of releasing the starch granules readily from the protein matrix of soft wheat. However, it must be noted that in a recent publication Sulaiman et al.[364] expressed the view that the hypothesis that variation in endosperm texture is controlled by variation in the level of friabilin associated with starch granules is likely to be an oversimplification.

A more detailed study of wheat germ proteins using modern separation techniques resulted in the detection of special proteins having hemagglutinating properties and demonstrated their tendency to bind to receptors on the cell membranes. These proteins, called wheat germ agglutinins or lectins, were studied by several research workers.[365-367] A review about lectins in higher plants is given by Lis and Sharen.[368]

Bracciali et al.[369] investigated the immunochemical behavior of a purified soft wheat lectin. They found that the fraction with a molecular weight of 40 kDa obtained from durum wheat germ showed an immunological pattern of identity with the lectin from soft wheat germ. Furthermore, they were unable to detect any immunological differences between soft wheat lectin and durum wheat lectin. It appears that lectins of Triticae are immunologically identical. Lectins are encoded by group 1 chromosomes.[367]

Summarizing our knowledge about cytoplasmic proteins of wheat, it must be noted that cytoplasm contains hundreds and hundreds (if not thousands) of biologically active proteins. Their full knowledge requires an enormous amount of further research work which is correlated more with general plant physiology than with today's problems of cereal processing.

VI. NUTRITIVE VALUE OF WHEAT PROTEINS AND WHEAT PROTEIN PREPARATIONS

As noted in the general discussion of cereal proteins (see preceding chapter), the total wheat protein and especially the storage proteins of endosperm are poor in lysine, and therefore their biological value is relatively low. Nevertheless, because in mixed diets (feed mixtures) the wheat protein may be easily supplemented with proteins having a complementary amino acid composition (higher lysine content and lower amount of sulfur-containing proteins), the real value of the wheat protein in nutrition (feeding) is higher than may be calculated from the amino acid composition. While discussing the nutritional value of gluten proteins it must be mentioned that a small part of the population is sensitive to particular gliadin components of wheat. The disease (called celiac disease or gluten-sensitive enteropathy) is characterized by malabsorption of nutrients as a consequence of damage to the absorptive epithelial cells that line the small intestine.

The cytoplasmic proteins of wheat generally have a better amino acid composition from the point of view of nutritional value because their lysine content is higher and the glutamic acid (glutamine) content is lower than that of the gluten proteins. Some of the albumin components in wheat have special amino acid compositions. For example, albumins 13A and 13B, isolated by Feillet and Nimmo,[370] contain practically no phenylalanine (see Table 34). Probably such protein preparations could be used in special diets for people having inherited disorders of amino acid metabolism.

TABLE 34
Amino Acid Composition of Some Water-Soluble Proteins of Wheat (mol/10^5 g Protein)

Amino Acid	Albumin 13A[a]	Albumin 13B[a]	Albumin[b]
Lysine	23	48	46
Histidine	14	1	3
Arginine	56	53	52
Threonine	25	24	21
Serine	56	66	62
Aspartic acid	55	70	70
Glutamic acid	106	95	101
Glycine	75	75	76
Alanine	26	76	70
Valine	72	101	104
Leucine	74	68	72
Isoleucine	23	16	15
Proline	69	88	71
Tyrosine	36	29	31
Phenylalanine	16	—	2
Tryptophan	16	35	28
Cystine	66	54	75
Methionine	21	17	21

[a] From Feillet and Nimmo.[370]
[b] From Ewart.[162]

The growing demand for proteins in the food industry and also in some other fields resulted in an increase in the production of plant protein preparations, concentrates, and isolates. Among these products the cereal proteins play a growing role. The use of plant protein concentrates has some significant advantages. Some of these may be summarized as follows:

1. Their protein content is high, and therefore they might well be used for protein enrichment and for production of new foods with high protein content.
2. The protein content may be accurately regulated and uniform quality guaranteed.
3. The problems of storage and transport of concentrates generally may be more easily solved than those of other raw materials having a low protein content.

4. During the procedure for the production of concentrates it is possible to eliminate some components which are not desirable (enzyme inhibitors, glycosides, etc.).

One of the best-known cereal protein concentrates is the vital gluten produced in many countries of the world. Total production of vital gluten has been estimated to be about 300,000 tons/year.[371] The largest utilizer of vital gluten is the baking industry, but it is also used in breakfast foods, pet foods, meat analogs, processed meat, and other foods. The quality of vital gluten is generally characterized by protein content (normally 75 to 80%), water absorption (vital gluten of good quality absorbs 1.5 to 2 times its own weight, and this absorption remains constant under any conditions), and the velocity of swelling (the maximal water absorption and swelling must be achieved in 20 to 60 s). The production of other protein preparations from wheat is not yet significant.

The procedures used for the production of protein preparations from wheat generally may be classified as follows: (1) air (dry) processing, (2) wet processing using water or water solutions, and (3) procedures using nonaqueous solvents.

The air classification of flours, based on the density differences of starch and storage wheat protein particles, is widely used and permits the production of preparations with a 20 to 25% enrichment of protein content. The wet processes are mainly connected with starch production. Generally, wheat flour dough is produced and the starch and gluten are separated by washing. The remaining wet gluten is dried under mild conditions.[379,389,390]

In the old processes the water-soluble proteins were lost and a great amount of wastewater was formed. The newer procedures try to save all the protein and other components of wheat, producing not only starch and vital gluten, but also other protein preparations (germ, soluble proteins) and fiber.

The production of wheat protein concentrates using flotation methods with organic solvents is at this time only in the experimental stage; no industrial uses are known.

Among the chemically modified gluten preparations the succinylated and acylated products may be important because of better solubility and higher swelling and water-absorbing capacity. The enzymatically degraded gluten preparations (hydrolyzed gluten) also may be used in the production of some special foods[371] and meat flavors.

REFERENCES

1. Kasarda, D. D., Bernardin, J. E., and Nimmo, C. C., Wheat proteins, in *Advances in Cereal Science and Technology,* Vol. 1, Pomeranz, Y., Ed., American Association of Cereal Chemists, St. Paul, MN, 1976, 158.
2. Wrigley, C. W. and Bietz, J. A., Proteins and amino acids, in *Wheat: Chemistry and Technology,* 3rd ed., Vol. 1, Pomeranz, Y., Ed., American Association of Cereal Chemists, St. Paul, MN, 1988, 159.

3. Tatham, A. S., Shewry, P. R., and Belton, P. S., Structural studies of cereal prolamins including wheat gluten, in *Advances in Cereal Science and Technology,* Vol. 10, Pomeranz, Y., Ed., American Association of Cereal Chemists, St. Paul, MN, 1990, 1.
4. Kreis, M., Shewry, P. R., Forde, B. G., Forde, J., and Miflin B. J., Structure and evolution of seed storage proteins and their genes with particular reference to those of wheat, barley and rye, in *Oxford Surveys of Plant Molecular and Cell Biology,* Vol. 2, Miflin, B. J., Ed., Oxford University Press, Oxford, 1985, 253.
5. Wrigley, C. W., Autran, J. C., and Bushuk, W., Identification of cereal varieties by gel electrophoresis of the grain proteins, in *Advances in Cereal Science and Technology,* Vol. 5, Pomeranz, Y., Ed., American Association of Cereal Chemists, St. Paul, MN, 1982, 211.
6. Fox, P. F. and Mulvihill, D. M., Enzymes in wheat, flour and bread, in *Advances in Cereal Science and Technology,* Vol. 5, Pomeranz, Y., Ed., American Association of Cereal Chemists, St. Paul, MN, 1982, 107.
7. Wrigley, C. W. and Shepard, K. W., Electrofocusing of grain proteins from wheat genotypes, *Ann. N.Y. Acad. Sci.,* 209, 154, 1973.
8. Kaczkowski, J. and Tkachuk, R., Wheat glutenins, *Ann. Technol. Agric.,* 29, 107, 1980.
9. Woychik, J. H., Boundy, J. A., and Dimler, R. J., Starch gel electrophoresis of wheat gluten proteins with concentrated urea, *Arch. Biochem. Biophys.,* 94, 477, 1961.
10. Jones, R. W., Taylor, N. W., and Senti, F. R., Electrophoresis and fractionation of wheat gluten, *Arch. Biochem. Biophys.,* 84, 363, 1959.
11. Lee, J. W. and McRitchie, F., The effect of gluten protein fractions on dough properties, *Cereal Chem.,* 48, 620, 1971.
12. Simmonds, D. H. and Wrigley, C. W., The effect on the solubility and molecular weight range of wheat gluten and storage proteins, *Cereal Chem.,* 49, 317, 1972.
13. Simmonds, D. H. and Orth, R. A., Structure and composition of cereal proteins as related to their industrial utilization, in *Industrial Uses of Cereals,* Pomeranz, Y., Ed., American Association of Cereal Chemists, St. Paul, MN, 1973, 51.
14. Bietz, J. A. and Wall, J. S., Wheat gluten subunits: molecular weights determined by sodium-dodecyl-sulphate polyacrylamide gel electrophoresis, *Cereal Chem.,* 49, 416, 1972.
15. Meredith, O. B. and Wren, J. J., Determination of molecular weight distribution in wheat flour proteins by extraction and gel filtration in a dissociating medium, *Cereal Chem.,* 43, 169, 1966.
16. Orth, R. A. and Bushuk, W., Studies on glutenin. I. Comparison of preparative methods, *Cereal Chem.,* 50, 106, 1973.
17. Kobrehel, K. and Bushuk, W., Studies of glutenin. X. Effects of fatty acids and their sodium salt on solubility in water, *Cereal Chem.,* 54, 833, 1977.
18. Kobrehel, K. and Bushuk, W., Studies of glutenin. XI. Note on glutenin solubilization with supernatants in water, *Cereal Chem.,* 55, 1060, 1978.
19. Wasik, R. J., Daoust, H., and Martin, C., Studies on glutenin solubilized in high concentrations of sodium stearate, *Cereal Chem.,* 56, 90, 1979.
20. Hamauzu, Z., Khan, K., and Bushuk, W., Studies of glutenin. XIV. Gel filtration and sodium-dodecyl-sulphate electrophoresis of glutenin solubilized in sodium stearate, *Cereal Chem.,* 56, 513, 1979.
21. Kobrehel, K., Extraction of wheat proteins with salts of fatty acids and their electrophoretic characterization, *Ann. Technol. Agric.,* 29, 125, 1980.

22. Graveland, A., Bongers, P., and Bosveld, P., Extraction and fractionation of wheat flour proteins, *J. Sci. Food Agric.,* 30, 71, 1979.
23. Graveland, A., Extraction of wheat proteins by sodium dodecyl sulphate, *Ann. Technol. Agric.,* 29, 113, 1980.
24. Graveland, A., Bosveld, P., Lichtendonk, W. J., Moonen, H. E. E., and Schepstra, A., Extraction and fractionation of wheat flour proteins, *J. Sci. Food Agric.,* 33, 1117, 1982.
25. Bushuk, W., Khan, K., and McMaster G., Functional glutenin: a complex of covalently and noncovalently linked components, *Ann. Technol. Agric.,* 29, 279, 1980.
26. Feillet, P., Fevre, E., and Jeanjean, M. F., Recherche d'un nouveau test d'appreciation de la force boulangere des blés tendres, résultats preliminaires, *Bull. Anc. Eleves Ec. Meun. ENSMIC,* 271, 22, 1976.
27. Jeanjean, M. F. and Feillet, P., Eine neue biochemische Methode zur Ermittlung des Backfähigkeit von Weichweizen, *Getreide Mehl Brot,* 33, 127, 1979.
28. Jeanjean, M. F. and Feillet, P., Properties of wheat gel proteins, *Ann. Technol. Agric.,* 29, 295, 1980.
29. Landry, J. and Moureaux, T., Heterogenité des glutélines du grain de mais: extraction séléctive et composition en acides aminé des trois fractions isolée, *Bull. Soc. Chim. Biol.,* 52, 1021, 1970.
30. Ryadchikow, V. G., Zima, V. G., Zhmakina, O. A., Lebedev, A. V., and Philipas, T. B., Studies of wheat flour glutenins by modified Landry-Moureaux method and gliadins by isoelectric focusing, *Ann. Technol. Agric.,* 29, 321, 1980.
31. Haff, L. A. and Easterday, R. L., Sephacryl gels: physical properties and evaluation of performance in filtration, *J. Liq. Chromatogr.,* 1, 811, 1978.
32. Haff, L. A., Fractionation of water insoluble proteins using Sephacryl S-200 in formamide, *Prep. Biochem.,* 8, 99, 1978.
33. Preston, K. R., Gel filtration of wheat gluten proteins on Sephacryl S-300, *Cereal Chem.,* 59, 73, 1982.
34. Skerrit, H.I., Immonochemistry of cereal grain storage proteins, in *Advances in Cereal Science and Technology,* Vol. 9, Pomeranz, Y., Ed., American Association of Cereal Chemists, St. Paul, MN, 1988, 263.
35. Örsi, F., Pallagi, E., and Lásztity, R., Investigation of wheat proteins by HPLC, in *Gluten Proteins,* Lásztity, R. and Békés, F., Eds., World Scientific, Singapore, 1987, 141.
36. Huebner, F. R. and Bietz, J. A., Separation of wheat gliadins by preparative reversed-phase high performance liquid chromatography, *Cereal Chem.,* 61, 544, 1984.
37. Huebner, F. R., Christianson, D. D., Nelsen, T. C., and Bietz, J. A., Gliadin and glutenin analysis by SE-HPLC for wheat classification, in *Gluten Proteins,* Bushuk, W. and Tkachuk, R., Eds., American Association of Cereal Chemists, St. Paul, MN, 1990, 145.
38. Huebner, F. R. and Bietz, J. A., Detection of quality differences among wheats by high performance liquid chromatography, *J. Chromatogr.,* 327, 333, 1985.
39. Bietz, J. A., Analysis of wheat gluten proteins by reversed phase high-performance liquid chromatography: techniques and applications, in *Gluten Proteins,* Graveland, A. and Moonen, J. H. E., Eds., TNO, Wageningen, 1985, 1.
40. Elton, G. A. H. and Ewart, J. A. D., Starch gel electrophoresis of wheat proteins, *Nature (London),* 187, 600, 1960.
41. Elton, G. A. H. and Ewart, J. A. D., Starch gel electrophoresis of cereal proteins, *J. Sci. Food Agric.,* 13, 12, 1962.

42. Woychik, J. H., Boundy, J. A., and Dimler, R. J., Starch gel electrophoresis of wheat gluten proteins with concentrated urea, *Arch. Biochem. Biophys.*, 94, 477, 1961.
43. Wrigley, C. W., Gel electrofocusing — a technique for analysing multiple protein samples by isoelectric focusing, *Sci. Foods,* 15, 17, 1968.
44. Wrigley, C. W., Protein mapping by combined gel electrofocusing and electrophoresis: application to the study of genotypic variation in wheat gliadins, *Biochem. Genet.*, 4, 509, 1970.
45. Bietz, J. A. and Wall, J. S., Wheat gluten subunits: molecular weights determined by sodium-dodecyl-sulphate polyacrylamide gel electrophoresis, *Cereal Chem.*, 49, 416, 1972.
46. Orth, R. A. and Bushuk, W., Studies on glutenin. II. Relation of variety, location of growth and baking quality to molecular weight distribution of subunits, *Cereal Chem.*, 50, 191, 1973.
47. Tkachuk, R. and Mellish, V. J., Use of two-dimensional electrophoresis procedure to characterize wheat proteins, in *Gluten Proteins,* Lásztity, R. and Békés, F., Eds., World Scientific, Singapore, 1987, 111.
48. Bietz, J. A., Fractionation of wheat gluten proteins by capillary electrophoresis, in *Gluten Proteins,* Association of Cereal Research, Detmold, Germany, 1993, 404.
49. Bietz, J. A., Capillary electrophoresis of wheat proteins: optimization and use in varietal identification, *Cereal Foods World,* 37, 555, 1992.
50. Sozinov, A. A. and Poperelya, F. A., Polymorphism of prolamins and selection (in Russian), *Dokl. Vses. Akad. Skh. Nauk,* 10, 21, 1979.
51. Wrigley, C. W., du Cros, D. L., Archer, J. J., Downie, P. G., and Roxbourgh, C. M., The sulphur content of wheat — endosperm protein and its relevance to grain quality, *Aust. J. Plant Physiol.*, 7, 755, 1980.
52. Almgard, G. and Clapham, D., Swedish wheat cultivars distinguished by content of gliadins and isozymes, *Swed. J. Agric. Res.*, 7, 137, 1977.
53. Bushuk, W. and Zillman, R. R., Wheat cultivar identification by gliadin electrophero-grams. I. Apparatus, method and nomenclature, *Can. J. Plant Sci.*, 58, 505, 1978.
54. Autran, J. C. and Bourdet, A., Possibilities d'un controle variétal qualitatif et quantitatif dans les lots de blés commerciaux, *C.R. Acad. Agric.*, 61, 66, 1975.
55. Ellis, J. R. S. and Beminster, C. H., The identification of U.K. wheat varieties by starch gel electrophoresis of gliadin proteins, *J. Natl. Inst. Agric. Bot.*, 14, 221, 1977.
56. Autran, J. C., L'identification des varietées de blé, *Bull. Anc. Eleves Ec. Fr. Meun.*, 256, 163, 1973.
57. Wrigley, C. W. and Shephard, K. W., Identification of Australian wheat cultivars by laboratory procedures. Examination of pure samples of grain, *Aust. J. Exp. Agric. Anim. Husb.*, 14, 796, 1974.
58. Sozinov, A. A. and Poperelya, F. A., Vertical electrophoresis of alcohol soluble proteins of endosperm in starch gel as a method for studies of genetic characteristics of wheat (in Russian), *Dokl. Vses. Akad. Skh. Nauk,* 2, 9, 1971.
59. Nehéz, R. and Nagy, M., Prolaminok gélelektroforézisének alkalmazása gabona-fajták nemesitésére és genetikai leírására (in Hungarian), *Növénytermelés,* 28, 263, 1979.
60. Glattes, H., Klaushofer, H., and Danzer, D., Bedeutung und Methoden der Identifizierung von Weizensorten. II. Mitteilung Identifizierung österreichischer Mahlweizen mit Hilfe Stärke-gelelectrophorese, *Ernahrung,* 4, 244, 1980.

61. Autran, J. C., Berrier, R., Jeanjean, M. F., Jou, P., and Kobrehel, J., Emploi de l'electrophorése dans les filieres cereales. Possibilitiés et limites, *Ind. Cereales,* 8, 13, 1981.
62. Du Cros, D. L. and Wrigley, C. W., Improved electrophoretic methods for identifying cereal varieties, *J. Sci. Food Agric.,* 30, 785, 1979.
63. Tkachuk, R. and Mettish, J., Wheat cultivar identification by high voltage gel electrophoresis, *Ann. Technol. Agric.,* 29, 207, 1980.
64. Konarev, V. G., Gavrilyuk, I. P., and Gubareva, N. K., The method of cultivar identification of wheat grain meal (in Russian), *Bull. Discovery Invention Rep.,* 507271, 11, 1975.
65. Wrigley, C. W., The genetic and chemical significance of varietal differences in gluten composition, *Ann. Technol. Agric.,* 29, 213, 1980.
66. Glattes, H., Klaushofer, H., and Danzer, D., Bedeutung und Methoden der Identifizierung von Weizensorten. III. Mitteilung Identifizierung Österreichischer Weizen mit Hilfe der Polyacrylamidgel-Elektrophorese, PAGE Methode, *Ernahrung,* 4, 545, 1980.
67. Bushuk, W., Rerie, W., and Zillmann, R. R., Procedure Manual for Polyacrylamide Gel Electrophoresis of Giadins as a Basis for Wheat Cultivar Identification, Department of Plant Science, University of Manitoba, Winnipeg, 1979.
68. Du Cros, D. L., Lawrance, G. J., Miskelly, D., and Wrigley, C. W., Systematic Identification of Australian Wheat Varieties by Laboratory Methods, Tech. Publ. No. 7, CSIRO Wheat Research Unit, North Ryde, Australia, 1980.
69. Konarev, V. G., Yakubziner, M. M., Trofimov, V. M., Skays, A. Y., Gavrilyuk, I. P., Gubareva, N. K., and Chernoburova, A. D., The determination of cultivars of wheat and barley grain by protein formulas (in Russian), *Vestn. Skh. Nauki,* 6, 124, 1976.
70. Konarev, V. G., Gavrilyuk, I. P., and Gubareva, N. K., Gliadin polymorphism and its use in the identifying varieties of and registration of genetic resources with regard to wheat and other cereals (in Russian), *Vestn. Skh. Nauki,* 7, 84, 1977.
71. Gubareva, N. K., Gavrilyuk, I. P., and Chernoburova, A. D., Determination of the identity and the cultivar purity of wheat grain according to electrophoretic patterns of the gliadins. Experimental methods and catelogue of cultivar electropherograms, *Dokl. Vses. Akad. Skh. Nauk,* 6, 1, 1975.
72. Gubareva, N. K., Rudenko, M. I., and Chernoburova, A. D., Comparative analysis of cultivars of durum wheat by gliadin electrophoretic spectra (in Russian), *Trudy Prikl. Bot. Genet. Sel.,* 63, 24, 1979.
73. Sapirsten, H. D. and Bushuk, W., Computer-aided analysis of gliadin electropherograms. II. Wheat cultivar identification and class comparisons, *Cereal Chem.,* 62, 377, 1985.
74. Lookhart, G. L., Jones, V. L., Hall, S. B., and Finney, K. F., An improved method for standardizing polyacrylamide gel electrophoresis of wheat gliadin proteins, *Cereal Chem.,* 59, 178, 1982,
75. Jones, B. L., Lookhart, G. L., Halls, S. E., and Finney, F. K., Identification of wheat cultivars by gliadin electrophoresis: electropherograms of the 88 wheat cultivars most commonly grown in the United States in 1979, *Cereal Chem.,* 59, 181, 1982.
76. Wrigley, C. W., Robinson, P. J., and Williams, W. T., Association between electrophoretic patterns of gliadin proteins and quality characterization of wheat, *J. Sci. Food Agric.,* 32, 433, 1981.

77. Wrigley, C. W. and McCausland, J., Variety identification by laboratory methods, in Instruction Manual for Barley, Wheat and Other Cereals, Tech. Publ. No. 4, CSIRO Wheat Research Unit, North Ryde, Australia, 1977.
78. Sozinov, A. A. and Poperelya, F. A., Genetic classification of prolamines and its use for plant breeding, *Ann. Technol. Agric.,* 29, 229, 1980.
79. Lookhart, G. L., Cox, T. S., and Ching, O. K., Statistical analyses of gliadin reversed-phase high-performance liquid chromatography patterns of hard red spring and hard red winter wheat cultivars grown in a common environment: classification indices, *Cereal Chem.,* 70, 430, 1993.
80. Marchylo, B. A., Hatcher, D. W., and Kruger, J. E., Identification of wheat cultivars by reversed-phase high-performance chromatography of storage proteins, *Cereal Chem.,* 65, 28, 1988.
81. Bietz, J. A., Analysis of wheat gluten protein by reversed phase high-performance liquid chromatography techniques and applications, in *Gluten Proteins,* Graveland, A. and Moonen, J. H. E., Eds., TNO, Wageningen, 1985.
82. Bietz, J. A. and Cobb, L. A., Improved procedures for rapid wheat varietial identification by reserved-phase high-performance liquid chromatography of gliadins, *Cereal Chem.,* 62, 332, 1985.
83. Shewry, P. R. and Miflin, B. J., Seed storage proteins of economically important cereals, in *Advances in Cereal Science and Technology,* Vol. 7, Pomeranz, Y., Ed., American Association of Cereal Chemists, St. Paul, MN, 1985.
84. Kasarda, D. D., Structure and properties of α-gliadins, *Ann. Technol. Agric.,* 29, 151, 1980.
85. Platt, S. G. and Kasarda, D. D., Separation and characterization of α-gliadin fractions, *Biochim. Biophys. Acta,* 243, 407, 1971.
86. Huebner, F. R., Rothfuss, J. A., and Wall, J. S., Isolation and chemical comparison of different γ-gliadins from hard red winter flour, *Cereal Chem.,* 44, 221, 1967.
87. Booth, M. R., Isolation of further components of wheat gliadins, *J. Sci. Food Agric.,* 21, 185, 1970.
88. Charbonnier, L., Isolation and characterization of ω-gliadin fractions, *Biochim. Biophys. Acta,* 359, 142, 1974.
89. Charbonnier, L., Tercé-Laforgue, Th., and Mossé, J., Some physicochemical properties of *Triticum vulgare* β-, γ- and ω-gliadins, *Ann. Technol. Agric.,* 29, 175, 1980.
90. Booth, M. R. and Ewart, J. A. D., Studies on four components of wheat gliadins, *Biochim. Biophys. Acta,* 181, 226, 1969.
91. Kasarda, D. D., Da-Roza, D. A., and Ohms, J. I., N-terminal sequence of α_2-gliadin, *Biochim. Biophys. Acta,* 351, 290, 1974.
92. Autran, J. C., Lew, E. J. L., Nimmo, C. C., and Kasarda, D. D., N-terminal amino acid sequencing of prolamins from wheat and related species, *Nature (London),* 282, 527, 1979.
93. Bietz, J. A., Huebner, F. R., Saderson, J. E., and Wall, J. S., Wheat gliadin homology through N-terminal amino acid sequence analysis, *Cereal Chem.,* 54, 1070, 1977.
94. Patey, A. L., Evans, D. J., Tiplady, R., Byfield, P. G. H., and Matthews, E. W., Sequence comparison of γ-gliadin and coeliac toxic α-gliadin, *Lancet,* 2, 718, 1975.
95. Bernardin, J. E., Kasarda, D. D., and Mecham, D. K., Preparation and characterization of α-gliadin, *J. Biol. Chem.,* 242, 445, 1967.

96. Thompson, W. P. and Murray, M. G., Sequence organization in pea and bean DNA and a model for genomic evolution, in *The Plant Genome. Proc 4th John Innes Symp.*, Davies, D.R. and Hopwood, D.A., Eds., The John Innes Charity, Norwich, England, 1980, 31.
97. Garcia Olmedo, F., Carbonero, P., and Jones, B. L., Chromosomal locations of genes that control wheat endosperm proteins, in *Advances in Cereal Science and Technology,* Vol. 5, Pomeranz, Y., Ed., American Association of Cereal Chemists, St. Paul, MN, 1982, 1.
98. Kasarda, D. D., Okita, T. W., Bernardin, J. E., Baecker, P. A., Nimmo, C. C., Lew, E. J. L., Dieter, M. D., and Greene, F., Nucleic acid (cDNA) and amino acid sequences of α-type gliadins from wheat *(Triticum aestivum), Proc. Natl. Acad. Sci. U.S.A.,* 81, 4712, 1984.
99. Bartels, D., Altosaar, I., Harberd, N. P., Barker, R. F., and Thompson, R. D., Molecular analysis of γ-gliadins gene families at the complex Gli-1 locus of bread wheat *(T. aestivum), Theor. Appl. Genet.,* 72, 845, 1986.
100. Sheetes, K. and Hedgcoth, C., Nucleotide sequence of α-gliadin gene: comparisons with other γ-gliadin sequences show the structure of γ-gliadin genes and the general primary structure of γ-gliadins, *Plant. Sci.,* 57, 141, 1988.
101. Neill, J. D., Litts, J. C., Anderson, O. D., Greene, F. C., and Stilles, I. J., Expression of a wheat α-gliadin gene in *Saccharomyces cerevisiae, Gene,* 55, 303, 1987.
102. Greene, F. C., In vitro synthesis of wheat *(Triticum aestivum)* storage proteins, *Plant Physiol.,* 68, 778, 1981.
103. Scheets, K. and Hedgcoth, C., Expression of a wheat α-gliadin in *Saccharomyces cerevisiae* from a yeast ADH 1 promoter, *J. Agric. Food Chem.,* 37, 389, 1989.
104. Halford, N. G., Forde, J., Shewry, P. R., and Kreis, M., Functional analysis of the upstream regions of a silent and an expressed member of family of wheat seed protein genes in transgenic tobacco, *Plant. Sci.,* 62, 207, 1989.
105. Lásztity, R., Recent results in cereal protein research, *Period. Polytech.* (Techn. Univ. Budapest) 16, 331, 1972.
106. Chen, Y. H., Yang, J. T., and Chau, K. H., Determination of the helix and β-form of proteins in aqueous solution by circular dichroism, *Biochemistry,* 13, 3350, 1974.
107. Luer, C. A. and Wong, K. P., Conformation of *Escherichia coli* ribosomal protein L_7/L_{12} in solution: hydrodynamic, spectroscopic and conformation prediction studies, *Biochemistry,* 18, 2019, 1979.
108. Kasarda, D. D., Bernardin, J. E., and Thomas, R. S., Reversible aggregation of α-gliadin to fibrils, *Science,* 155, 203, 1967.
109. Greene, F. C. and Kasarda, D. D., Apolar interactions of α-gliadin: binding of 2-toluidinylnaphthalene-6-sulphonate, *Cereal Chem.,* 58, 601, 1971.
110. Popineau, Y. and Godon, B., Surface hydrophobicity of gliadin components, *Cereal Chem.,* 59, 55, 1982.
111. Popineau, Y. and Godon, B., Application de la chromatographie d'interaction hydrophobe au fractionnement des prolamines de blés tendres, *C.R. Acad. Sci. Paris Ser. D.,* 287, 251, 1978.
112. Caldwell, K. A., The fractionation and purification of gliadins by hydrophobic interaction chromatography, *J. Sci. Food Agric.,* 30, 185, 1979.
113. Chung, K. H. and Pomeranz, Y., Acid soluble proteins of wheat flours. II. Binding to hydrophobic gels, *Cereal Chem.,* 56, 196, 1979.

114. Anderson, O. D., Greene, F. C., and Litts, J. C., Structure of the α-gene gliadin gene family from the bread wheat cultivar Cheyenne, in *Gluten Proteins,* Bushuk, W. and Tkachuk, R., Eds., American Association of Cereal Chemists, St. Paul, MN, 1990, 640.
115. Tatham, A. S., Shewry, P. R., and Field, J. M., Conformational studies of the repetitive domains of the cereal proteins, in *Gluten Proteins,* Bushuk, W. and Tkachuk, R., Eds., American Association of Cereal Chemists, St. Paul, MN, 1990, 376.
116. Purcell, J. M., Kasarda, D. D., and Wu, C. S. C., Secondary structures of wheat α- and β-gliadin proteins. Fourier transform infrared spectroscopy, *J. Cereal Sci.,* 7, 21, 1988.
117. Tatham, A. S., Miflin, B. J., and Shewry, P. R., The β-turn conformation in wheat gluten proteins: relationship to gluten elasticity, *Cereal Chem.,* 62, 405, 1985.
118. Popineau, Y. and Pineau, F., Changes of conformation and surface hydrophobicity of gliadins, *Lebensm. Wiss. Technol.,* 21, 113, 1988.
119. Tatham, A. S. and Shewry, P. R., The conformation of wheat gluten proteins. The secondary structures and thermal stabilities of α-, β-, and ω-gliadins, *J. Cereal Sci.,* 3, 103, 1985.
120. Metakowski, E. V., Vaccino, P., Accerbi, M., Redaelli, R., and Pogna, E., Polymorphism and spontaneous mutations at the gliadin-coding loci, in *Gluten Proteins,* Association for Cereal Research (Germany), Detmold, 1993, 218.
121. Bushuk, W., Khan, K., and McMaster, G. J., Functional glutenin: a complex of covalently and noncovalently linked components, *Ann. Technol. Agric.,* 29, 279, 1980.
122. McMaster, G. J., Association of Carbohydrate and Protein in Wheat Gluten, Ph.D. thesis, University of Manitoba, Winnipeg, 1982.
123. Chung, O. K. and Tsen, C. C., Changes in lipid binding and distribution during baking, *Cereal Chem.,* 52, 533, 1975.
124. Lásztity, R., Békés, F., Nedelkovits, J., and Varga, J., Investigation of the complex protein of wheat, *Acta Chim. Acad. Sci. Hung.,* 101, 281, 1979.
125. Békés, F., Zawistowska, U., and Bushuk, W., Protein-lipid complexes in the gliadin fraction, *Cereal Chem.,* 60, 371, 1983.
126. Békés, F., Zawistowska, U., and Bushuk, W., Lipid mediated aggregation of gliadin, *Cereal Chem.,* 60, 379, 1983.
127. Frazier, P. J., Shearing, K. M., Daniels, N. W. R., and Eggit, P. W. R., The ligolin lipid complex in gluten, in *Gluten Proteins,* Graveland, A. and Moonen, J.H.E., Eds., TNO, Wageningen, 1985, 91.
128. Bushuk, W., Békés, F., McMaster, G. J., and Zawistowska, V., Carbohydrate and lipid complexes with gliadin and glutenin, in *Gluten Proteins,* Graveland, A. and Moonen, J.H.E., Eds., TNO, Wageningen, 1985, 101.
129. Lásztity, R., Békés, F., Örsi, F., Smied, I., and Kárpáti, M., Protein-lipid and protein-carbohydrate interactions in the gluten complex, in *Gluten Proteins,* Lásztity, R. and Békés, F., Eds., World Scientific, Singapore, 1987, 343.
130. Békés, F., Gupta, R. B., Batey, I. L., Gras, P. W., and McRitchie, F., Lipid mediated aggregates of gluten proteins and their relations to functional properties, in *Gluten Proteins,* Bushuk, W. and Tkachuk, R., Eds., American Association of Cereal Chemists, St. Paul, MN, 1990, 170.
131. Paternotte, T. A., Orsel, R., and Hamer, R. J., Interactions between flour proteins and flour lipids at the liquid/air interface, in *Gluten Proteins,* Association of Cereal Research (Germany), Detmold, 1993, 207.

132. Zawistowska, V., Békés, F., and Bushuk, W., Gluten proteins with high affinity to flour lipids, *Cereal Chem.,* 62, 284, 1985.
133. Hamer, R. J., van Ort, M. G., Harritsen, A., Weegels, P. L., and Prieto, J. A., New methods to understand interactions in wheat flour doughs, interactions between gliadins and flour lipids, in *Gluten Proteins,* Bushuk, W. and Tkachuk, R., Eds., American Association of Cereal Chemists, St. Paul, MN, 1990, 296.
134. Chen, J., Khan, K., Shelton, D. R., and D'Appolonia, B. L., Isolation and fractionation of carbohydrate-containing proteins from wheat gluten, *Cereal Chem.,* 69, 475, 1992.
135. Chen, J., Shelton, D. R., D'Appolonia, B. L., and Khan, K., Structural characterization of the carbohydrate portion of a glycopeptide from wheat gluten, *Cereal Chem.,* 69, 481, 1992.
136. Beckwith, A. C., Nielsen, H. C., Wall, J. S., and Huebner, F. R., Isolation and characterization of a high molecular weight protein from wheat gliadin, *Cereal Chem.,* 43, 14, 1966.
137. Bietz, J. A. and Wall, J. S., Identity of high molecular weight gliadin and ethanol-soluble glutenin subunits of wheat: relation to gluten structure, *Cereal Chem.,* 57, 415, 1980.
138. Jos, J., Charbonnier, L., Mougenot, J., and Rey, J., Isolation and characterization of the toxic fraction of wheat gliadin in coeliac disease, in *Perspectives in Coeliac Disease,* McNicholl, B. and McCarthy, C.P., Eds., MTP Press, Lancaster, 1979, 75.
139. Bushuk, W., Nomenclature, in *Gluten Proteins,* Bushuk, W. and Tkachuk, R., Eds., American Association of Cereal Chemists, St. Paul, MN, 1990, 781.
140. Orth, R. A. and Bushuk, W., Studies on glutenin. I. Comparison of preparative methods, *Cereal Chem.,* 50, 106, 1973.
141. Bietz, J. A. and Wall, J. S., The effect of various extractants on the subunit composition and association of wheat glutenin, *Cereal Chem.,* 52, 145, 1975.
142. Mecham, D. K., Sokol, H. A, and Pence, J. W., Extractable protein and hydration characteristics of flours and doughs in dilute acid, *Cereal Chem.,* 39, 81, 1962.
143. Mecham, D. K., Cole, E. W., and Ng, H., Solubilizing effect of mercurie chloride on the gel protein of wheat flour, *Cereal Chem.,* 49, 62, 1972.
144. Huebner, F. R. and Wall, J. S., Fractionation and quantitative differences of glutenin from wheat varieties varying in baking quality, *Cereal Chem.,* 53, 258, 1976.
145. Woychik, J. H., Huebner, F. R., and Dimler, R. J., Reduction and starch-gel electrophoresis of wheat gliadin and glutenin, *Arch. Biochem. Biophys.,* 105, 151, 1964.
146. Payne, P. I. and Corfield, K. G., Subunit composition of wheat glutenin proteins, isolated by gel filtration in a dissociating medium, *Planta,* 145, 83, 1979.
147. Bietz, J. A. and Huebner, F. R., Structure of glutenin: achievements at the Northern Regional Research Center, *Ann. Technol. Agric.,* 29, 249, 1980.
148. Bushuk, W., Khan, K., and McMaster, G., Functional glutenin: a complex of covalently and noncovalently linked components, *Ann. Technol. Agric.,* 29, 279, 1980.
149. McRitchie, F., du Cros, D. L., and Wrigley, C. W., Flour polypeptides related to wheat quality, in *Advances in Cereal Science and Technology,* Vol. 10, Pomeranz, Y., Ed., American Association of Cereal Chemists, St. Paul, MN, 1990, 79.
150. Ng, P. K. and Bushuk, W., Concerning the nomenclature of high molecular weight glutenin subunits, *J. Cereal Sci.,* 9, 53, 1989.
151. Shewry, P. R., Halford, N. G., and Tatham, A. S., High molecular weight subunits of wheat glutenin, *J. Cereal Sci.,* 15, 105, 1992.

152. Jackson, E. A., Holt, L. M., and Payne, P. I., Characterization of high molecular weight gliadin and low molecular weight glutenin subunits of wheat endosperm by two dimensional electrophoresis and the chromosomal location of their controlling genes, *Theor. Appl. Genet.,* 66, 29, 1983.
153. Payne, P. I. and Lawrence, G. J., Catalogue of alleles for the complex gene loci, Glu-Al, Glu-B1 and Glu-D1, which code for high-molecular-weight subunits of glutenin in hexaploid wheat, *Cereal Res. Commun.,* 11, 29, 1983.
154. Wasik, R. J. and Bushuk, W., Studies of glutenin. V. Note on additional preparative methods, *Cereal Chem.,* 51, 112, 1974.
155. Wu, Y. W. and Dimler, R. J., Hydrogen ion equilibria of wheat gluten, *Arch. Biochem. Biophys.,* 102, 230, 1963.
156. Wu, Y. V. and Dimler, R. J., Hydrogen ion equilibria of wheat gluten in guanidine-hydrochloride solutions, *Arch. Biochem. Biophys.,* 108, 490, 1964.
157. Bietz, J. A. and Wall, J. S., Isolation and characterization of gliadinlike subunits from glutenin, *Cereal Chem.,* 50, 537, 1973.
158. Huebner, F. R. and Wall, J. S., Wheat glutenin subunits. I. Preparative separation by gel-filtration and ion exchange chromatography, *Cereal Chem.,* 51, 228, 1974.
159. Huebner, F. R., Donaldson, G. L., and Wall, J. S., Wheat glutenin subunits. II. Compositional differences, *Cereal Chem.,* 51, 240, 1974.
160. Shewry, P. R., Field, J. M., Faulke, A. J., Parmar, S., Miflin, B. J., Dietler, M. D., Lew, E. J. L., and Kasarda, D. D., Purification and N-amino sequence analysis of high molecular weight (HMW) gluten polypeptides of wheat, *Biochim. Biophys. Acta,* 788, 23, 1984.
161. Belitz, H. D., Kim, J. J., Kieffer, R., Seilmeier, W., Werbeck, V., and Wieser, H., Separation and characterization of reduced glutelins from different wheat varieties and importance of the gliadin/glutenin ratio for the strength of gluten, in *Gluten Proteins,* Association for Cereal Research (Germany), Detmold, 1993, 189.
162. Ewart, J. A. P., A hypothesis for the structure and rheology of glutenin, *J. Sci. Food Agric.,* 19, 617, 1968.
163. Lásztity, R., Nedelkovits, J., and Varga, J., The structure of the high molecular weight protein components of gluten, paper presented at the IUPAC Symposium, Riga, Latvia, 1970.
164. Bushuk, W. and Wrigley, C. W., Glutenin in developing wheat grain, *Cereal Chem.,* 48, 448, 1971.
165. Bushuk, W., Molecular structure of bread wheat glutenin, in *Gluten Proteins,* Association for Cereal Research (Germany), Detmold, 1993, 5.
166. Graveland, A., Bosveld, P., Lichtendonk, W. J., Marseille, J. F., Moonen, J. H. E., and Sheepstra, A., A model for the molecular structure of the glutenins from wheat flour, *J. Cereal Sci.,* 3, 1, 1985.
167. Kasarda, O. D., Glutenin structure in relation to wheat quality, in *Wheat is Unique,* Pomeranz, Y., Ed., American Association of Cereal Chemists, St. Paul, MN, 1989, 277.
168. Gao, L., Ng, P. K. W., and Bushuk, W., Structure of glutenin based on farinograph and electrophoretic results, *Cereal Chem.,* 69, 452, 1992.
169. Anderson, O. D., Halford, N. G., Forde, J., Xip, R. E., Shewry, P. R., and Greene, F. C., Structure and analysis of the high-molecular-weight glutenin genes from *Triticum aestivum* L., v. Cheyenne, in *Proc. 7th Int. Wheat Genetics Symp.,* Institute for Plant Science Research, Cambridge, 1988, 699.

170. Margiotta, B., Colaprico, G., Turchetta, T., and Lafiandra, D., Studies of allelic variants of high molecular weight glutenin subunits by reversed-phase high performance liquid chromatography, in *Gluten Proteins,* Association for Cereal Research (Germany), Detmold, 1993, 319.
171. Tilley, K. A., Lookhart, G. L., and Hoseney, R. C., Biochemical and structural differences among high molecular weight glutenin subunits, in *Gluten Proteins,* Association for Cereal Research (Germany), Detmold, 1993, 26.
172. Werner, W. E., Adalsteins, A. E., and Kasarda, D. D., Composition of high-molecular-weight glutenin subunit dimers formed by partial reduction of residue glutenin, *Cereal Chem.,* 69, 535, 1992.
173. Masci, S., Lafiandra, D., Porceddu, E., Ellen, J., Lew, L., Peggy Tato, J., and Kasarda, D. D., D-Glutenin subunits: N-terminal sequences and evidence for the presence of cysteine, *Cereal Chem.,* 70, 581, 1993.
174. Kazemie, M. and Bushuk, W., Identification of a unique group of high molecular weight proteins in some wheat grain, *Cereal Chem.,* 69, 103, 1992.
175. Kazemie, M. and Bushuk, W., Presence of K-proteins in developing wheat grain, *Cereal Chem.,* 69, 103, 1992.
176. Okita, T. W., Cheesbrough, V., and Reeves, C. D., Evolution and heterogeneity of the α,β-type and the γ-type gliadin DNA sequences, *J. Biol. Chem.,* 260, 8203, 1985.
177. Colot, V., Bartels, P., Thompson, R., and Flavell, R., Molecular characterization of an active wheat LMW glutenin gene and its relation to other wheat and barley prolamin genes, *Mol. Gen. Genet.,* 216, 81, 1989.
178. Cassidy, B. G. and Dvorák, J., Molecular characterization of low molecular weight glutenin cDNA clone from *Triticum durum, Theor. Appl. Genet.,* 81, 653, 1991.
179. Ellen, J., Lew, L., Kuzmicky, D. D., and Kasarda, D. D., Characterization of low molecular weight glutenin subunits by reversed-phase high-performance liquid chromatography, sodium dodecyl sulfate-polyacrylamide gel electrophoresis, and N-terminal amino acid sequencing, *Cereal Chem.,* 69, 508, 1992.
180. Anderson, O. D., Cassidy, B., Steffen, J., Dvorák, J., and Greene, F. C., Structure of the high- and low-molecular-weight gene families of the homologue group-1 chromosomes of the hexaploid bread wheat cultivar Cheyenne, in *Gluten Proteins,* Bushuk, W. and Tkachuk, R., Eds., American Association of Cereal Chemists, St. Paul, MN, 1990, 512.
181. Pomeranz, Y., Interaction between lipids and gluten proteins, *Ann. Technol. Agric.,* 29, 385, 1980.
182. Bushuk, W., Békés, F., McMaster, G. J., and Zawistowska, U., Carbohydrate and lipid complexes with gliadin and glutenin, in *Gluten Proteins,* Graveland, A. and Moonen, J.H.E., Eds., TNO, Wageningen, 1985, 101.
183. Chen, J., Khan, K., Shelton, D. R., and D'Appolonia, B. L., Isolation and fractionation of carbohydrate-containing proteins from wheat gluten, *Cereal Chem.,* 69, 475, 1992.
184. Chen, J., Shelton, D. R., D'Appolonia, B. L., and Khan, K., Structural characterization of the carbohydrate portion of a glycopeptide from wheat gluten, *Cereal Chem.,* 69, 481, 1992.
185. Tilley, K. A., Lookhart, G. L., Hoseney, R. C., and Mawhinney, T. P., Evidence for glycosilation of glutenins, in *Gluten Proteins,* Association for Cereal Research (Germany), Detmold, 1993, 14.
186. Feillet, P., Wheat proteins, evaluation and measurement of wheat quality, in *Cereals for Food and Beverages, Recent Progress in Cereal Chemistry,* Inglett, G. E. and Munck, L., Eds., Academic Press, New York, 1980, 183.

187. Orth, R. A. and Bushuk, W., A comparative study of the proteins of wheats of diverse baking quality, *Cereal Chem.,* 49, 268, 1972.
188. Lásztity, R., Correlation between the chemical structure and rheological properties of gluten, *Period. Polytech.* (Techn. Univ. Budapest), 26, 3, 1982.
189. Holme, J. and Briggs, D. R., Studies on the physical nature of gliadin, *Cereal Chem.,* 36, 321, 1959.
190. Cunningham, D. K., Geddes, W. F., and Anderson, T. A., Preparation and chemical characteristics of the cohesive proteins of wheat, barley, rye and oats, *Cereal Chem.,* 32, 91, 1955.
191. Beckwith, A. C., Wall, J. S., and Dimler, R. I., Amide groups as interaction sites in wheat gluten proteins: effect of amide-ester conversion, *Arch. Biochem. Biophys.,* 103, 319, 1963.
192. McRitchie, F., The fractionation and properties of gluten proteins, *J. Macromol. Sci. Chem.,* 6, 823, 1972.
193. McRitchie, F., Conversion of a weak flour to a strong one by increasing the proportion of its high molecular weight gluten protein, *J. Sci. Food Agric.,* 24, 1325, 1973.
194. McRitchie, F., Differences in baking quality between wheat flours, *J. Food Technol.,* 13, 187, 1978.
195. Preston, K. R. and Tipples, K. H., Effects of acid-soluble and acid-insoluble gluten proteins on the rheological and baking properties of wheat flours, *Cereal Chem.,* 57, 314, 1980.
196. Hamada, A. S., McDonald, C. E., and Sibbit, L. D., Relationship of protein fractions of spring wheat flour to baking quality, *Cereal Chem.,* 59, 296, 1982.
197. Doekes, J. G. and Wennekes, L. M. J., Effect of nitrogen fertilization on quantity and composition of wheat flour protein, *Cereal Chem.,* 59, 276, 1982.
198. Lásztity, R., Varga, J., Örsi, F., and Ragasits, L., The effect of the fertilizers on the proteins distribution and technological quality of wheat, in *Gluten Proteins,* Graveland, A. and Moonen, J.E.H., Eds., TNO, Wageningen, 1984, 69.
199. Ragasits, Z. and Varga, J., A búza minõségében mûtrágya hatására bekövetkezett változás vizsgálata Osborne-és gélkromatográfiás módszerekkel, *Növénytermelés,* 27, 131, 1978.
200. Doekes, G. J., Electrophoresis of grain proteins as an aid in wheat breeding, in Proc. 5th Cereal and Bread Congress, Dresden, 1970.
201. Damidaux, R., Autran, J. C., Grignac, P., and Feillet, P., Mise en évidence de relations applicables en sélection entre l'electrophorégramme des gliadines et les propriétìs viscoelastiques du gluten de *Triticum durum, Desf. C.R. Acad. Sci. Paris Ser. D.,* 287, 701, 1978.
202. Sozinov, A. A. and Poperelya, F. A., Genetic classification of prolamins and its use for plant breeding, *Ann. Technol. Agric.,* 29, 229, 1980.
203. Sozinov, A. A., Blocks of cereal storage proteins as genetic markers, in *Gluten Proteins,* Graveland, A. and Moonen, J.H.E., Eds., TNO, Wageningen, 1984, 121.
204. Sasek, A., Stehno, Z., Cerny, J., Bartos, P., and Bradova, J., Gliadin lines in a model set of polymorphic common wheat varieties — populations, *Sci. Agric. Bohemoslov.,* 18, 87, 1985.
205. Nehéz, R., Experiences of gliadin gel electrophoresis in wheat breeding, in *Gluten Proteins,* Lásztity, R. and Békés, F, Eds., World Scientific, Singapore, 1987, 161.

206. Branlard, G., Dardevet, M., Nieto-Taladriz, M. T., and Khelifi, D., Allelic diversity of the omega gliadins as revealed by SDS-PAGE, their possible implication in quality variation, in *Gluten Proteins,* Association for Cereal Research (Germany), Detmold, 1993, 234.
207. Rath, C., Odenbach, W., Gerstenkorn, P., and Weipert, D., Gliadin, HMW- and LMW-glutenin subunit patterns in two sets of inbred backcross lines of winter wheat and their relation to baking quality, in *Gluten Proteins,* Association for Cereal Research (Germany), Detmold, 1993, 270.
208. Wasik, R. J. and Bushuk, W., Sodium-dodecyl-sulphate polyacrylamide gel electrophoresis of reduced glutenin of durum wheats of different sphagetti-making, *Cereal Chem.,* 52, 328, 1975.
209. Payne, P. I., Corfield, K. G., and Blackman, J. A., Identification of a high-molecular-weight subunit of glutenin whose presence correlates with bread-making quality in wheats of related pedigree, *Theor. Appl. Genet.,* 55, 153, 1979.
210. Bournouf, T. and Bouriquet, R., Glutenin subunits of genetically related European hexaploid wheat cultivars: their relation to bread-making quality, *Theor. Appl. Genet.,* 58, 107, 1980.
211. Payne, P. I., The genetical basis of breadmaking quality of wheat, *Aspects Appl. Biol.,* 15, 79, 1987.
212. Kolster, P. and Vereijken, J. W., Evaluating HMW glutenin subunits to improve bread-making quality of wheat, *Cereal Foods World,* 38, 76, 1993.
213. Marchylo, B. A., Lukow, O. M., and Kruger, J. E., Quantitative variation in high molecular weight subunit 7 in some Canadian wheats, *J. Cereal Sci.,* 15, 29, 1992.
214. Khelifi, D. and Branlard, G., The effects of HMW- and LMW subunits of glutenin and of gliadins on the technological quality of progeny from four crosses between poor breadmaking quality and strong wheat cultivars, *J. Cereal Sci.,* 16, 195, 1992.
215. Feillet, P., Aith-Mouh, O., Kobrehel, K., and Autran, J. C., The role of low molecular weight glutenin proteins in the determination of cooking quality of pasta products. An overview, *Cereal Chem.,* 66, 26, 1989.
216. Békés, F. and Gras, P. W., Effects of individual HMW glutenin subunit on mixing properties, in *Gluten Proteins,* Association for Cereal Research (Germany), Detmold, 1993, 161.
217. Bloksma, A. H., Thiol and disulphide groups in dough rheology, *Cereal Chem.,* 52(3,11), 170r, 1975.
218. Greenwood, C. T. and Ewart, J. A. D., Hypothesis for the structure of glutenin in relation to rheological properties of gluten and dough, *Cereal Chem.,* 52(3,11), 146r, 1975.
219. Beckwith, A. C., Wall, J. S., and Jordan, R. W., Reversible reduction and reoxidation of the disulphide bonds in wheat gliadin, *Arch. Biochem. Biophys.,* 112, 16, 1965.
220. Beckwith, A. C. and Wall, J. S., Reduction and reoxydation of wheat glutenin, *Biochim. Biophys. Acta,* 130, 155, 1966.
221. Bloksma, A. H., The relation between the thiol and disulphide contents of dough and its rheological properties, *Cereal Chem.,* 49, 104, 1972.
222. Bloksma, A. H., Rheology and chemistry of dough, in *Wheat Chemistry and Technology,* Vol. 1, 2nd ed., Pomeranz, Y., Ed., American Association of Cereal Chemists, St. Paul, MN, 523, 1980.
223. Telegdy Kováts, L. and Lásztity, R., Die Bedeutung und Rolle der Sulphydrilgruppen in der Weizenchemie und Weizenverarbeitung, *Period. Polytechn.* (Techn. Univ. Budapest), 9, 253, 1965.

224. Lásztity, R., Investigation of the rheological properties of gluten. II. Viscoelastic properties of chemically modified gluten, *Acta Chim. Acad. Sci. Hung.*, 62, 75, 1969.
225. Dronzek, B. and Bushuk, W., A note on the formation of free radicals during mixing, *Cereal Chem.*, 45, 286, 1968.
226. Bloksma, A. H., Oxidation by molecular oxygen of thiol groups in unleavened doughs from normal and defatted wheat flours, *J. Sci. Food Agric.*, 14, 529, 1963.
227. Mecham, D. K. and Knapp, C., The sulfhydril content of doughs mixed under nitrogen, *Cereal Chem.*, 43, 226, 1966.
228. Grosch, W. and Sarwin, R., Quantification of free and protein bound glutathione in wheat flours and doughs, in *Gluten Proteins,* Association for Cereal Research (Germany), Detmold, 1993, 356.
229. Kobrehel, K., Nimbona, C., Buchanan, B. B., Bergmann, D., Wong, J. J., and Yee, B. C., Thioredoxin-linked reduction of wheat storage proteins. II. Technological consequences, in *Gluten Proteins,* Association for Cereal Research (Germany), Detmold, 1993, 381.
230. Tao, H. P., Adalsteins, A. E., and Kasarda, D. D., Intermolecular disulfide bonds link specific high molecular weight glutenin subunits in wheat endosperm, *Biochim. Biophys. Acta,* 1159, 13, 1992.
231. Köhler, P., Belitz, H. D., and Wieser, H., Disulfide bonds in wheat gluten, in *Gluten Proteins,* Association for Cereal Research (Germany), Detmold, 1993, 79.
232. Weegels, P. L., Hamer, R. J., and Schofield, D. J., Depolymerisation and polymerisation of individual glutenin subunits *in situ* in dough — implications for the structure of gluten, in *Gluten Proteins,* Association for Cereal Research (Germany), Detmold, 1993, 57.
233. Pomeranz, Y., Relation between chemical composition and bread-making potentialities of wheat flour, in *Advances in Food Research,* Vol. 16, Chichester, C. O., Mrak, E. M., and Stewart, G. F., Eds., Academic Press, New York, 1968, 335.
234. Jankiewicz, M. and Pomeranz, Y., Comparison of the effect of N-ethylmaleimide and urea on rheological properties of dough, *Cereal Chem.*, 42, 37, 1965.
235. Vakar, A., Pumpyanskii, A. J., and Semenova, L. V., The influence of D_2O on the physical properties of gluten and wheat dough (in Russian), *Prikl. Biochim. Mikrobiol.*, 1, 25, 1965.
236. Nierle, W. and El Baya, A. W., Functionality of wheat gluten in baking, in *Gluten Proteins,* Bushuk, W. and Tkachuk, E., Eds., American Association of Cereal Chemists, St. Paul, MN, 1990, 42.
237. Batey, I. L., Chemical modification a probe of gluten structure, *Ann. Technol. Agric.*, 29, 363, 1980.
238. Batey, I. L., Chemical modification of lysine residues in wheat gluten with potassium cyanate, *J. Cereal Sci.*, 1, 71, 1983.
239. Mita, T. and Matsumoto, H., Flow properties of aqueous gluten methyl ester dispersion, *Cereal Chem.*, 58, 57, 1981.
240. Mueller, H. G., Hlynka, I., and Kuzina, F. D., Effects of some organic solvents on extensigraph characteristics of dough, *Cereal Chem.*, 42, 303, 1965.
241. Ponte, J. G., Titcomb, S. T., and Cotton, R. H., Dough improving effects of some aliphatic hydrocarbons. I. Baking and physical dough studies, *Cereal Chem.*, 41, 203, 1964.
242. Ponte, J. G., Titcomb, S. T., De Stefanis, V. A., and Cotton, R. H., Effect of hexane in doughs made with different flours with and without added fat, *Cereal Chem.*, 43, 475, 1966.

243. Ponte, J. G., De Stefanis, V. A., Titcomb, S. T., and Cotton, R. H., Study on gluten properties as influenced by certain organic solvents, *Cereal Chem.,* 44, 211, 1967.
244. Kaczkowski, J., Ko, S. S., and Pior, H., Gliadin hydrophobicity and breadmaking potential, in *Gluten Proteins,* Bushuk, W. and Tkachuk, R., Eds., American Association of Cereal Chemists, St. Paul, MN, 1990, 66.
245. Popineau, Y., Fractionation of acetic acid soluble proteins from wheat gluten by hydrophobic interaction chromatography. Evidence for different behavior of gliadin and glutenin proteins, *J. Cereal Sci.,* 3, 29, 1985.
246. Wall, J. S., The role of wheat proteins in determining baking quality, in *Recent Advances in the Biochemistry of Cereals,* Laidman, D. L. and Jones, R. G. W., Eds., Academic Press, New York, 1979, 275.
247. Singh, N. K. and Shepherd, K. W., The structure and genetic control of a new class of disulfide-linked proteins in wheat endosperm, *Theor. Appl. Genet.,* 71, 79, 1985.
248. Sing, N. K. and Shepherd, K. W., Solubility behavior, synthesis, degradation and subcellular location of a new class of disulfide-linked proteins in wheat endosperm, *Aust. J. Plant Physiol.,* 14, 245, 1987.
249. Bechtel, D. B., Wilson, J. D., and Shewry, P. R., Immunochemical localization of the wheat storage protein triticin in developing endosperm tissue, *Cereal Chem.,* 68, 573, 1991.
250. Simmonds, D. H. and O'Brien, T. P., Morphological and biochemical development of the wheat endosperm, in *Advances in Cereal Science and Technology,* Vol. 4, Pomeranz, Y., Ed., American Association of Cereal Chemists, St. Paul, MN, 1980, 5.
251. Anderson, J. A., *Enzymes and Their Role in Wheat Technology,* Interscience, New York, 1946.
252. Rohrlich, M., *Getreideenzyme,* Paul Parey, Berlin, 1969.
253. Reed, G. and Thorn, J. A., Enzymes, in *Wheat: Chemistry and Technology,* Pomeranz, Y., Ed., American Association of Cereal Chemists, St. Paul, MN, 1971, 453.
254. Kruger, J. E., Changes in the amylases of hard red spring wheat during growth and maturation, *Cereal Chem.,* 49, 391, 1972.
255. Marchylo, B., Kruger, J. E., and Irvine, G. N., α-Amylase from immature hard red spring wheat. I. Purification and some chemical and physical properties, *Cereal Chem.,* 53, 157, 1976.
256. Sargeant, J. G., α-Amylase isoenzymes and starch degradation, *Cereal Res. Commun.,* 8, 77, 1980.
257. Meredith, P. and Pomeranz, Y., Sprouted grain, in *Advances in Cereal Science and Technology,* Vol. 7, Pomeranz, Y., Ed., American Association of Cereal Chemists, St. Paul, MN, 1985, 239.
258. Gale, M. E., Alpha-amylase genes in wheat, in *3rd Int. Symp. Pre-Harvest Sprouting in Cereals,* Kruger, J.E. and LaBerge, O.E., Eds., Westview Press, Boulder, CO, 1983, 105.
259. Rowsell, E. V. and Goad, D. J., The constituent of wheat binding latent-amylase, *Biochem. J.,* 84, 73, 1962.
260. Tipples, K. H. and Tkachuk, R., Wheat β-amylase. I. Isolation, *Cereal Chem.,* 42, 111, 1965.
261. Tkachuk, R. and Tipples, K. H., Wheat β-amylases. II. Characterization, *Cereal Chem.,* 43, 62, 1966.
262. Kruger, J. E., Changes in the amylases of hard red spring wheat during growth and maturation, *Cereal Chem.,* 49, 379, 1972.

263. Kruger, J. E., On the relationship between free and latent β-amylases in wheat, *Cereal Chem.,* 47, 79, 1970.
264. Kruger, J. E., Modification of wheat β-amylase by proteolytic enzymes, *Cereal Chem.,* 56, 298, 1979.
265. Kaminski, E. and Bushuk, W., Wheat proteases. I. Separation and detection by starch-gel electrophoresis, *Cereal Chem.,* 46, 317, 1969.
266. Skupin, J. and Warchalewski, J., Isolation and properties of protease A from wheat grain, *J. Food Sci. Agric.,* 22, 11, 1971.
267. Salgó, A. and Lásztity, R., Die Protease des Weizens und ihre Technologische Bedeutung, in *Bericht 8. Tagung Internationale Probleme der modernen Getreidechemie und Getreideverarbeitung,* Bergholz, Rehbrücke, 1980.
268. Kruger, J. E., Changes in the levels of proteolytic enzymes from hard red spring wheat during growth and maturation, *Cereal Chem.,* 50, 122, 1973.
269. Kruger, J. E. and Preston, K., The nature and role of proteolytic enzymes during early germination, *Cereal Res. Commun.,* 4, 213, 1976.
270. Prentice, N., Burger, W. C., Kastenschmidt, J., and Huddle, J. D., The distribution of acidic and neutral peptidases in barley and wheat kernels, *Plant Physiol.,* 20, 361, 1967.
271. Prentice, N., Burger, W. C., Kastenschmidt, J., and Moeller, M., Peptide hydrolase in wheat embryo, *Phytochemistry,* 9, 41, 1970.
272. Preston, K. R. and Kruger, J. E., Purification and properties of two proteolytic enzymes with carboxypeptidase activity in germinated wheat, *Plant Physiol,* 58, 516, 1976.
273. Preston, K. R. and Kruger, J. E., Specifity of two isolated wheat carboxypeptidases, *Phytochemistry,* 16, 525, 1977.
274. Kruger, J. E. and Preston, K. R., Changes in aminopeptidases of wheat kernels during growth and maturation, *Cereal Chem.,* 55, 360, 1978.
275. Salgó, A., Investigation of Wheat Proteases (in Hungarian), Ph.D. thesis, Technical University of Budapest, Budapest, Hungary, 1981.
276. Zawistowska, U., Sangster, K., Zawistowski, J., Lang-Staff, J., and Friesen, A. D., Immobilized metal affinity chromatography of wheat α-amylases, *Cereal Chem.,* 65, 413, 1988.
277. Kneen, E. and Sandstedt, R. M., An amylase inhibitor from certain cereals, *J. Am. Chem. Soc.,* 65, 1247, 1943.
278. Petrucci, T., Tomasi, M., Cantagalli, P., and Silano, V., Comparison of wheat albumin inhibitors of α-amylase and trypsin, *Phytochemistry,* 13, 2487, 1974.
279. Buonocore, V., Petrucci, T., and Silano, V., Wheat protein inhibitors of α-amylase, *Phytochemistry,* 16, 811, 1977.
280. Belitz, H. D. and Weder, J. K. P., Protein inhibitors of hydrolases occurring in foodstuffs, in Proc. EUROFOOD TOX II. Interdisciplinary Conference on Natural Toxicants in Food, Institute of Toxicology, Zürich, 1986, 92.
281. Buonocore, V., Gramenzi, E., Pace, W., Petrucci, T., Pocrio, E., and Silano, V., Interaction of wheat monomeric and dimeric protein inhibitors with α-amylase from yellow mealworm (*Tenetbrio molitor* L. larva), *Biochem. J.,* 187, 637, 1980.
282. Granum, P. E., Studies on α-amylase inhibitors in foods, *Food Chem.,* 4, 173, 1979.
283. Hochstrasser, K. and Werle, E., Purification of trypsin inhibitors from germ of wheat and rye seeds, location of the active centers, *Z. Physiol. Chem.,* 350, 249, 1969.
284. Mikola, J. and Kirsi, M., Differences between endospermal and embryonal trypsin inhibitors in barley, wheat and rye, *Acta Chem. Scand.,* 26, 787, 1972.

285. Mitsunaga, T., Isolation and characterization of trypsin inhibitors from wheat germ, *J. Nutr. Sci. Vitaminol.*, 25, 43, 1979.
286. Chang, C. R. and Tsen, C. C., Isolation of trypsin inhibitors from rye, triticale and wheat samples, *Cereal Chem.*, 58, 207, 1981.
287. Chang, C. R. and Tsen, C. C., Characterization and heat stability of trypsin inhibitors from rye, triticale and wheat samples, *Cereal Chem.*, 58, 211, 1981.
288. Boisen, S. and Djurtoft, R., Trypsin inhibitor from wheat endosperm, purification and characterization, *Cereal Chem.*, 58, 460, 1981.
289. Trufanov, V. A. and Kichatinova, V. S., Disulfide reductase and thiol oxidase activity of the maturing wheat grain (in Russian), *Prikl. Biokhim. Mikrobiol.*, 25, 361, 1989.
290. Laskowski, J. M. and Kato, I., Protein inhibitors of proteinases, *Annu. Rev. Biochem.*, 49, 593, 1980.
291. Kruger, J. E. and Marchylo, B., Note on the presence of debranching enzymes in immature wheat kernels, *Cereal Chem.*, 55, 529, 1978.
292. Marshall, J. J., Starch degrading enzymes, old and new, *Staerke*, 27, 377, 1975.
293. Lee, J. W. and Ronalds, J. A., Glycosidases and glycanases of wheat flour doughs, *J. Sci. Food Agric.*, 23, 199, 1972.
294. Sullivan, B., Esterases in relation to milling and baking, in *Enzymes and Their Role in Wheat Technology*, Vol. 1, Anderson, J. A., Ed., Interscience, New York, 1946, 153.
295. Acker, L., Phospholipases of cereals, in *Advances in Cereal Science and Technology*, Vol. 7, Pomeranz, Y., Ed., American Association of Cereal Chemists, St. Paul, MN, 1985, 85.
296. Lásztity, R. and Lásztity, Lj., Phytic acid in cereal technology, in *Advances in Cereal Science and Technology*, Vol. 10, Pomeranz, Y., Ed., American Association of Cereal Chemists, St. Paul, MN, 1990, 309.
297. Guss, P. L., Richardson, T., and Stahmann, M. A., The oxidation-reduction enzymes of wheat. III. Isoenzymes of lipoxidase in wheat fractions and soyabean, *Cereal Chem.*, 44, 607, 1967.
298. Hale, S., Richardson, T., von Elbe, J. H., and Hagedorn, D. J., Isoenzymes of lipoxydase, *Lipids*, 4, 209, 1969.
299. Faubion, J. M. and Hoseney, R. C., Lipoxygenase: its biochemistry and role in breadmaking, *Cereal Chem.*, 58, 175, 1981.
300. Lamkin, W. M., Miller, B. S., Nelson, S. W., Traylor, D. D., and Lee, M. S., Polyphenol oxidase activities of hard red winter, soft red winter, hard red spring, white common, club and durum wheat cultivars, *Cereal Chem.*, 58, 27, 1981.
301. Marsh, D. R. and Galliard, T., Measurements of polyphenol oxidase activity in wheat-milling fractions, *J. Cereal Sci.*, 4, 241, 1986.
302. McCallum, J. A. and Walker, J. R., o-Diphenolase activity, phenolic content and colour of New Zealand wheats, flours and milling streams, *J. Cereal Sci.*, 12, 83, 1990.
303. Hatcher, D. W. and Kruger, J. E., Distribution of polyphenoloxidase in flour mill-streams of Canadian common wheat classes milled at three extraction rates, *Cereal Chem.*, 70, 51, 1993.
304. Kruger, J. E. and La Berge, D. E., Changes in peroxidase activity and peroxidase isoenzyme patterns of wheat during kernel growth and maturation, *Cereal Chem.*, 51, 345, 1974.
305. Kruger, J. E. and La Berge, D. E., Changes in peroxidase activity and peroxidase isoenzymes of wheat during germination, *Cereal Chem.*, 51, 578, 1974.
306. Kruger, J. E., Changes in the catalases of wheat during kernel growth and maturation, *Cereal Chem.*, 54, 820, 1977.

307. Kobrehel, K., Laignelet, B., and Feillet, P., Study of some factors of macaroni brownness, *Cereal Chem.,* 51, 671, 1974.
308. Elkassabany, M., Hoseney, R. C., and Seib, P. A., Ascorbic acid as an oxidant in wheat flour. I. Conversion to dehydroascorbic acid, *Cereal Chem.,* 57, 85, 1980.
309. Walther, C. and Grosch, W., Substrate specifity of the glutathione dehydrogenase (dehydroascorbate) from wheat flour, *J. Cereal Sci.,* 5, 299, 1987.
310. Rohrlich, M., Glutaminsäure Dekarboxylase in Getreide, *Getreide Mehl,* 7, 89, 1957.
311. Salgó, A. and Feller, U., Inactivation and stabilization of glucose-6-phosphate dehydrogenase in extracts from germinating wheat, in *Gluten Proteins,* Lásztity, R. and Békés, F., Eds., World Scientific, Singapore, 1987, 538.
312. Balls, A. K. and Hale, V. S., A sulfur bearing constituent of the petroleum ether extract of wheat flour, *Cereal Chem.,* 17, 243, 1940.
313. Békés, F. and Smied, I., Assay into the protein lipid complexes of wheat flour soluble in petroleum ether, *Acta Aliment.,* 10, 229, 1981.
314. Redman, D. G. and Fisher, N., Fractionation and comparison of purothionin and globulin components of wheat, *J. Sci. Food Agric.,* 19, 651, 1968.
315. Mak, A. S. and Jones, B. L., The amino acid sequence of wheat purothionin, *Can. J. Biochem.,* 54, 835, 1976.
316. Jones, B. L. and Mak, S. A., Amino acid sequences of two α-purothionins of hexaploid wheat, *Cereal Chem.,* 54, 511, 1977.
317. Ohtani, J., Okada, T., Kogahiyami, M., and Yoshizuma, A., Amino acid sequence of purothionin A, a lethal toxic protein for brewer's yeast from wheat, *Agric. Biol. Chem.,* 39, 2269, 1975.
318. Redman, D. G. and Fisher, N., Purothionin analogues from barley flour, *J. Sci. Food Agric.,* 20, 427, 1969.
319. Ozaki, Y., Wada, K., Hase, T., Matsubara, H., Nakanishi, T., and Yoshizumi, H., Amino-acid sequence of a purothionin homologue from barley flour, *J. Biochem.,* 87, 549, 1980.
320. Békés, F., Study of purothionin analogues of certain cereals, *Acta Aliment.,* 10, 343, 1981.
321. Békés, F. and Lásztity, R., Comparative analysis of the primary structure of grain thionins, *Acta Aliment.,* 10, 357, 1981.
322. Hernandez-Lucas, C., Carbonero, P., and Garcia-Olmedo, F., Identification and purification of purothionin homologue from rye *(Secale cereale), J. Agric. Food Chem.,* 26, 794, 1978.
323. Békés, F. and Lásztity, R., Isolation and determination of amino acid sequence of avenothionin, a new purothionin analogue from oat, *Cereal Chem.,* 58, 360, 1981.
324. Garcia-Olmedo, F., Carbonero, P., and Jones, B. L., Chromosomal locations that control wheat endosperm proteins, in *Advances in Cereal Science and Technology,* Vol. 4, Pomeranz, Y., Ed., American Association of Cereal Chemists, St. Paul, MN, 1982, 1.
325. Samuelsson, G., Mistletoe toxins, *Syst. Zool.,* 22, 566, 1973.
326. Samuelsson, G. and Petterson, B. H., The amino acid sequence of viscotoxin-B from the European misletoe (*Viscum album* L., Loranthaceae), *Eur. J. Biochem.,* 21, 86, 1971.
327. Békés, F., A study of purothionin isolated from the petroleum-ether extract of wheat flour, *Acta Aliment.,* 6, 39, 1977.

328. Carbonero, P., Garcia-Olmedo, F., and Hernandez-Lucas, C., External association of hordothionin with protein bodies in mature barley, *J. Agric. Food Chem.,* 28, 399, 1980.
329. Monge, R. S., Delibes, A., Hernandez-Lucas, C., Carbonero, P., and Garcia-Olmedo, F., Homologous chromosomal location of the genes encoding thionins in wheat and rye, *Theor. Appl. Genet.,* 54, 61, 1979.
330. Coulson, E. J., Harris, T. H., and Axelrod, B., Effect on small laboratory animals of the infection of the crystalline hydrochloride of a sulfur protein from wheat flour, *Cereal Chem.,* 19, 301, 1942.
331. Balls, S. A. K. and Hale, W. S., The inhibitory effect of a prolamin from wheat flour on the fermentation of wheat maches, *Cereal Chem.,* 21, 74, 1944.
332. Stuart, L. S. and Harris, T. H., Bactericidal and fungicidal properties of a crystalline protein isolated from unbleached wheat flour, *Cereal Chem.,* 19, 288, 1942.
333. Fernandez de Caleya, R., Gonzalez-Pascual, B., Garcia-Olmedo, F., and Carbanero, P., Susceptibility of phytopathogenic bacteria to wheat purothionins in vitro, *Appl. Microbiol.,* 23, 998, 1972.
334. Okada, T., Yoshizumu, M., and Terashima, Y., A lethal substance for brewer's yeast in wheat and barley. I. Assay of toxicity in various grains and sensitivity of various yeast strains, *Agric. Biol. Chem.,* 34, 1089, 1970.
335. Okada, T., Yoshizumi, M., and Terashima, Y., A lethal substance for brewer's yeast in wheat and barley. II. Isolation and some properties of toxic principle, *Agric. Biol. Chem.,* 34, 1095, 1970.
336. Okada, T. and Yoshizumi, M., The mode of action of toxic protein in wheat and barley on brewer's yeast, *Agric. Biol. Chem.,* 37, 2289, 1973.
337. Carrasco, L., Vasquez, D., Hernandez-Lucas, C., Carbonero, P., and Garcia-Olmedo, F., Thionins: plant peptides that modify membrane permeability in cultured mammalian cells, *Eur. J. Biochem.,* 116, 185, 1981.
338. Jones, B. L. and Meredith, P., Inactivation of alpha-amylase activity by purothionins, *Cereal Chem.,* 59, 321, 1982.
339. Johnson, T. C., Wada, K., Buchanan, B. B., and Holmgren, A., Reduction of purothionin by the wheat seed thioredoxin system and potential function as a secondary thiol messenger in redox control, *Plant Physiol.,* 85, 446, 1987.
340. Hoseney, R. C. and Pomeranz, Y., Functional (bread-making) and biochemical properties of wheat flour components. VII. Petroleum ether-soluble lipoproteins of wheat flour, *Cereal Chem.,* 47, 153, 1970.
341. Hernandez-Lucas, C., Fernandez de Caleya, R., Carbonero, P., and Garcia-Olmedo, F., Reconstitution of petroleum ether-soluble wheat lipopurothionin by building of DGDG to the chloroform-soluble form, *J. Agric. Food Chem.,* 25, 1287, 1977.
342. Mak, A. S. and Jones, B. L., Separation and characterization of chimotryptic peptides from α- and β-purothionins of wheat, *J. Sci. Food Agric.,* 27, 205, 1976.
343. Meredith, P., Lammonds, H. G., and Frazer, A. C., Examination of wheat gluten by partial solubility methods. I. Partition by organic solvent, *J. Food Sci. Agric.,* 11, 320, 1960.
344. Garcia-Olmedo, F. and Garcia-Faure, R., A new method for the estimation of common wheat (*T. aestivum* L.) in pasta products, *Lebensm. Wiss. Technol.,* 2, 94, 1969.
345. Garcia-Olmedo, F. and Carbonero, P., Homologous protein synthesis controlled by homologous chromosomes in wheat, *Phytochemistry,* 9, 1945, 1970.
346. Redman, D. G. and Ewart, J. A. D., Characterization of three wheat proteins found in chloroform-methanol extracts of flour, *J. Sci. Food Agric.,* 24, 629, 1973.

347. Rodriguez-Loperena, M. A., Aragoncillo, C., Carbonero, P., and Garcia-Olmedo, F., Heterogenity of wheat endosperm proteolipids (CM-proteins), *Phytochemistry,* 14, 1219, 1975.
348. Salcedo, G., Rodriguez-Loperena, M. A., and Aragoncillo, C., Relationship among LMW hydrophobic proteins from wheat endosperm, *Phytochemistry,* 17, 1491, 1978.
349. Prada, J., Sanchez-Monge, R., Salcedo, G., and Aragoncillo, C., Isolation of the major low molecular weight gliadins from wheat, *Plant Sci. Lett.,* 25, 281, 1982.
350. Salcedo, G., Prada, J., and Aragoncillo, C., Low molecular weight gliadinlike proteins from wheat endosperm, *Phytochemistry,* 18, 725, 1979.
351. Salcedo, G., Prada, J., Sanchez-Monge, R., and Aragoncillo, C., Aneuploid analysis of low molecular weight gliadins from wheat, *Theor. Appl. Genet.,* 56, 65, 1980.
352. Salcedo, G., Aragoncillo, C., Rodriguez-Loperena, M. A., Carbonero, P., an Garcia-Olmedo, F., Differential allelic expression at a locus encoding an endosperm protein in tetraploid wheat, *(T. turgidum), Genetics,* 89, 147, 1978.
353. Molchanova, M. I., Belova, T. E., Dubstova, G. N., and Nechaev, A. P., Comparative study of lipid-protein complexes isolated from wheat grain and chloroplast lamellar system, *Prikl. Biochim. Mikrobiol.,* 18, 477, 1983.
354. Shewry, P. R., Lafiandra, D., Salcedo, F., Aragoncillo, C., and Garcia-Olmedo, F., N-terminal amino acid sequence of CM-soluble proteins and albumins, from endosperm of wheat, barley, and related species, *FEBS Lett.,* 175, 359, 1984.
355. Gautier, M. F., Alary, R., Kobrehel, K., and Joudrier, P., Chloroform-methanol-soluble proteins are the main components of *Triticum durum* sulfur rich glutenin fractions, *Cereal Chem.,* 66, 535, 1989.
356. Hussein, K. F. R. and Stegemann, H., Comparison of proteins from wheat kernels by various electrophoretic methods in polyacrylamide, *Z. Acker Pflanzenbau,* 146, 68, 1978.
357. Nietsche, G. and Belitz, H. D., Elektroforetische Untersuchung wasserlöslicher Weizenproteine, *Getreide Mehl Brot,* 30, 213, 1976.
358. Ohms, P. J., Elektrophoretische Sortendiagnose von Getreide. Erkennung von Weizensorten mit A-Backqualitat um Verteilungsmuster der Reduzierten Albumin/Globulin-Fraktion, *Z. Lebensm. Unters. Forsch.,* 170, 27, 1980.
359. Figueron, J. D. C. and Khan, K., Albumin fraction from spring, winter, and soft wheats — protein and associated carbohydrate identified by gel filtration chromatography and gel electrophoresis, *Cereal Chem.,* 70, 689, 1993.
360. Clements, R. L., Polyacrylamide gel electrophoresis of salt-soluble proteins of soft wheats from eastern United States, *Cereal Chem.,* 67, 264, 1990.
361. Pogna, N. E., Redaelli, R., and Beretta, A. M., The water-soluble proteins of wheat: biochemical and immunological studies, in *Gluten Proteins,* Bushuk, W. and Tkachuk, R., Eds., American Association of Cereal Chemists, St. Paul, MN, 1990, 407.
362. Krattiger, A. F., Payne, P. I., Worland, A. J., and Law, N. C., Identification and chromosomal assignment of Alb-Al, a gene coding for HMW-albumins on the long arm chromosome 5A of wheat, in *Gluten Proteins,* Bushuk, W. and Tkachuk, R., Eds., American Association of Cereal Chemists, St. Paul, MN, 1990, 657.
363. Greenwell, P. and Schofield, J. D., A starch granule protein associated with endosperm softness in wheat, *Cereal Chem.,* 63, 379, 1986.
364. Sulaiman, S. D., Brennan, C. S., Vaughan, J. G., and Scofield, J. D., Studies on friabilin proteins from wheat, in *Gluten Proteins,* Association for Cereal Research (Germany), Detmold, 1993, 634.

365. Rice, R. H. and Etzler, M. E., Chemical modification and hybridization of wheat germ agglutinins, *Biochemistry,* 14, 4093, 1975.
366. Stinissen, N. M., Peumans, W. J., and Carlier, A. R., Occurrence and immunological relationship of lectins in gramineous species, *Planta,* 159, 105, 1983.
367. Stinissen, H. M., Peumans, W. J., Law, C. N., and Payne, P. I., Control of lecithins in *Triticum aestivum* and *Aegilops umbelludata* by homologous group 1 chromosomes, *Theor. Appl. Genet.,* 67, 53, 1983.
368. Lis, H. and Sharen, N., Lecithins in higher plants, in *The Biochemistry of Plants,* Vol. 6, Marcus, A., Ed., Academic Press, New York, 1981, 372.
369. Bracciali, A., Cantagalli, P., Pompucci, G., and Tarli, P., Note on the identical immunochemical behavior of a protein fraction from durum wheat germ and a purified lectin from soft wheat germ, *Cereal Chem.,* 57, 367, 1980.
370. Feillet, P. and Nimmo, C. C., Soluble proteins of wheat. III. Isolation and characterization of two albumins, ALB 13A and ALB 13B from flour, *Cereal Chem.,* 47, 447, 1970.
371. Hesser, J. H., Non food uses of wheat glutens challenges and opportunities of an emerging industry, in *Non Food Use of Cereals,* Lásztity, R. and Kárpáti, M., Eds., MÉTE, Budapest, 1994, 107.
372. Lásztity, R., A tészta feszültségrelaxációjának vizsgálata. II (in Hungarian), *Élelmiszervizsgalati Közl.,* 6, 120, 1960.
373. Lásztity, R., Investigation of the rheological properties of gluten. I. Viscoelastic properties of gluten, *Acta Chim. Acad. Sci. Hung.,* 53, 139, 1967.
374. Trufanov, V. A., Thioloxidase and disulfide reductase activities of wheat cell organelles (in Russian), *Prikl. Biokhim. Mikrobiol.,* 29, 728, 1993.
375. Pritchard, P. E. and Brock, C. J., The glutenin fraction of wheat protein: the importance of genetic background on its quantity and quality, *J. Sci. Food Agric.,* 65, 401, 1994.
376. Sasek, A., Cerny, I., Sykorova, S., and Kubanek, I., Construction of wheat genotypes with higher baking quality by electrophoresis of gliadin and HMW subunits of glutenin, *Sci. Agric. Bohemoslov.,* 21, 257, 1989.
377. Vapa, Lj., Dencic, S., Soltes-Rak, E., and Kevresan, S., Genetic variation in *Glu*-1 loci and bread-making quality in wheat, *Cereal Res. Commun.,* 23, 23, 1995.
378. Ewart, J. A. D., Amino acid analysis of glutenins and gliadins, *J. Sci. Food Agric.,* 18, 111, 1967.
379. Shewry, P. R., Miflin, B. J., Lew, E. J. L., and Kasarda, D. D., The preparation and characterization of an aggregated gliadin fraction of wheat, *J. Exp. Bot.,* 34, 1403, 1983.
380. Kasarda, D. D., Tao, H. P., Evans, P. K., Ada Isteins, A. E., and Yuen, S. W., Sequencing of a protein from a single spot of a 2-D gel pattern: N-terminal sequence of a major wheat LMW glutenin subunit, *J. Exp. Bot.,* 39, 899, 1988.
381. Tao, M. P. and Kasanda, D. D., Two dimensional gel mapping and N-terminal sequencing of LMW-glutenin subunits, *J. Exp. Bot.,* 40, 105, 1989.
382. Ewart, J. A. D., Isolation and characterization of wheat albumin, *J. Sci. Food Agric.,* 20, 730, 1969.
383. Andrews, J. L., Hay, R. L., Skerrit, J. H., and Sutton, K. H., HPLC and immunoassay-based glutenin subunit analysis: screening for dough properties in wheats grown under different environmental conditions, *J. Cereal Sci.,* 20, 203, 1994.

384. Bai, B. K., Czuchajowska, Z., and Pomeranz, Y., Comparison of polyphenoloxidase activities in wheat and flours from Australian and U.S. cultivars, *J. Cereal Sci.*, 19, 291. 1994.
385. Sreeramulo, G. and Singh, N. K., High M_r glutenin subunits of Indian wheat cultivars: association of subunits 5 ÷ 10 with the IBL/IRS wheat-rye translocation, *J. Cereal Sci.*, 20, 217, 1994.
386. Wrigley, C. W., *Identification of Food Grain Varieties,* Association of American Cereal Chemists, St. Paul, MN, 1995.
387. Lookhart, G. and Bean, S., A fast method for wheat cultivar differentiation using capillary zone electrophoresis, *Cereal Chem.*, 72, 42, 1995.
388. Ewart, J. A. D., Amino Acid analysis of gliadins and glutenins, *J. Sci. Food Agric.*, 18, 111, 1967.
389. Knight, E., *Wheat Starch and Gluten,* Leonard Hill, London, 1965.
390. Sarkki, M. L., Wheat Gluten, in *Cereals for Food and Beverages, Recent Progress in Cereal Chemistry,* Inglett, G. E. and Munck, L., Eds., Academic Press, New York, 1980, 155.

4 Rye and Triticale Proteins

I. INTRODUCTION

Rye is grown in some parts of Europe (Germany, Poland, Russia, and Scandinavian countries). It is consumed as rye bread or rye-wheat mixed bread. A significant portion of rye is used as feed or for industrial purposes (e.g., alcoholic beverages). World production of rye has been continuously decreasing in recent decades due to the lower yields in comparison to other cereals and limited demand for food purposes. The world production today is about 30 million tons per year.

Rye belongs to the genus *Secale* of the grass family Gramineae. Only *Secale cereale* L. is extensively cultivated, although several other species are known.[1] Only the diploid rye (2n = 14) with seven pairs of chromosomes is common in cultivation; the tetraploid rye is grown to a very limited extent in Europe. Both winter and spring rye are known; however, the winter crop is widely grown due to better yield and nutritional properties.

The mature rye grain is more slender than that of wheat, and it is grayish-yellow, brown, or somewhat greenish in color. The mature kernels have a wrinkled pericarp, which gives them a rough appearance. Like other cereals, the main morphological parts of the kernel are the pericarp, endosperm, and embryo. The starchy endosperm represents the bulk of the kernel.

Triticale, a new cereal species synthesized by combining the genomes of wheat (*Triticum durum* or *Triticum aestivum*) and rye (diploid), plays at this time a very small but slowly growing role in the cereal production of the world. As a result of efforts of Canadian, Polish, Russian, Hungarian, and other research workers today, triticale is on the threshold of being recognized as a new crop species and a promising commercial agricultural crop for the future.[2-5] The newer achievements in triticale utilization confirm the view that triticale might be successfully used in both human nutrition and animal feeding.

II. PROTEIN CONTENT, ITS DISTRIBUTIONS AND GROSS AMINO ACID COMPOSITION

Although there is wide variation in the protein content of the rye kernel, it has generally been confirmed that the protein content of rye grains is lower than that of wheat.[6-10] The distribution of proteins in the morphological parts of the kernel is similar to that of other cereals. The germ is richest in protein, and the starchy endosperm contains the lowest amount of proteins. The aleurone layer has an intermediate protein content. In Table 1 proportions of morphological parts of the rye grain are shown. The protein content of rye and some rye products are summarized in Table 2. In a more recent publication based on investigation of more than 100 samples in the period from 1969 to 1980 Golenkov[11] noted an average value of about 10.72% for Russian rye grains. Crude protein contents of Swedish rye varied between 9 and 11%.[12]

TABLE 1
Proportions of the Morphological Parts of Rye Grain (%)[7]

Morphological Part	Variety			
	Vjatka	Avangard	Kazanskaya	Commercial
Pericarp	11.14	11.65	13.00	11.37
Aleurone layer	10.86	11.91	12.10	12.20
Embryo	1.45	1.53	1.63	1.80
Scutellum	1.99	2.09	2.11	1.73
Endosperm	74.56	72.82	71.16	72.90

TABLE 2
Protein Content of Rye Grain and Some Rye Products (%)[10]

Product	Protein Content	Product (percent extraction)	Protein Content
Rye kernel	19.0	Flour (60%)	5.7
Fine bran	13.0	Flour (75%)	6.6
Coarse bran	17.5	Flour (85%)	8.0
Germ	35.2	Flour (100%)	9.0

The protein content of triticale varies widely depending on the variety and environmental conditions. Zilinsky and Borlaug[13] reported protein contents of 12.8 to 17.9% for 191 lines of triticale grown at CIMMYT (International Center for Maize and Wheat Improvement, Mexico City, Mexico) from 1959 to 1970. In a catalogue published by Konarev[14,36] the protein contents of 272 triticale samples (143 hexaploid and 129 octaploid varieties) are summarized. The data varied between 13.7 and 23.6%. A total of 80 samples of winter triticale grown in Sweden showed protein contents ranging from 9.4 to 17%.[12]

The internal morphology of the triticale kernel as discerned by both light and electron microscopy closely resembles that of its parental species. On the basis of investigations of the ultrastructure of triticale kernels from early stages of development to maturity, only one major difference is noted in the structure of the aleurone layer of wheat and triticale kernels.[15,16] The aleurone layer of triticale is much more irregular in shape than that of wheat.

Most of the research workers have characterized the proteins of rye and triticale using the Osborne solubility fractionation technique, separating albumins, globulins, prolamins, and glutelins from the endosperm. Other solvents or procedures are rarely used. If classic Osborne fractions are investigated it can be generally stated that rye endosperm contains a high proportion of water- and salt-soluble proteins. Triticale has a middle position between wheat and rye (see Table 3).

TABLE 3
Proportion of Proteins in Fractions Extracted by Various Solvents (% of Total Protein)

Fraction	Triticale[a]	Rye[b]	Rye[a]	Rye[c]	Hard Red Spring Wheat[b]
Albumin	26.4	34.7	15.2	49	11.9
Globulin	6.5	10.7	18.5	21	5.2
Prolamin	24.4	19.0	40.2	ND	28.5
Acetic acid soluble	17.3	9.4	ND	39	16.6
Residue	19.0	20.6	ND	ND	14.0
Nitrogen	93.6	94.0			96.2

Note: ND, not determined.

[a] From Ljubarszkij.[7]
[b] From Chen and Bushuk.[34]
[c] From Örsi and Lásztity.[20]

Graveland et al. fractionated the rye proteins using a combined procedure based on SDS solubility and centrifugation.[23,24] SDS-insoluble glycoproteins and gel proteins I, SDS-soluble and 70% alcohol-insoluble gel proteins II, glutelins and globulins, SDS-soluble and 70% alcohol-soluble gel proteins III, secalins, and albumins were separated.

The amino acid composition of total protein in rye and triticale is very similar to that of wheat. The most important difference which may be noted is the slightly higher lysine content in rye protein and, to a lesser extent, in triticale protein. Most amino acid composition data[11,18,19,21,29] show that the lysine content of triticale is higher than that of durum and common wheats, but lower than that of rye. The amino acid compositions of different triticale flours as compared with wheat and rye flours and the amino acid compositions of different parts of the triticale grains are demonstrated in Tables 4 and 5. The amino acid compositions of Osborne's fractions of rye proteins are shown in Table 6.

TABLE 4
Amino Acid Composition of Rye, Tricitale, and Wheat Flours (g Amino Acid/100 g Protein)

Amino Acid	Rye	Triticale[a]	Triticale[b]	Hard Red Wheat
Lysine	3.49	2.80	2.50	2.10
Histidine	2.14	2.34	2.09	2.31
Ammonia	3.40	3.25	3.78	4.06
Arginine	4.55	4.77	3.88	3.67
Aspartic acid	6.82	5.67	6.36	3.43
Threonine	3.26	3.05	2.85	2.51
Serine	4.11	4.37	3.96	4.07
Glutamic acid	30.51	32.91	36.00	40.53
Proline	15.29	14.18	12.50	12.54
Glycine	3.82	3.87	3.66	3.60
Alanine	4.06	3.55	3.31	2.88
Cystine	2.65	3.22	2.43	2.49
Valine	5.22	4.93	4.73	4.34
Methionine	2.15	2.25	1.68	1.70
Isoleucine	4.21	4.37	4.19	3.94
Leucine	6.65	7.55	7.29	7.11
Tyrosine	2.16	2.81	2.70	2.48
Phenylalanine	5.16	4.98	4.94	6.09
Tryptophan	ND	ND	0.99	ND

Note: ND, not determined.

[a] From Tsen.[3]
[b] From Seyed Rasheeduddin and McDonald.[22]

III. STORAGE PROTEINS OF RYE AND TRITICALE

A. Low Molecular Weight Storage Proteins

The low molecular weight storage proteins of rye nearly correspond to the alcohol-soluble portion of endosperm proteins according to the classification system of Osborne. Rye gliadin, rye prolamin, and secalin are the names used for this group of proteins.

Among the endosperm proteins of rye the low molecular weight storage proteins (secalins) were investigated thoroughly. The results of the early investigations are summarized in the review of Simmonds and Campbell.[6]

TABLE 5
Amino Acid Composition of Triticale Grain and Some Milling By-Products (g Amino Acid/16 g Nitrogen)

Amino Acid	Triticale Grain[a]	Rye[b]	Shorts	Triticale Bran
Lysine	3.31	3.8	4.70	4.88
Histidine	2.40	3.4	2.94	2.81
Ammonia	3.19		2.81	2.71
Arginine	5.25	5.0	7.07	7.08
Tryptophan	1.11	1.9	1.05	0.12
Aspartic acid	6.87		8.25	8.44
Threonine	3.20	3.9	3.51	3.56
Serine	4.82	6.8	4.36	4.38
Glutamic acid	32.2	38.2	24.0	23.6
Proline	10.3	ND	7.14	7.11
Glycine	4.44	ND	5.18	5.15
Alanine	4.07	ND	4.88	5.14
Cystine	2.97	ND	3.00	3.20
Valine	4.52	6.8	4.74	4.83
Methionine	1.63	1.9	1.44	1.53
Isoleucine	3.70	6.4	3.65	3.62
Leucine	6.98	9.2	6.79	6.86
Tyrosine	2.84	1.0	2.72	2.75
Phenylalanine	4.94	6.9	4.36	4.35

Note: ND, not determined.

[a] From Sayed Rasheeduddin and McDonald.[22]
[b] From Ljubarskij.[7]

Of the more recent work the investigations of Preston and Woodbury[25] may be mentioned. The low molecular weight storage proteins (secalins) of rye were fractionated by gel filtration chromatography. Using Sephadex G-100 gels four fractions were obtained, with molecular weights of about 100, 44, 27, and 10 kDa. The fraction with the highest molecular weight contained the greatest glutamic acid (glutamine) content. On the other hand, the lower molecular weight fractions resembled globulin and albumin fractions in their amino acid composition. Using SDS-PAGE the heterogeneity of the fractions was observed. Some changes in the electrophoretic patterns were observed after reduction of the disulfide bonds.

In a more recent study Charbonnier et al.[26] reported on the investigation of rye prolamins. The solubility and extractability of this group of proteins and the separation by ion-exchange chromatography on sulfopropyl-Sephadex C-50 and gel filtration on Sephadex G-100 were investigated. They also determined molecular

TABLE 6
Amino Acid Composition of Endosperm Proteins and Rye Flour

Amino Acid	mol %				Flour[b] (g/100 g protein)
	Albumins[a]	Globulins[a]	Gliadins[a]	Glutelins[a]	
Lysine	2.1	4.3	0.7	2.0	3.49
Histidine	1.5	2.1	1.3	1.3	2.14
Arginine	2.6	4.8	1.5	1.7	4.55
Aspartic acid	4.1	7.5	2.1	2.7	6.82
Threonine	3.2	4.0	2.0	2.5	3.6
Serine	5.1	5.5	4.9	5.3	4.11
Glutamic acid	27.7	16.4	36.7	33.7	30.51
Proline	16.6	6.5	20.3	16.6	15.29
Glycine	4.3	8.1	2.3	7.2	3.82
Alanine	4.5	7.4	2.5	3.4	4.06
Valine	10.5	14.0	9.6	9.4	5.22
Methionine	1.3	1.7	1.1	1.0	2.15
Isoleucine	3.5	3.9	3.2	2.3	4.21
Lycucine	6.6	7.6	5.9	5.2	6.65
Tyrosine	1.6	2.2	1.0	2.3	2.16
Phenylalanine	4.6	3.5	4.6	3.4	5.16
Cystine	UD	UD	UD	UD	2.65

Note: UD, undetermined.

[a] From Preston and Woodbury.[25]
[b] From Tsen.[3]

weights, amino acid compositions, and N-terminal amino acids of the isolated fractions. For the characterization of the fractions obtained by chromatographic procedures, starch gel electrophoresis was applied.

It has been stated that 60% (v/v) ethanol is the most specific solvent for the extraction of the low molecular weight storage proteins (secalins) of the rye endosperm. The defatting of rye meal before extraction with water-saturated 1-butanol resulted in a 40% loss of secalin yield. Using chromatography on Sephacryl 200 four fractions were separated. The first two fractions, having higher molecular weight, were named C secalins; the remaining fractions, with lower molecular weight, were termed B and A secalins. Ten fractions were separated if sulfopropyl-Sephadex C-50 columns were used. Like ω-gliadins of wheat, C secalins have high glutamic acid (glutamine) and proline content and are practically free of sulfur-containing amino acids. The B secalins were found to be similar to α-, β-, and γ-gliadins of wheat. It was supposed that these secalins are probably only noxious for gluten-sensitive people. The secalins with the lowest molecular weight (A secalins) contain practically no lysine or histidine. Some data on amino acid composition of protein fractions are given in Table 7.

TABLE 7
Amino Acid Composition of Some Secalin Fractions (Residues per 1000 Residues in Secalin Fractions)[26]

Amino Acid	Secalin Fractions C	B2	B3	B7	B8	A4	A5
Tryptophan	0	3	2	3	4	5	6
Lysine	4	7	7	7	8	0	2
Histidine	5	11	10	16	17	0	1
Arginine	18	14	18	16	16	33	32
Aspartic acid (asparagine)	4	20	26	27	27	22	29
Threonine	10	24	31	26	27	79	73
Serine	44	52	53	51	52	74	75
Glutamic acid (glutamine)	436	378	355	344	340	257	264
Proline	288	208	177	191	189	73	81
Glycine	12	23	23	24	24	60	58
Alanine	5	24	27	27	27	64	63
Cystine	1	24	28	27	28	86	78
Valine	12	39	47	44	44	57	53
Methionine	0	11	16	16	15	46	37
Isoleucine	41	45	55	56	55	51	53
Leucine	38	62	71	71	72	47	49
Tyrosine	13	6	7	6	7	27	25
Phenylalanine	69	49	47	48	48	19	21

A more effective separation of low molecular weight rye storage proteins became possible with the use of the gel electrophoresis technique. It was found that gel electrophoresis patterns show differences between varieties, and it was suggested that the secalin components are genetically similar to the wheat gliadin components. The electrophoretic techniques described for wheat variety identification[27] can be applied to rye without any significant modification.[28] Genetic analysis revealed that secalins are coded by chromosome 1R and partly by chromosome 2R (in wild types, 6R). Each of the loci encoding polypeptides of storage proteins is complex. This fact explains the large amount of variation in electrophoresis banding patterns between cultivars. Electrophoretic analysis of rye proteins reveals several distinct polypeptides ranging in size from about 10 to 100 kDa. The nomenclature of components of secalin (rye gliadin) is based on nomenclature generally accepted for wheat gliadins. β-, γ-, and ω-secalins are distinguished according to mobility. The α-type gliadins are missing in rye. Reviews about genetic and electrophoretic properties of rye prolamins were published by Shewry and Miflin,[30] Kreis et al.,[31] and Tatham et al.[32]

A comprehensive study of variations in electrophoretic spectra of rye cultivars was realized by Konarev et al.[33] A total of 50 rye cultivars (diploid and tetraploid) grown in different parts of Russia were studied; 7600 single kernel samples were investigated, and 242 variations in electrophoretic patterns were observed, with β-, γ-, and ω-gliadins being present (α-gliadins did not occur). The overwhelming majority of samples showed a triplet of ω-gliadins (according to the nomenclature of Konarev, ω 234). Occurrence of bands 4 and 5, belonging to the β-group, is also frequent. The variability of the spectra is related to changes in bands β 1-3, γ 1-5, and ω 5-9. Most typical spectra are summarized in Table 8.

TABLE 8
Most Typical Electrophoretic Spectra of Alcohol-Soluble Storage Proteins of Rye Cultivars Grown in Russia[33]

Type of Spectrum	Protein Formula β	γ	ω	Frequency (Percent of Total Number of Samples)
62	45	—	234578	14.9
140	345	—	23458	10.1
71	45	5	234578	9.0
144	345	1	23457	7.2
158	345	15	234578	6.3
161	345	5	23458	3.7
64	45	1	234578	3.6
83	45	45	234578	2.0
164	345	45	23458	2.8
79	45	15	234578	1.7
109	345	145	234578	2.0
63	45	—	1234578	1.4
159	345	15	1234578	1.5
69	45	4	234578	1.3
15	5	—	23457	1.1
145	345	1	123457	1.1
142	345	1	347	1.0
206	1345	—	23457	2.9
209	345	4	2345	1.1

To date only the N-terminal amino acid sequences and the possible structure of the polypeptides have been studied (for a review see Reference 32). The data collected to date confirm the high degree of similarity of γ- and ω-secalins to the corresponding γ- and ω-gliadins of wheat.

The γ-secalins are sulfur-rich polypeptides with relatively compact conformation and high thermostability. The nonrepetitive domain near the C-terminus is helical, and in the repetitive N-terminal domain the occurrence of β-turns is typical. The 75-kDa γ-secalins differ from the other type of γ-gliadins in that they form polymers stabilized by interchain disulfide bonds. The 40-kDa γ-secalins are generally monomeric; the disulfide bonds are intramolecular.

The ω-secalins belong to the sulfur-poor group of prolamins, exhibiting great similarly to the ω-gliadins of wheat. Only short N-terminal amino acid sequences of ω-secalins are known. The sequences are similar to those of ω-gliadin of wheat, with short nonrepetitive domains followed by several repeated peptides. Although ω-secalins have not yet been studied in detail, the far-UV CD spectrum indicates a high degree of structural similarity to ω-gliadins.

It is suggested that the ω-secalins are rod-shaped molecules with a secondary structure based predominantly on repetitive β-turns.

The genome of octaploid triticale contains all DNAs coding for wheat and rye polypeptides. Hence, triticale proteins may contain all the polypeptides of its parental species, but only these polypeptides. On the basis of a detailed comparison of the electrophoretic patterns of wheat, rye, and triticale protein fractions it was confirmed that triticale endosperm proteins do not contain any protein bands that are not present in the patterns of equivalent fractions of the parents.[34-36] In Figure 1, electrophoretic patterns of wheat variety Bezostaya-1, of rye variety C-2, and those of the corresponding octaploid triticale (AD SOS 10-70) are shown.

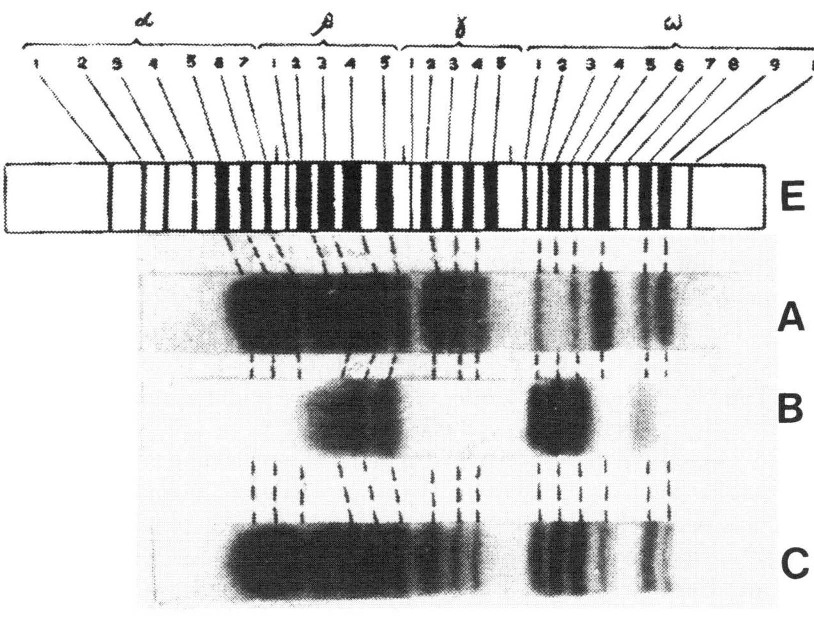

FIGURE 1 Electrophoretic spectra of (A) wheat variety Bezostaya-1, (B) rye variety C-2, and (C) corresponding triticale (AD SOS 10-70); E is etalon. (From Konarev, V.G., Ed. in World Collection Catalogue, No. 216 (in Russian) V.I.R., Leningrad, 1978. With permission.)

B. High Molecular Weight Storage Proteins

The structure of the high molecular weight storage proteins of rye has not been investigated as thoroughly as that of wheat. The rye flour does not form gluten, and therefore the rheological properties of rye flour doughs are influenced to a lesser extent by endosperm proteins. Rye flour doughs have viscoplastic properties which are determined primarily by polysaccharides and amylase enzyme complexes and only to a lesser extent by rye proteins. In the breeding programs of rye production the determination of protein content and amino acid composition is primarily used for the evaluation of the nutritive (feeding) value of the cultivars. The control of baking value is realized mostly through complex evaluation by test baking or determination of the properties of the starch-amylase system.

The high molecular weight storage proteins of rye (rye glutenin, rye glutelin) are composed of polypeptides linked with disulfide bonds. After reduction of the disulfide bonds different subunits may be obtained. The subunits exhibiting electrophoretic characteristics similar to those of high molecular weight (HMW) glutenin subunits of wheat were named HMW secalins or HMW subunits of rye glutenin. SDS-PAGE of single seeds from commercial varieties of rye reveals a variable number of HMW secalin bands.[37]

When homozygous inbred lines are analyzed, only one or two bands are usually present.[37] These have mobilities in the same range as the HMW subunits of wheat. The amino acid composition of the HMW rye glutenin subunits is characterized by high glycine and relatively low proline content. Glutamate accounts for between 30 and 39% of the total residues. About 90% of carboxyl groups are amidated. Only partial N-terminal amino acid sequences of HMW subunits are known. Shewry et al.[38] reported that N-terminal amino acid sequences indicate that d-hordein of barley and HMW secalins of rye are homologous with HMW glutenin subunits of wheat.

Belitz et al.[39] hydrolyzed wheat, barley, and rye prolamins and glutelins with chymotrypsin. The resulting peptide mixtures were separated into pure compounds by gel filtration, ion exchange, and RP-HPLC. The amino acid composition and amino acid sequence of characteristic peptides were determined. A repeat motif based on the tetrapeptide PQQP has been found in all proteins investigated. Differences were found in the hydrophobicity distribution of peptides of wheat, rye, and barley.

The full molecular structure of HMW subunits of rye glutenin is not yet known. Nevertheless, the comparison of known sequences with other subunits suggests that they can be divided into two structural domains: a nonrepetitive domain and a second one containing repetitive blocks of amino acids.

As discussed in Chapter 3, the polymeric protein wheat glutenin contains not only HMW subunits but LMW subunits, too. Rye glutenin does not appear to have LMW subunits.

The properties of triticale storage proteins are generally intermediate to those of the parents.[22] The most information about the proteins of the endosperm has been achieved by gel electrophoretic separation procedures. Both the low (prolamins, triticalins) and high molecular weight storage protein (glutenin) subunits were thoroughly investigated by several authors. Reviews of the results were given by Larter et al.[4] and Bushuk and Larter.[2]

It was found that the three soluble protein fractions of triticale did not contain any protein bands that were not present in the patterns of equivalent fractions of the parents. Investigation of glutenin subunits also showed[40] that all of the major subunits of the two parents were present in the triticale glutenin. The amino acid compositions of glutenins isolated from triticale and from its parental species showed great similarities.[11] Some data are summarized in Table 9. All results mentioned above suggest that the endosperm proteins of triticale are a mixture of the proteins of the two parental species.

TABLE 9
Amino Acid Composition of Rye, Triticale, and Wheat Glutenin (g Amino Acid/100 g Protein)

Amino Acid	Rye[a]	Triticale	Durum Wheat	Wheat
Lysine	3.98	3.50	3.37	2.1
Histidine	2.42	2.41	2.42	1.9
Ammonia	3.39	3.51	3.51	ND
Arginine	5.06	5.05	5.68	3.8
Aspartic acid	6.32	6.02	5.94	4.8
Threonine	3.58	3.45	3.31	3.8
Serine	5.24	5.29	5.37	5.2
Glutamic acid	29.23	30.87	30.67	39.7
Proline	12.24	11.78	10.39	12.6
Glycine	4.98	5.05	4.85	5.3
Alanine	4.29	4.08	4.07	3.9
Valine	5.19	5.06	4.96	4.8
Methionine	1.66	1.53	1.64	1.5
Isoleucine	3.66	3.71	3.81	3.9
Leucine	7.37	7.28	7.46	5.1
Tyrosine	3.86	4.11	4.00	3.8
Phenylalanine	4.96	4.61	4.68	4.4

Note: ND, not determined.

[a] From Bushuk, W., Proteins of triticale. Chemical and physical characteristics, in *Triticale: First Man-Made Cereal*, Tgen, C. C., Ed., American Association of Cereal Chemists, St. Paul, MN, 1974, 128.

IV. METABOLICALLY ACTIVE PROTEINS

A. Enzymes

Like other cereal grains, rye and triticale are relatively rich in enzymes. From a technological point of view the most important enzyme groups are amylases and proteases. Generally rye and triticale have high α-amylase activity. The greater part of the activity is located in the pericarp and the smaller part in the endosperm. The amylase activity and distribution vary depending on the variety as well as agronomic and climatic conditions. Spring and winter triticale, grown at different locations in a given crop year and at the same location during consecutive crop years, showed marked differences in α-amylase activity.

The activity of α- and β-amylases of triticale and its products was investigated by Golenkov and Kalinitchenko.[48] It was reported that the amylase activity of triticale was higher than that of wheat and also rye.

Rye belongs to the group of cereals most sensitive to field sprouting. This fact is sometimes correlated with big losses caused by rainy weather during harvesting periods. It was reported that a correlation might be found between α-amylase activity and sensitivity to field sprouting. It was also stated that the level of α-amylase activity is highly determined by genetic factors. Cultivars having low α-amylase activity are also characterized by good resistance to field sprouting; therefore, in the breeding programs of rye great attention is paid to the control of α-amylase activity.

Relatively little work was done in more detailed investigation of the structure of rye and triticale amylases. In an early publication it was reported that significant differences were found in amino acid composition and electrophoretic mobility of the α-amylases of wheat, triticale, and rye, suggesting that the triticale α-amylase is a new enzyme and not just a mixture of the amylases present in the parents. However, the molecular weights were similar and the kinetic properties of the α-amylase of triticale were intermediate between those of the α-amylases of the parental species. The heterogeneity of α-amylases of triticale was revealed by Silvanovich and Hill.[52]

Polymorphism of amylases from rye endosperm was studied by Lapinsky and Masojc.[56,57] Recent reviews of cereal amylases were published by Hill and McGregor[58] and Kruger et al.[59] From the perspective of the possible use of rye flour from sprouted grain in bread making, the observation that rye α-amylase activity may be effectively inhibited by barley α-amylase inhibitor is interesting.[60]

Both rye and triticale possess considerable proteinase activity; this is generally much higher than that of the wheat grains. The proteolytic activity is in great part located in the bran fractions. The flours (and endosperm) contain much lower activity. More types of enzymes and isoenzymes are present with a pH optimum ranging from 3.8 to near neutral.

Several years ago Madl and Tsen[53,54] reported the results of well-organized, exhaustive work concerning triticale proteases and their comparison with those of wheat and rye. The proteolytic enzymes of triticale and rye were extracted using sodium acetate buffer. After extraction the proteases were separated by gel chromatography (Bio-Gel P-60) and affinity chromatography on Sepharose-hemoglobin columns. Five fractions showing proteolytic activity were separated, with molecular weights of about 10 to 15, 15 to 28, 30 to 35, 35 to 65, and 70 kDa, respectively, suggesting the presence of at least two proteolytic enzymes and their dimers. The heat stability of the proteases was intermediate between enzymes of low and high heat resistance. The values obtained are similar to those reported from wheat proteases.[55] Chemical modifications of the enzymes connected with kinetic studies gave results suggesting the role of thiol groups in the active centers of the enzymes.

An additional study of the possible active centers should be necessary because the presence of enzymes having other active centers has not been excluded. It might also be mentioned that modification of the thiol groups is not involved in the active center, but the influencing of the tertiary structure may also cause a change in enzyme activity. Investigations of wheat protease[55] resulted in the separation of proteolytically active protein fractions which were inhibited by serine reagents and EDTA. These findings suggest the presence of serine enzymes and metal-containing proteolytic enzymes, too.

The presence of natural enzyme inhibitors in raw soya has been well known for some time. With the development of techniques for protein and enzyme separation and isolation more and more naturally occurring enzyme inhibitors have also been detected in different cereals. From the point of view of the use of rye and triticale as food and feed the inhibitors, amylases and proteases are the most important.

The presence of α-amylase inhibitors — which inhibit a number of different α-amylases, but not those of wheat — was first recognized by Kneen and Sandstedt.[61] Later a series of α-amylase inhibitors were isolated from the albumin fraction of wheat and their genetic control was studied. The results of these investigations were reviewed by Kasarda et al.[62] and Garcia-Olmedo et al.[63] The presence of α-amylase inhibitors in rye and triticale has not yet been investigated. Nevertheless, the fact that both tetra- and hexaploid wheats contain α-amylase inhibitors suggests that such types of proteins also occur in triticale.

The trypsin and trypsin inhibitors of rye and triticale were exhaustively investigated by Madl and Tsen.[64] The trypsin-inhibiting activity of rye flour has been found to be extremely high and that of wheat flour quite low. The activity of triticale flour was intermediate in comparison with that of the parental species. They suggested that the triticale inhibitor content might be inherited from the rye. The molecular weight of the trypsin inhibitor (based on the separation on Bio-Gel P-60 columns) was in the range of 10 to 14 kDa, with the highest activity at 10,000 trypsin unit inhibition (TUI) per milliliter. The gel electrophoresis investigations revealed the heterogeneity of fractions containing trypsin inhibitors. On the basis of the evaluation of gel electrophoresis patterns, Madl and Tsen[64] concluded that at least four and possibly as many as seven of the proteins of the trypsin-inhibitory protein fraction were active trypsin inhibitors. Kinetic measurements were also made. They indicated that classical noncompetitive inhibition was exhibited by the triticale trypsin inhibitor.

More recently Chang and Tsen[65,66] reported on the investigation of wheat, rye, and triticale protein inhibitors. The inhibitors were isolated using affinity chromatography (on trypsin-bound Sepharose gel), CM-cellulose ion-exchange chromatography, and gel filtration chromatography. Three trypsin inhibitors having molecular weights of 44, 17, and 5.3 kDa have been isolated from rye samples. In the triticale samples only two types of inhibitor molecules (molecular weights of 19.5 and 5.4 kDa) were found. Among the trypsin inhibitors mentioned above, the occurrence of rye inhibitor 17 kDa and triticale inhibitor 19.5 kDa is more frequent. All the inhibitors contained small amounts of carbohydrates. The amino acid compositions confirmed the similarities of the inhibitors from rye and triticale. Relatively high amounts of glutamic acid, leucine, and glycine are characteristic for both types of proteins. The contents of methionine and tryptophan are very low (0.3 and 0.6 to 0.99%, respectively).

The heat stability of the trypsin inhibitors was also studied.[65,66] The heat stability of triticale trypsin inhibitors was found to be the highest. Heating at 100°C for 1 h inactivated 7% of the activity of trypsin inhibitor from triticale, 35% of that from rye, and 71% of that from a hard red winter wheat.

Chymotrypsin-inhibiting activity of rye, triticale, and wheat flour extracts was reported by Madl and Tsen.[64] The inhibitor activities of different wheat, rye, and triticale samples varied widely. Some data are shown in Table 10.

TABLE 10
Chymotrypsin Inhibitor Activities in Extracts from Triticale, Wheat, and Rye Flours[64]

Cereal	CUI/ml
Triticale	
MT-1	75.0
MT-2	91.5
MT-3	102.5
MT-4	61.5
MT-5	58.0
KT	51.0
Wheat	
AW	95.5
CW	82.5
EW	42.0
Rye	
RR-2	88.0
MR	73.3

Note: CUI = chymotrypsin unit inhibition.

The molecular weight of the inhibitor was found to be about 20 kDa. The protein fractions obtained by separation with chromatographic methods all showed heterogeneity when investigated with gel electrophoresis. On the basis of the evaluation of electrophoretic patterns, Madl and Tsen[64] concluded that at least three, and possibly four, chymotrypsin-inhibiting proteins were present in the fifth protein fractions from an extract of MT-3 triticale. Kinetic experiments have shown that chymotrypsin inhibitor acts as a competitive inhibitor.

Of the other enzymes the redox enzymes are the most interesting. The darkening of rye flour doughs is connected with the activity of tyrosinases[10] and is one of the quality factors in evaluating rye flours. Although the polyphenol oxidases of wheat were extensively investigated,[67] practically no work was done on the investigation of this type of enzyme in rye and triticale. Peroxidase isoenzymes and catalases of triticale were investigated by Noll.[44]

B. Other Proteins

It has been known since 1940 that from the petroleum ether extract of wheat flour a low molecular weight protein rich in lysine and sulfur-containing amino acids may be isolated (called purothionin).[68] Later similar proteins — thionins and purothionin analogues — were isolated from barley,[69] oat,[70,71] and rye.[71,72] The rye thionin named secalethionin differs from thionins of other cereal grains because it does not contain α-thionin components. To date only β-secalethionin has been isolated and identified. The primary structure of β-secalethionin (see Figure 2) shows great similarity to that of other thionins. The lipid protein complex of the secalethionin named liposecalethionin might also be isolated. The composition of the complex is also similar to that of lipopurothionin.

Rye contains some low molecular weight proteins related to CM proteins.[30]

Other proteins of rye and triticale belonging to the albumin and globulin group (according to the classification of Osborne) have not yet been studied in detail.

V. NUTRITIVE VALUE OF RYE AND TRITICALE PROTEINS AND PROTEIN CONCENTRATES

The relatively higher lysine content of rye proteins has been known for some time. Since lysine is the first limiting amino acid in cereals, the higher lysine content of rye flour proteins results in a higher nutritive value. Triticale protein also has a lysine content higher than that of wheat, but lower than that of rye. The nutritive (biological) value of triticale proteins was exhaustively investigated due to the great research program connected with the production, chemistry, and food and feed uses of triticale. Some results of this investigation are summarized by Kies and Fox[73] and Bushuk and Larter.[2] Human and mouse bioassay tests reported by these authors indicate that the quality of the triticale protein is superior to wheat protein quality

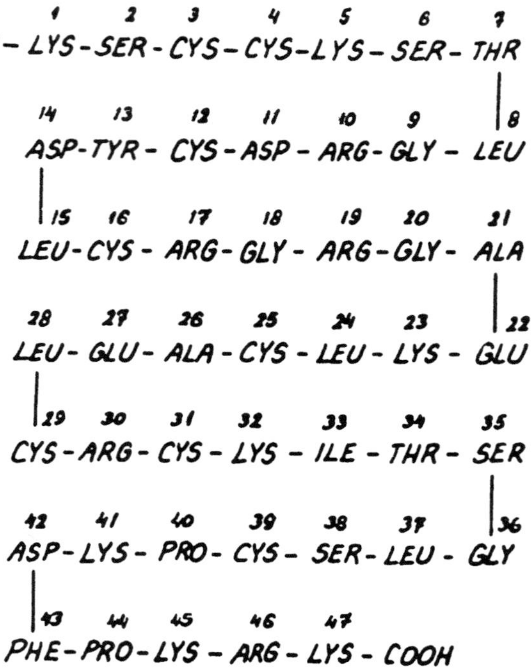

FIGURE 2 Primary structure of β-secalethionin. (From Békés, F. and Lásztity, R., *Acta Aliment.,* 10, 357, 1981. With permission.)

in the materials tested. The same conclusion was made more recently by Netchajev[74] and even more recently by Sharif et al.[78]

Vaidehi and Wakefield[75] studied the nutritive value of the protein of chapatis made from triticale flour and triticale/wheat flour blends. Albino rats were used as bioassay animals. The protein efficiency ratio (PER) values of two triticale cultivars (T-1 and T-2) were 2.00 and 1.54, respectively, significantly higher than the PER of wheat. They concluded that triticale could replace part of the wheat in the human diet.

The production of protein concentrates from triticale may be realized in different ways. Anderson et al.[76] used the Martin process[77], a technocological procedure frequently used in wheat starch-gluten production, to obtain starch and gluten from triticale flours. They recovered 17% of the flour as dried gluten. The preparation obtained had a protein content of about 70%.* It was concluded on the basis of wet milling studies that triticale is a good source of protein-rich supplements for food products.

Air classification also may be used for production of protein-enriched flour fractions. The protein shift for triticale flour was considerably higher than that for spring and winter wheat flours.[77] It was also found that air classification did not selectively concentrate specific protein classes in different fractions.[77]

* Commercial gluten preparations always contain other components — mainly starch, fiber, and ash.

REFERENCES

1. Evans, L. E. and Scoles, G. J., Cytogenesis, plant breeding and agronomy, in *Rye: Production Chemistry and Technology,* Bushuk, W., Ed., American Association of Cereal Chemists, St. Paul, MN, 1976, 13.
2. Bushuk, W. and Larter, E. N., Triticale: production, chemistry and technology, in *Advances in Cereal Science and Technology,* Vol. 3, Pomeranz, Y., Ed., American Association of Cereal Chemists, St. Paul, MN, 1978, 115.
3. Tsen, C. C., *Triticale: First Man-Made Cereal,* American Association of Cereal Chemists, St. Paul, MN, 1974.
4. Larter, E. N., Gustafson, J. P., Kaltsikes, P. J., and Bushuk, W., Twenty-Five Years of Triticale Research at the University of Manitoba, Department of Plant Science, University of Manitoba, Winnipeg, 1980.
5. Kiss, A., *Triticale a homok új gabonája,* Mezõgazdasági Kiadó, Budapest, 1968.
6. Simmonds, D. H. and Campbell, W. P., Morphology and chemistry of the rye grain, in *Rye: Production Chemistry and Technology,* Bushuk, W., Ed., American Association of Cereal Chemists, St. Paul, MN, 1976, 63.
7. Ljubarszkij, L. N., *Rozh,* Izd. Tech. Ekonom. Literatury, Moscow, 1956.
8. Kent, M. L., *Technology of Cereals,* Pergamon Press, Oxford, 1975.
9. Jankiewicz, M., *Bialka w Technologiji Zboz,* Wydawnictwo Przemyslu Legkiego i Spozywczego, Warsaw, 1968.
10. Auerman, L. J. *Technologija Chlebopetchenyja,* Izd. Pistchewaya Prom, Moscow, 1972.
11. Golenkov, V. F., Comparative amino acid composition of proteins of wheat, rye and triticale grain, in *Amino Acid Composition and Biological Value of Cereal Proteins,* Lásztity, R. and Hidvégi, M., Eds., Reidel, Dordrecht, 1985, 349.
12. Graham, H., Aman, P., and Pettersson, D., Variation in composition of Swedish cereal grains, in *Cereal Science and Technology, Proc. 23rd Nordic Cereal Congress,* Munck, L., Ed., Danish Cereal Society, Copenhagen, 1988, 87.
13. Zilinsky, F. J. and Borlaug, N. E., Progress in Developing Triticale as an Economic Crop, Res. Bull. No. 17, CIMMYT, 1971, 1.
14. Konarev, V. G., Ed., Protein, lysine and 5-alkylresorcinol content of winter triticale, Catalogue of World Collection of Allunion Institute of Plant Production, No. 332 (in Russian), V. I. R., Leningrad, 1982.
15. Simmonds, D. H., The structure of the developing and mature triticale kernel, in *Triticale: First Man-Made Cereal,* Tsen, C.C., Ed., American Association of Cereal Chemists, St. Paul, MN, 1974, 105.
16. Lorenz, K., Yetter, M., and Saunders, R. M., Scanning electron microscopy of maturing triticale, wheat and rye, *Cereal Chem.,* 55, 66, 1975.
17. Chen, C. H. and Bushuk, W., Nature of proteins in triticale and its parental species. I. Solubility characteristics and amino acid composition of endosperm protein, *Can. J. Plant. Sci.,* 50, 9, 1970.
18. Villegas, E., McDonald, C. E., and Gilles, K. A., Variability in the lysine content of wheat, rye and triticale protein, *Cereal Chem.,* 47, 746, 1970.
19. Ruchman, J. E., Uscheile, F. P., Jr., and Qualset, C. C., Protein, lysine and grain yields of triticale and wheat as influenced by genotype, *J. Agric. Food Chem.,* 21, 697, 1973.
20. Örsi, F. and Lásztity, R., Comparative study of proteins of some rye and triticale cultivars grown in Hungary using HPGLC, *Acta Aliment.,* 22, 107, 1993.
21. Nehés, R., Bioenergetic aspects of amino acid production in cereals, in *Amino Acid Composition and Biological Value of Cereal Proteins,* Lásztity, R. and Hidvegi, M., Eds., Reidel Publishers, Dordrecht, 1985, 357.

22. Seyed Rasheeduddin, A. and McDonald, C. E., Amino acid composition, protein fractions and baking quality of triticale, in *Triticale: First Man-Made Cereal,* Tsen, C. E., Ed., American Association of Cereal Chemists, St. Paul, MN, 1974, 137.
23. Graveland, A., Extraction of wheat proteins with sodium dodecyl sulphate, *Ann. Technol. Agric.,* 29, 113, 1980.
24. Graveland, A., Bosveld, P., Lichtendonk, W. J., Moonen, J. H. E., and Sheepstra, A., Extraction and fractionation of wheat flour proteins, *J. Sci. Food Agric.,* 33, 1117, 1982.
25. Preston, K. R. and Woodbury, W., Amino acid composition and subunit structure of rye gliadin proteins fractionated by gel filtration, *Cereal Chem.,* 52, 719, 1975.
26. Charbonnier, L., Tercé Laforgue, Th., and Mossé, J., Rye prolamins, extractability separation and characterization, *J. Agric. Food Chem.,* 29, 968, 1981.
27. Wrigley, C. W., Autran, J. C., and Bushuk, W., Identification of cereal varieties by gel electrophoresis of the grain protein, in *Advances in Cereal Science and Technology,* Vol. 5, Pomeranz, Y., Ed., American Association of Cereal Chemists, St. Paul, MN, 1982, 211.
28. Du Cros, D. L. and Wrigley, C. W., Improved electrophoretic methods for identifying cereal varieties, *J. Sci. Food Agric.,* 30, 785, 1979.
29. Lásztity, R., Lásztity, B., Hidvégi, M., and Sarkadi, L., Effect of fertilizers on yield, protein content and amino acid composition of winter cereals, *Period. Polytech. (Budapest),* 36, 26, 1992.
30. Shewry, P. R. and Miflin, B. J., Seed storage proteins of economically important cereals, in *Advances in Cereal Science and Technology,* Vol. 7, Pomeranz, Y., Ed., American Association of Cereal Chemists, St. Paul, MN, 1985, 1.
31. Kreis, M., Shewry, P. R., Forde, B. G., Forde, J., and Miflin, B. J., Structure and evolution of seed storage proteins and their genes with particular reference to those of wheat barley and rye, in *Oxford Surveys of Plant Molecular and Cell Biology,* Vol. 2, Miflin, B. J., Ed., Oxford University Press, Oxford, 1985, 253.
32. Tatham, A. S., Shewry, P. R., and Belton, P. S., Structural studies of cereal prolamins, including wheat gluten, in *Advances in Cereal Science and Technology,* Vol. 10, Pomeranz, Y., Ed., American Association of Cereal Chemists, St. Paul, MN, 1990, 1.
33. Konarev, V. G., Peneva, T. I., and Lubo-Lesnichenko, I. F., Analysis of populations of cultivated rye populations based on gliadin electrophoretic spectra (in Russian), *Seljkohozaystvennaya Biologiya,* No. 1, 43, 1983.
34. Chen, C. H. and Bushuk, W., Nature of proteins in triticale and its parental species. II. Gel filtration and disc electrophoresis results, *Can. J. Plant Sci.,* 50, 15, 1969.
35. Chen, C. H. and Bushuk, W., Nature of proteins in triticale and its parental species. III. A comparison of their electrophoretic patterns, *Can. J. Plant Sci.,* 50, 25, 1969.
36. Konarev, V. G., Ed., Triticale (in Russian), *Catalogue of World Collection No. 216,* V.I.R., Leningrad, 1978.
37. Shewry, P. R., Parmar, S., and Miflin, B. J., Extraction, separation and polymorphism of the prolamin storage proteins (secalins) of rye, *Cereal Chem.,* 60, 1, 1983.
38. Shewry, P. R., Tatham, A. S., Pappin, D. J., and Keen, J., N-terminal amino acid sequences show that D-hordein of barley and high molecular weight (HMW) secalins of rye are homologous with HMW glutenin subunits of wheat, *Cereal Chem.,* 65, 510, 1988.
39. Belitz, H. D., Seilmeier, W., and Wieser, H., Comparative characterization of prolamin and glutelin fractions from wheat, rye, barley and maize by peptide patterns and by partial amino acid sequences, in *Gluten Proteins,* Graveland, A. and Moonen, J.H.E., Eds., TNO, Wageningen, 1984, 21.

40. Orth, R. A., Dronzek, B. L., and Bushuk, W., Studies of glutenin. VII. Inheritance of its physicochemical factors in triticale, *Cereal Chem.,* 50, 142, 1973.
41. Klassen, A. H. and Hill, R. D., Comparison of starch from triticale and its parental species, *Cereal Chem.,* 48, 647, 1971.
42. Berry, C. P., D'Appolonia, B. L., and Gilles, K. A., The characterization of triticale starch and its comparison with starches of rye, durum and HRS wheat, *Cereal Chem.,* 48, 415, 1971.
43. Hill, R. D., Klassen, A. J., and Dedio, W., Metabolic factors influencing kernel development in triticale, in Proc. Int. Symp., McIntyre, and Campbell, M., Eds., International Development Research Center, Ottawa, Ontario, Canada, 149, 1979.
44. Noll, J. S., Changes in the Proteins and Carbohydrates of Developing Cereal Grains and Their Relationship to Kernel Shrivelling in Triticale, Ph.D. thesis, University of Manitoba, Winnipeg, 1977.
45. Dedio, W., Simmonds, D. H., Hill, R. D., and Shealy, M., Distribution of α-amylase in the triticale kernel during development, *Can. J. Plant Sci.,* 55, 29, 1975.
46. Lorenz, K., Triticale — a promising new cereal grain for the baking industry?, *Baker's Dig.,* 48, 30, 1974.
47. Welsh, J. and Lorenz, K., Environmental effects on utilization and agronomic performance of Colorado grown triticales, in *Triticale: First Man-Made Cereal,* Tsen., C.C., Ed., American Association of Cereal Chemists, St. Paul, MN, 1974, 258.
48. Golenkov, B. F. and Kalinitchenko, V. A., Features of the complex of carbohydrate-amylase in triticale and its products, paper presented at the 6th Int. Cereal and Bread Congress, Winnipeg, 1978.
49. Salunkhe, D. K., Chavan, J. K., and Kadam, S. S., *Postharvest Biotechnology of Cereals,* CRC Press, Boca Raton, FL, 1985.
50. Meredith, P. and Pomeranz, Y., Sprouted grain, in *Advances in Cereal Science and Technology,* Vol. 7, Pomeranz, Y., Ed., American Association of Cereal Chemists, St. Paul, MN, 1985, 239.
51. Lee, W. Y. and Unrau, A. M., Alpha-amylase of a synthetic cereal species, *J. Agric. Food Chem.,* 17, 1306, 1969.
52. Silvanovich, M. P. and Hill, R. D., Alpha-amylases from triticale purification and characterization, *Cereal Chem.,* 54, 1270, 1977.
53. Madl, R. L. and Tsen, C. C., Proteolytic activity in triticale, *Cereal Chem.,* 50, 215, 1973.
54. Madl, R. L. and Tsen, C. C., The proteolytic enzyme system, in *Triticale: First Man-Made Cereal,* Tsen, C. C., Ed., American Association of Cereal Chemists, St. Paul, MN, 1974, 157.
55. Lásztity, R. and Salgó, A., Die Proteasen des Weizens und ihre Technologische Bedeutung, in *Bericht 8. Tagung Internationale Probleme der Modernen Getreideverarbeitung und Getreidechemie,* Institut für Getreideverarbeitung, Bergholz-Rehbrücke, 1980, 77.
56. Lapinski, M. and Masojc, P., Polymorphism of amylases from rye endosperm. I. Variability of the electrophoretic pattern of amylases from inbred lines, *Genet. Pol.,* 24, 131, 1983.
57. Masojc, P. and Lapinski, M., Polymorphism of amylases from rye endosperm. II. Intra- and intercultivar variability of electrophoretic pattern of amylases, *Genet. Pol.,* 25, 17, 1984.
58. Hill, R. D. and McGregor, A. W., Cereal alpha-amylases in grain research and technology, in *Advances in Cereal Science and Technology,* Vol. 9, Pomeranz, Y., Ed., American Association of Cereal Chemists, St. Paul, MN, 1988.

59. Kruger, J. E., Lineback, D., and Stauffer, C. E., *Enzymes and Their Role in Cereal Technology,* American Association of Cereal Chemists, St. Paul, MN, 1987.
60. Törrönen, A., Leisola, M., and Haarasilta, S., Inhibition of rye α-amylase activity by barley α-amylase inhibitor, *Cereal Chem.,* 69, 355, 1992.
61. Kneen, E. and Sandstedt, R. M., An amylase inhibitor from certain cereals, *J. Am. Chem. Soc.,* 65, 1247, 1943.
62. Kasarda, D. D., Bernardin, J. E., and Nimmo, C. C., Wheat proteins, in *Advances in Cereal Science and Technology,* Vol. 2, Pomeranz, Y., Ed., American Association of Cereal Chemists, St. Paul, MN, 1976.
63. Garcia-Olmedo, F., Carbonero, P., and Jones, B. L., Chromosomal locations of genes that control wheat endosperm proteins, in *Advances in Cereal Science and Technology,* Vol. 5, Pomeranz, Y., Ed., American Association of Cereal Chemists, St. Paul., MN, 1982, 1.
64. Madl, R. L. and Tsen, C. C., Trypsin and chymotryspin inhibitors of triticale, in *Triticale: First Man-Made Cereal,* Tsen, C. C., Ed., American Association of Cereal Chemists, St. Paul, MN, 1974, 168.
65. Chang, C. R. and Tsen, C. C., Isolation of trypsin inhibitors from rye, triticale and wheat samples, *Cereal Chem.,* 58, 207, 1981.
66. Chang, C. R. and Tsen, C. C., Characterization and heat stability of trypsin inhibitors from rye, triticale and wheat samples, *Cereal Chem.,* 58, 211, 1981.
67. Lamkin, W. M., Miller, B. S., Nelson, S. W., Traylor, D. D., and Lee, S. M., Polyphenol oxidase activities of hard red winter, soft red winter, hard red spring, white common, club and durum wheat cultivars, *Cereal Chem.,* 58, 27, 1981.
68. Balls, A. K. and Hale, W. S., A sulfur bearing constituent of the petroleum ether extract of wheat flour, *Cereal Chem.,* 17, 243, 1940.
69. Redman, D. G. and Fisher, N., Purothionin analogues from barley flour, *J. Sci. Food Agric.,* 20, 427, 1969.
70. Békés, F. and Lásztity, R., Isolation and determination of amino acid sequence of avenothionin, a new purothionin analogue from oat, *Cereal Chem.,* 58, 360, 1981.
71. Békés, F. and Lásztity, R., Comparative analysis of the primary structure of grain thionins, *Acta Aliment.,* 10, 357, 1981.
72. Hernandez-Lucas, C. Q., Carbonero, P., and Garcia-Olmedo, F., Identification and purification of a purothionin homologue from rye (*Secale cereale* L.), *J. Agric. Food Chem.,* 26, 794, 1978.
73. Kies, C. and Fox, H. M., Triticale and human nutrition, in *Triticale: First Man-Made Cereal,* Tsen, C. C., Ed., American Association of Cereal Chemists, St. Paul, MN, 1974, 202.
74. Netchajev, A. P., Untersuchung der Chemischen Zusammensetzung der Triticale, in *Bericht 8. Tagung Internationale Probleme der Modernen Getreidechemie und Getreideverarbeitung,* Institut für Getreideverarbeitung, Bergholz-Rehbrücke, 1980, 224.
75. Vaidehi, M. P. and Wakefield, L. M., Protein quality of chapatis prepared with various blends of triticale and wheat flours, *Nutr. Rep. Int.,* 16, 349, 1977.
76. Anderson, R. A., Stringfellow, A. C., and Griffin, E. L., Jr., Preliminary processing studies reveal triticale properties, *North-West. Miller,* 279, 10, 1972.
77. Knight, J. W., *Chemistry of Wheat Starch and Gluten and Their Conversion Products,* Lennard Hill, London, 1965.
78. Sharif, G., Vohra, P., and Qualse, C. D., Further studies on the nutritional evaluation of wheat, triticale and rice grains using the red flour beetle, *Cereal Chem.,* 58, 86, 1981.

5 Barley Proteins

I. INTRODUCTION, GENERAL CHARACTERIZATION OF THE BARLEY PROTEINS

Barley ranks fourth in production among the cereal grains. About two thirds of the production is used in animal feeds. A great part of the barley is raw material for the brewing industry. Only a small proportion is used for human consumption and is prepared by a dehulling process.

Most cultivated barleys are covered. The kernel of covered barley consists of the caryopsis and the flowering glumes (or husks). The husks consist of two membranous sheets that completely enclose the caryopsis. One of the husks (the lemina) is drawn out into a long awn. In some countries naked (huskless) barley is also produced. The caryopsis is a one-seeded fruit in which the outer pericarp layers enclose the aleurone layer, the starchy endosperm, and the embryo. The husk makes up from 7 to 25% of the grain, and the proportions of embryo and endosperm (including the aleurone layer) are 3 and 77%, respectively (calculated based on a husk content of 13%).[1,2] The protein content of the embryo is the highest (over 30%) and that of the endosperm is the lowest. The aleurone layer of barley differs from that of other cereals. The aleurone layer of most cereal grains is a single layer and that of barley is at least two cells thick. The aleurone cells contain granules composed of proteins and are much richer in protein than are the cells of endosperm. In the endosperm of barley individual protein bodies may be recognized, but the dominant component of these cells is starch.

The protein content of the covered barley is 8 to 13% (calculated as $N \times 6.25$). The protein content is highly influenced by the level of nitrogen fertilization.[3-7] In the experiments of Kirkman et al.,[7] e.g., the protein content of two barley cultivars was increased from 7.87 to 12.94% by increasing the level of nitrogen fertilization.

The proteins of barley endosperm in the early works were classified on the basis of solubility. Albumins, globulins, prolamins (hordeins), and glutelins were distinguished. Generally the amount of albumins is relatively low (3 to 5% of the total protein), and a considerable quantity of globulins (10 to 20% of the total protein) occurs in the endosperm. The main components of the proteins are hordein (35 to 45%) and glutelin (35 to 45%). The distribution of the proteins between the different solubility fractions depends on variety and also the agronomic (N fertilization) conditions.[4,7,8] In the more recent publications, classification according to the biological role of the proteins is widely accepted and used. As with the classification of wheat proteins, barley storage proteins (hordein and glutelin) and barley cytoplasmic (or metabolically active) proteins (albumins and globulins) are also distinguished. The studies of protein synthesis in the maturing grains have shown that hordein and glutelin are synthesized in the later stages of the grain and deposited in the protein bodies and protein matrix. The albumin fraction is synthesized early in grain development. The biosynthesis of the globulin fractions has an intermediate position. Storage proteins are probably also components of the salt-soluble fraction.

The proportions of different protein fractions generally change with increasing total protein content of the barley grains. The amount of storage proteins and especially that of hordein increased markedly with increasing total protein content. There are only small increases in the total amounts of the other protein fractions. In an experiment of Kirkman et al.[7] the hordein content of a barley variety increased from 36 to 49%, expressed as a percentage of the total protein content. The relative increase of the hordein fraction is dependent on the variety. In the high-lysine barley mutants the hordein fraction does not increase disproportionately with increasing total protein content.[7]

The amino acid composition of the total protein of barley is similar to that of other cereal grains. High glutamic acid (glutamine) and proline content, relatively low amounts of basic amino acids, and considerable cystine content characterize the barley proteins. Some data on the amino acid composition of barley proteins are shown in Table 1. The amino acid composition of the total protein shows some

TABLE 1
Amino Acid Composition of the Barley Proteins

Amino Acid	Normal Barley[9]	Normal Barley[17]	High-Lysine Mutant KVL 468[17]	High-Lysine Mutant 1508[17]
Lysine	3.5	3.50	3.76	5.35
Histidine	2.1	2.25	2.33	2.77
Arginine	4.4	4.82	5.13	7.05
Aspartic acid	6.1	5.28	5.56	8.29
Threonine	3.5	3.33	3.57	4.33
Serine	4.2	4.19	4.37	4.77
Glutamic acid	24.6	24.37	23.45	17.02
Proline	10.9	11.56	11.06	7.25
Glycine	4.2	3.79	4.02	5.63
Alanine	4.1	3.65	4.12	5.08
Cystine	2.5	2.12	2.20	2.07
Valine	5.4	5.27	5.05	5.77
Ietethionine	1.6	1.73	1.85	2.16
Isoleucine	3.8	3.68	3.53	3.57
Leucine	6.9	7.19	6.94	6.91
Tyrosinc	2.5	3.47	3.59	3.70
Phenylalanine	5.1	5.27	5.28	4.38
Tryptophan	1.4	1.33	1.45	1.61

Note: Values are in g/16 g nitrogen.

changes depending on the level of nitrogen fertilization and the total protein content. Several authors reported that increases in the nitrogen content of barley seed resulting from increased nitrogen fertilization led to a decrease in the relative lysine content of the grain proteins.[3-8,10-12] It was concluded that the decreased relative lysine content of the whole grain was due to the increased synthesis of hordein.[7] The latter protein fraction is poor in lysine.[13] Selection of cereal varieties of improved protein quality, based on a screening program for elevated grain lysine levels, has led to the recognition of the maize high-lysine lines opaque-2 and floury-2. The first high-lysine line to be recognized in barley was Hyproly, screened from the world barley collection. The investigation of the ultrastructure of the high-lysine barley and also the study of the distribution of the protein between different fractions revealed that the higher lysine content correlated with a lower hordein content of the barley seeds.[14-16]

About 15 years ago a new hybrid of wheat and wild barley *(Hordeum chilense)* was obtained[142] and named tritordeum. From the beginning this amphiploid has shown promising characteristics as a new crop, so because of its high protein content Cubero et al.[143] suggested that tritordeum could be used as a protein source crop. Later studies showed that the protein contents of tritordeum and of wheat are not significantly different when the grain yields are similar.[144]

II. STRUCTURE AND COMPOSITION OF THE BARLEY STORAGE PROTEINS

A. Low Molecular Weight Storage Proteins (Hordeins)

According to the classification system used in this book, the low molecular weight storage proteins of barley, also called hordeins, represent a group of proteins extractable with 70% ethanol (without reducing agents). Isopropanol (55% v/v) also may be used.[18] Researchers working in the field of biochemistry and genetics of cereal storage proteins also include in the group of hordeins the polypeptides obtained after reduction of disulfide bonds of high molecular weight storage proteins (barley glutelins), named D-hordeins.[19] A possible means of isolating the hordeins is mechanical separation of the protein bodies of endosperm. The latter are formed from hordein molecules.[18,20] The hordeins are the main protein fraction in barley and have a great influence on the technological and nutritional quality of this grain.[21,22]

The hordein fraction extracted from barley is a mixture of different proteins. Various methods may be used for the separation of subgroups or individual components. Among the most powerful separation methods are gel electrophoresis,[7,23,24] two-dimensional gel electrophoresis,[18] and RP-HPLC. Using these methods the alcohol-soluble endosperm protein fraction may be separated into 15 to 20 distinct polypeptide bands (spots). The polypeptides may be classified according to molecular weight (electrophoretic mobility) into different groups. The majority of researchers distinguish group B and group C hordeins. A third group, with the lowest molecular weight, is also mentioned — the A group of hordeins.[25-27] This group differs in amino acid composition and is partly soluble in salt solutions (and is probably not a storage protein). The number and distribution of the electrophoretic bands are characteristic for the variety and therefore may be used for barley variety identification. A full range of electrophoretic methods have been applied to barley variety identification.[28-38] Recent developments in separation techniques suggest that RP-HPLC, capillary electrophoresis,[39] and immunochemical methods may be effectively used also.[40] A review of immunochemical methods in cereal research and technology has been published by Vaog and Munck.[41]

Bietz[42] reported on the gel electrophoresis investigation of hordein treated with β-mercaptoethanol and its *S*-pyridylethyl (PE) derivative. PAGE of PE-hordein revealed a heterogeneous banding pattern. When compared to wheat gliadin, PE-hordein had three intense bands corresponding to ω-gliadin, two to four faint bands in the γ-gliadin region, and four to five medium bands corresponding in mobility to β-gliadins. SDS-PAGE revealed five major bands in PE-hordein. The apparent molecular weights were the following: 32, 38, 47.4, 53.2, and 65.6 kDa. The SDS-PAGE pattern was quite similar to that obtained by other research workers.[22,36,43,44]

The quantity of hordein components is also dependent on growing conditions. Kirkman et al.[7] found that the percentage of amide nitrogen in the barley grains strongly and positively correlated with total nitrogen content and percentage of hordein in total protein. A negative correlation has been found between lysine content and amide content. This fact explains why amide content may be used as a selection criterion for barley lines which are low in hordein and therefore presumably richer in lysine. The lysine content of the hordein and salt-soluble proteins was constant over the whole range of seed nitrogen. A small decrease was observed in the lysine content of the residual fraction. Hordein was separated by SDS-PAGE into two groups (C- and B-hordeins). A low molecular weight fraction might also be separated, commonly called A-hordein.

The results of Kirkman et al.[7] showed that C-hordein increased from approximately 13 to 18.5% of the fraction. The increase in the quantity of B-hordein with the growing amount of total nitrogen in grain was not so great as for C-hordeins. This resulted in a decrease in the ratio of B- and C-hordeins from 6.7 to 4.4. There were, however, no apparent changes in the relative amounts of polypeptides present within either group. The quantity of A-hordein in the fractions was too low to be determined accurately.

Some selected data concerning the amino acid composition of total hordein are summarized in Table 2. Characteristic are the low lysine content and the high proportions of glutamic acid, glutamine, and proline.

The investigation of amino acid sequences of hordein started in the late 1970s. Data about N-terminal sequences of hordein polypeptides were published by Shewry et al.,[45-47] Schmitt and Svendsen,[48] and Bietz.[42] These independently determined sequences were either identical or similar and suggested a high degree of homology with prolamins of other cereals. As a result of progress on the genetics of barley proteins it was revealed that the genes coding for hordein proteins are located in chromosome 5. The polypeptides are coded by separate but linked loci, called Hor-1

TABLE 2
Amino Acid Composition of Hordeins (mol%)

Amino Acid	ω-Gliadin (*Triticum monococcuam*)	Hordein (Normal Barley)[a]	Hordein (High-Lysine barley)[a]	Hordein C[b]
Lysine	0.13	0.5	1.0	0.0
Histidine	0.56	1.0	0.8	0.60
Arginine	1.08	2.0	2.1	0.84
Aspartic acid	1.18	1.6	3.4	0.83
Threonine	1.05	2.0	2.9	0.99
Serine	4.89	4.2	5.1	2.61
Glutamic acid	45.2	34.7	31.2	41.1
Proline	26.2	23.0	19.0	31.9
Glycine	0.89	2.5	5.4	0.41
Alanine	1.57	2.4	3.8	0.69
Cysteine	Trace	1.6	0.2	Trace
Valine	0.80	4.6	4.9	1.11
Methionine	0.13	0.9	1.0	0.22
Isoleucine	2.22	3.8	3.4	3.02
Leucine	4.70	6.9	7.8	4.31
Tyrosine	1.17	2.4	2.3	2.29
Phenylalanine	8.09	5.9	5.1	9.03

[a] From Brandt.[14]
[b] From Shewry et al.[45]

and Hor-2. It was suggested that each locus is a complex multigenic family derived from the duplication and divergence of a single ancestral gene. Results of genetic studies and techniques of molecular biology opened another way to investigate the structure of hordein homologs using fine structure analysis of the hordein loci employing cloned double-stranded DNA sequences which code for hordein polypeptides. As a first step toward analysis of the hordein structural genes, hordein polypeptides were synthesized *in vitro* with barley polyribosomes.[49,50] A cell-free protein synthesizing system was employed containing ribosomal subunits and transfer DNA, with all the additional factors essential for protein biosynthesis being provided by wheat germ extract or rabbit reticulocyte lysate. The newly synthesized hordein polypeptides were detected by inclusion of ^{35}S-labeled methionine in the cell-free system and autoradiography of the translation products on SDS-PAGE.

The second stage in these studies has involved the production of cDNA probes complementary to hordein mRNA, which can be used to localize the hordein structural genes. The results of early research in this field were reviewed by Cameron-Mills et al.[18] and Forde et al.[51]

On the basis of recent investigations a more detailed picture about polypeptides included in the barley hordein has been provided. With regard to classification, it is now generally accepted that hordein polypeptides may be divided into B and C groups.

The B-hordeins (called also sulfur-rich hordeins due to their relatively high amount of sulfur-containing amino acids) are presented as a mixture of monomers with intramolecular disulfide bonds, but they may form disulfide-stabilized aggregates, too.[52] B-hordeins are encoded by a single structural locus (Hor-2) located on the short arm of chromosome 5. Using SDS-PAGE the B-hordein fraction may be separated into various components with molecular weights of 36 to 45 kDa. The faster major band is called B1-hordein and the slowest major band B3-hordein.[19] Only minor differences in amino acid composition of purified components were observed (Table 3). High proline content (about 20%) and glutamic acid (glutamine) content (30 to 35 mol%) is typical. Two-dimensional electrophoresis (isoelectric focusing [IEF]/SDS-PAGE) analysis of B-hordein fractions from eight European cultivars with different structural alleles of the Hor-2 locus revealed a total of 47 major polypeptides.[53] The number of individual polypeptides present in varieties varied from 8 to 16. The individual polypeptides also varied in their contribution to the total B-fractions, from about 1% to over 40%. The polypeptides were classified into three groups (groups I, II, and III) on the basis of their cyanogen bromide cleavage patterns. Group III was present in all eight cultivars, and seven of these also had polypeptides of one of the other two groups. Polypeptides of all three classes were not found together in any cultivar. Results of studies published by Kreis et al.[54] suggested that the Hor-2 locus consists of two subfamilies of genes that code for structurally distinct groups of polypeptides. Based on comparative studies of wheat, rye, and barley proteins Shewry et al.[55] classified the sulfur-rich hordein polypeptides into group B and group γ hordeins. All of these studies confirm the view that hordein polypeptides belonging to group B (sulfur-rich hordeins) consist minimally of two distinct subgroups.

The first efforts to determine the amino acid sequence of B-hordein polypeptides were not successful. N-terminal amino acid sequences of B-hordein cannot be determined as this prolamin is resistant to Edman degradation.[56] Further research based on sequencing of genes coding for B-hordein polypeptides resulted in determination of the total primary structure of the B1 polypeptide. The sequenced Hor-2 gene of barley was devoid of introns and encoded a 271-amino acid-long B1-hordein polypeptide. The deduced amino acid sequence is shown in Figure 1. The N-terminal sequence (A) contains a putative signal peptide (19 amino acids). The remaining part of the coding sequence includes nine glutamine-proline blocks with the preferred core sequence PQQP, separated by one or two other residues, giving a glutamine-proline content of 78%. The second part (B) encodes 164 amino acids, 41% of which are glutamine + proline organized in scattered blocks. Seven cysteine residues are coded for by this portion of the gene. The last part (c) encodes the carboxy-terminal 35 amino acids, none of which are glutamine. Comparison of the gene with three other partial cDNA clones indicates that the charge polymorphism in the B1 polypeptide group is due to point mutations in the part of the gene corresponding to the carboxy-terminal half of the polypeptide. Comparison with the sequence of a second polypeptide gene (published by Forde et al.[61]) suggests that insertions or deletions

TABLE 3
Amino Acid Composition of B-Hordein Polypeptides (in mol%)

Amino Acid	Hordein B1[59]	Hordein B3[59]	Total Hordein[58]	γ-Wheat Gliadin[60]
Lysine	0.8	0.2	0.5	0.1
Histidine	1.6	1.4	2.1	1.5
Arginine	2.5	2.3	2.4	1.6
Aspartic acid	0.0	1.5	1.4	2.9
Threonine	2.0	2.3	2.1	1.7
Serine	4.3	5.1	4.7	5.3
Glutamic acid	32.0	35.1	35.4	41.7
Proline	20.8	21.6	20.6	15.1
Glycine	2.9	1.8	1.5	2.4
Alanine	2.5	2.6	2.2	3.4
Cysteine	2.2	2.2	2.5	1.8
Valine	6.3	5.7	5.6	3.8
Methionine	0.9	1.0	0.6	0.9
Isoleucine	4.1	4.4	4.1	3.9
Leucine	8.2	6.4	7.0	6.9
Tyrosine	2.3	2.2	2.5	3.1
Phenylalanine	5.1	4.1	4.8	3.7
Tryptophan	ND	ND	ND	0.2

Note: ND, not determined.

of glutamine-proline blocks in the amino-terminal domain are a major source of size polymorphisms in the B-hordein family.

The known amino acid sequences of B1- and B3-type polypeptides are about 80% homologous. The carboxy-terminal domain is proline poor and does not contain repeating units. The second domain toward the amino terminus contains octapeptide repeats (PQQPXPQQ).[62] The structural organization of typical B-hordein polypeptides is shown in Figure 2.

The C-hordeins (sulfur-poor hordeins) don't contain cysteine (methionine content is possible). They account for 10 to 20% of the total prolamin fraction of barley.[7] SDS-PAGE of C-hordein fractions from different barley cultivars reveals a variable number of major bands with molecular weights between 54 and 60 kDa. Minor bands, in some cases with lower (49 kDa) or higher (72 kDa) molecular weight, also may be present. The amino acid composition of C-hordeins (Table 4) is characterized by high glutamic acid (glutamine) and proline content. The phenylalanine content is also higher as in other storage proteins.

The first amino acid sequence data on C-hordeins were published by Shewry et al.[64] and Schmitt and Svendsen.[56] The investigated C-hordein polypeptides differed in molecular weight and their trypsin peptide maps, but not in their amino-terminal and carboxy-terminal amino acid sequences. Analysis of cDNA clones related to

A
Met Lys Thr Phe Leu Ileu Phe Ala Leu Leu Ala Ile Ala
Gln Pro Phe Pro Gln Gln Gln Ala Ile Thr Ser Thr Ala
Gln Pro Ile Pro Gln Gln Pro Gln Pro Tyr Pro Gln Gln
Gln Gln Pro Pro Phe Pro Gln Gln Pro Tyr Pro Gln Pro
Ala Phe Pro Gln Gln Pro Pro Phe Trp Pro Gln Gln Pro
Phe Pro Pro Gln Gln Pro Phe

B
Gly Leu Gln Gln Pro Ile Leu Ser Gln Gln Gln Pro Cys
Tyr Leu Gln Gly Gln Pro Leu Pro Thr Gln Gln Pro Thr
Gln Thr Leu Leu Gln Leu Gln Ile Pro Tyr Val Gln Pro
Leu Phe Val Lys Cys Pro Asn Leu Gln Gln Leu Ile Ser
Gln Gln Gln Cys Ser Pro Val Arg Met Pro Gln Le Ile
Val His Cys Ser Ser Gln Gln Leu Met Gln Ser Arg Ala
Leu Gln Gln Gln Cys Cys Gln Gln Leu Pro Gln Ile Pro
Tyr Val Ile Ala Arg Ile Ala Gln His Arg Phe Gln Gln
Ser Ile Phe Leu Gln Gln Gln Pro Gln Gln Ser Val Gln
Gln Gln Gln Gln Leu Gln Gln Gln Pro Gln Ser Ala Gln
Val Gly Gln Cys Tyr Phe Gln Gln Pro Gln Pro Gln Gln
Val Ser Gln Pro Val Gln Gln Pro Gln Gly Leu Gln Pro
Phe Leu Gln Pro His Gln Ile Ala Gln Leu

C
Gln Ala Thr Asn Ser Ile Ala Leu Arg Thr Leu Pro Thr
Pro Met Ile Asp Tyr Leu Pro Val Asn Val Asn Cys Met
Phe Gly Val Gly Thr Arg Val Gly Val

FIGURE 1 Deduced amino acid sequence heterogeneity of B1-hordein polypeptides. Sequences deduced from four different cDNAs are compared. A, B, and C are domains of the polypeptide; see text, pp. 164–165. (From Brandt, A., Montembault, A., and Cameron-Mills, V., *Carlsberg Res. Commun.*, 50, 333, 1985. With permission.)

C-hordein[62] showed that the major portion of the polypeptide chain consists of repeating octapeptide units. More recent studies (reviewed by Tatham et al.[65]) on the primary structure of C-hordein polypeptides confirmed that these polypeptides consist almost entirely of repeats mainly of the octapeptide motif PQQPFPQQ, but with some related pentapeptides (PQQPX) close to the amino terminus. These motifs

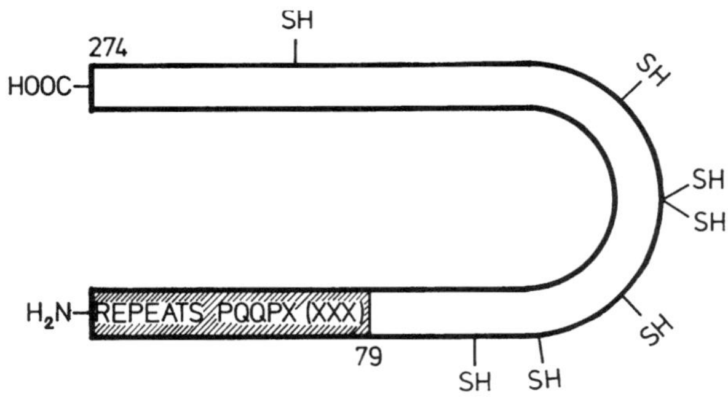

FIGURE 2 Structural organization of typical B1-hordein of barley.[65]

TABLE 4
Amino Acid Composition of C-Hordein (in mol%)

Amino Acid	C-Hordein[64] 1	2	3	Rye ω1-Secalin[66]	Wheat ω2-Gliadin[66]
Lysine	0.1	0.2	0.3	0.3	0.3
Histidine	0.8	1.1	1.1	0.5	0.8
Arginine	0.8	1.0	1.0	1.8	0.6
Aspartic acid	1.0	1.0	1.3	0.5	0.8
Threonine	0.9	1.4	1.3	1.0	1.7
Serine	3.0	3.3	3.3	4.1	5.9
Glutamic acid	38.9	38.3	38.1	42.9	42.8
Proline	32.5	30.9	30.5	30.6	29.1
Glycine	0.7	0.7	1.2	1.4	1.1
Alanine	0.7	0.9	1.0	0.6	0.6
Valine	1.3	1.0	1.2	1.0	0.4
Methionine	0.2	0.2	0.2	0.1	0
Isoleucine	3.2	2.8	2.7	2.4	1.6
Leucine	4.0	4.5	4.5	3.9	4.1
Tyrosine	2.0	2.2	2.2	1.4	1.5
Phenylalanine	8.6	9.3	9.5	7.4	8.9
Tryptophan	1.3	1.3	1.5	ND	ND

Note: ND, not determined.

are clearly related to those of B-hordeins (sulfur-rich prolamins), indicating a common evolutionary origin for at least these parts of proteins. The repeats in C-hordein are flanked by short, nonrepetitive N- and C-terminal domains of 12 and 7 residues, respectively (Figure 3). The latter contains a methionine residue that is probably the only sulfur-containing amino acid in the entire protein.

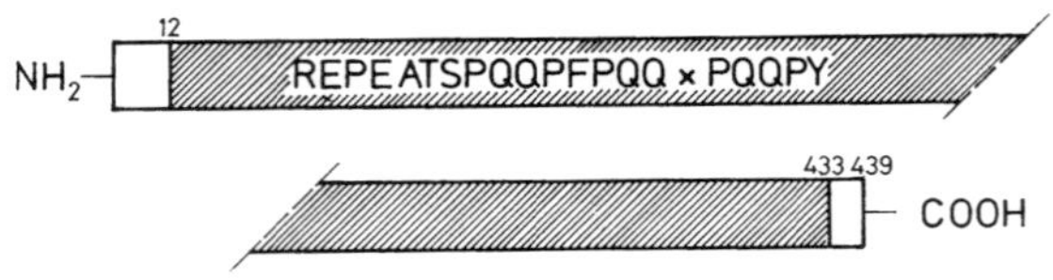

FIGURE 3 Structural organization of typical C-hordein of barley.[65]

The conformation of C-hordein molecules was also intensively studied. C-hordein of barley has been used as a model system for S-poor prolamins in general for several reasons. First, it is a single, structurally homogeneous group of proteins that can be treated as a single protein for physicochemical analysis. Second, it is relatively easy to prepare gram quantities from a mutant line of barley (Riso 56) from which the major B-hordeins are absent.

Amino acid sequencing, CD spectra, and hydrodynamic properties suggest that C-hordein molecules are rod shaped with an overwhelming amount of β-turns and a low level of α-helices and β-sheets, respectively.[65,67]

B. High Molecular Weight Storage Proteins (Glutelins)

The glutelin components of the storage proteins of barley were not investigated as exhaustively as the wheat glutenins. The HMW storage proteins of barley consist of polypeptides linked together with intermolecular disulfide bonds. They are not soluble in ethanol, but may be extracted with dilute sodium hydroxide or dilute acids. (Recently researchers studying the biochemistry and genetics of cereal proteins have used a classification which also includes the hordein polypeptides obtained by reduction of disulfide bonds of high molecular weight barley storage proteins. These polypeptides are called D-hordeins.)

Although the HMW storage proteins may be separated into subgroups using gel chromatography or different solvents,[68,69] the detailed study of their structure started with the splitting of disulfide bonds by reduction and separation of obtained polypeptides (subunits) using gel electrophoresis. In European cultivars of barley a single subunit (D-hordein, HMW subunit) may be observed on the electropherogram if SDS-PAGE separation is used.[70,71] A band with faster mobility, or sometimes two bands, may be present in other lines. D-hordein polypeptides appear to be encoded by a single structural locus (Hor-3) located on the long arm of chromosome 5.[72]

The amino acid composition of the total barley glutelins (Table 5) shows a high glutamic acid and proline content and a relatively high amount of glycine. These tendencies are better expressed in data on the amino acid composition of individual subunits (D-hordeins), as in Table 6. The glutamic acid (glutamine) content, and particularly the glycine content, is very high and the proline content is somewhat lower. A great similarity to the amino acid patterns of rye and wheat glutenin subunits (Table 6) may be observed.

TABLE 5
Amino Acid Composition of the Barley Glutelins (mol%)[14]

Amino Acid	Normal Barley (Bomi)	High Lysine (1508)
Lysine	2.2	4.4
Histidine	1.9	2.4
Arginine	3.2	4.8
Aspartic acid	4.2	7.5
Threonine	3.8	4.9
Serine	5.7	6.2
Glutamic acid	25.9	17.2
Proline	14.1	8.3
Glycine	6.3	9.4
Alanine	5.1	7.3
Cysteine	0.5	0.1
Valine	6.5	6.8
Methionine	1.3	1.7
Isoleucine	4.2	4.3
Leucine	8.2	8.1
Tyrosine	2.7	2.8
Phenylalanine	4.3	3.8

The structural organization of barley glutenin HMW subunits (D-hordeins) has not yet been intensively studied. However, preliminary N-terminal amino acid sequences[75] and far-UV CD spectra of D-hordein of barley, rye, and wheat glutenin subunits indicate that the three probably have very similar structure.

III. CYTOPLASMIC PROTEINS OF BARLEY

A. Albumins and Globulins

Cytoplasmic proteins of barley are treated mostly as albumins and globulins based on solubility. The amount of total salt-soluble proteins varies widely (10 to 35%). In the earlier work[76-79] the nonprotein nitrogen (free amino acids and peptides) was not calculated separately. This fact influenced the published data. In a more recent work, Rhodes and Gill[80] reported that the proportion of total salt-soluble proteins varied from 10.8 to 18% of the total protein in the normal genotypes and from 17.7 to 33% in those with high lysine. These data are in good agreement with the work of Miflin and Shewry.[81]

Compared to whole seed protein the albumins had higher proportions of lysine, threonine, methionine, and valine, but smaller proportions of phenylalanine, glutamic

TABLE 6
Amino Acid Composition of Subunits of High Molecular Weight (HMW) Storage Proteins of Barley, Rye, and Wheat (mol%)

Amino acid	D-Hordein[73]	Rye HMW Secalin[74]	Wheat Glutenin HMW Subunit 1A1[75]
ASP	1.3	1.3	1.0
THR	8.1	2.7	2.9
SER	9.7	5.0	6.3
GLU	29.6	34.0	37.1
PRO	11.6	13.7	16.5
GLY	15.7	16.5	14.7
ALA	2.5	6.4	2.5
CYS	1.5	1.4	0.8
VAL	4.5	2.8	2.4
MET	0.2	0.3	0.1
ILE	0.7	1.6	1.4
LEU	3.3	4.4	5.2
TYR	3.9	4.1	4.7
PHE	1.4	0.9	1.1
HIS	3.4	2.2	0.6
LYS	1.1	0.2	0.6
ARG	1.5	2.3	2.1

acid, and proline. The high-lysine lines had higher levels of lysine in the albumin proteins than the normal varieties. Some data about the amino acid composition of barley albumins are summarized in Table 7. The globulin fraction had generally higher proportions of lysine, leucine, and phenylalanine than the albumin fraction, but the threonine, methionine, glutamic acid, and proline proportions were lower. The variability in amino acid composition between genotypes was generally less in the globulins than in the albumins. Some data are given in Table 8.

Both the albumin and globulin fractions are heterogeneous and contain many polypeptide components. Data reported in the earlier publications noted a higher proportion of globulins in the cytoplasmic proteins.[82] More recent works[80,81] have found that albumins represent a higher proportion (8 to 12%) of the total protein than globulins (2 to 7%). Only several high-lysine mutants contained larger amounts of globulins (up to 17.8%). The electrophoretic patterns of the different varieties show many similarities, but characteristic differences also may be observed. It has been reported[83] that not only the hordeins but also the albumins of the barley grain are useful for variety identification. Taking into account the fact that many of the albumin components are in fact enzyme proteins, an additional staining for enzymatic activity also may be used in the identification of species and varieties.[83,84] Differences were found between high-lysine and normal varieties of the barley grains.

TABLE 7
Amino Acid Composition of Albumins of Barley (mol%)

Amino Acid	Normal (Bomi)[a]	High Lysine (1508)[a]	Normal (Ark Royal)[b]	High Lysine (Hiproly)[b]
Lysine	5.1	6.1	3.9	5.1
Histidine	1.9	1.9	—	—
Arginine	3.8	4.9	—	—
Aspartic acid	10.4	9.6	—	—
Threonine	4.6	5.0	3.9	4.7
Serine	5.4	5.9	—	—
Glutamic acid	14.5	11.5	13.8	13.7
Proline	7.3	6.0	7.3	8.1
Glycine	8.9	9.7	—	—
Alanine	10.6	9.8	—	—
Cysteine	0.5	0.5		
Valine	7.2	7.4	8.1	7.7
Methionine	1.9	2.1	1.6	1.5
Isoleucine	4.1	4.6	3.1	3.9
Leucine	7.9	9.3	7.4	6.1
Tyrosine	2.4	2.6	—	—
Phenylalanine	3.7	3.2	2.9	2.9

[a] From Brandt.[14]
[b] From Rhodes and Gill.[80]

The polypeptide composition was found[80] to be very similar for all genotypes, and differences existed mainly in the proportions of comparable subcomponents. The molecular weights of the components varied from 10 to 70 kDa.

B. Enzymes and Enzyme Inhibitors

1. Enzymes

In the mature unmalted grain the enzymes degrading polysaccharides (amylases, glucoamylases) and proteins (proteases, peptidases) are the most important components. The lipase activity of barley is low in comparison with that of oats and rice. Some oxidoreductases also may have a given practical importance.

During germination and malting a number of other enzymes are synthesized and play a role in the complex processes of malt production. In particular, enzymes degrading carbohydrates (barley endo-β-glucanase, exo-β-glucanase, cellobiase, laminaribiase, exoxylanase, arabinosidase, α- and β-amylase isoenzymes) and proteins (endopeptidase, carboxypeptidase, aminopeptidase, peptide hydrolase, etc.) are formed.

TABLE 8
Amino Acid Composition of Globulins of Barley (mol%)

	Normal		High Lysine	
Amino Acid	**Bomi[a]**	**Ark Royal[b]**	**1058[a]**	**Hiproly[b]**
Lysine	5.3	5.6	5.8	5.8
Histidine	1.7	—	2.2	—
Arginine	5.5	—	6.4	—
Aspartic acid	8.1	—	7.9	—
Threonine	4.4	3.9	4.5	4.0
Serine	5.4	—	4.7	—
Glutamic acid	15.5	10.7	12.7	11.2
Proline	9.3	4.6	6.7	5.1
Glycine	9.6	—	10.8	—
Alanine	7.9	—	8.4	—
Cysteine	0	—	0	—
Valine	7.6	7.2	5.3	6.2
Methionine	1.8	1.6	1.5	1.5
Isoleucine	3.8	3.9	3.5	3.5
Leucine	7.9	7.9	13.6	6.7
Tyrosine	2.8	—	2.7	—
Phenylalanine	3.6	3.5	3.5	3.5

[a] From Brandt.[14]
[b] From Rhodes and Gill.[80]

The amylases of barley were for some time the main object of investigation due to their importance during storage and malting of the barley grains. The β-amylases may be purified by successive fractionation on CM-cellulose, Sephadex, and DEAE-cellulose. At least four active components were separated. Some of them showed heterogeneity by gel electrophoretic investigation. The results suggest that the barley endosperm may contain as many as nine β-amylases. Further investigations are needed to elucidate the probable presence of dimers or other aggregates of the active enzymes. The α-amylases of barley and malt also may be separated by the gel electrophoresis technique. The α-amylase isoenzymes of several varieties of germinated barley were compared using isoelectric focusing techniques. Differences were detected between some varieties. The mature barley grains contained relatively small quantities of α-amylase. During germination a rapid increase was observed. Most of the research workers suggest that the *de novo* synthesis of α-amylases occurs in the aleurone layer. However, several more recent investigations[145-147] suggest that the site of initial α-amylase synthesis in germinating cereal grain is the embryo and not the aleurone layer or both.[148]

Several reviews concerning the role of amylases in cereal science and technology were published in the last decade.[86-88] Although both α- and β-amylases are present in barley grains, the research connected with barley amylases has concentrated on α-amylases playing an important role in the malting and brewing process.

β-Amylases of barley and malt were relatively poorly investigated.[89-92] Heterogeneity of the β-amylases in barley was studied by La Berge and Marchylo,[93] and Heygaard et al.[94] Hyproly barley variety and high-lysine lines derived from it had about four- to sixfold higher levels of β-amylase activity than normal genotypes. It was supposed that the 11-kDa subunit found in the albumin fraction of Hyproly might be an isoenzyme of β-amylase.

α-Amylases of barley were very intensively studied. The results of research work were summarized in review papers[86-88] and in a lot of other publications. The α-amylases were extracted and separated by gel eletrophoresis, isoelectric focusing, and other techniques.[95-98] All of these studies confirmed the heterogeneity of α-amylases.

Differences were observed between amylases of mature, immature, and germinated seeds.[99-101] The α-amylases are classified according to their electrophoretic mobility, pH optima, immunochemical properties, and isoelectric point. Isoelectric focusing showed that germinated barley (two- and six-rowed) contained multiple forms of α-amylases that could be divided into low (pI $\leq$ 5.5) and high pI (pI $\geq$ 5.8)[98] enzymes. Differences were observed between different cereals.

The protein-degrading enzymes of barley were also investigated. Proteolytic activity of mature, unmalted barley is quite low. Malted or field-sprouted grain is richer in protein-degrading enzymes. Early research work concerning the proteases and malt was reviewed by Burger.[102] More recent results are summarized by Palmer,[103] Meredith and Pomeranz,[99] and Kruger et al.[87]

Peroxidase isoenzymes in the mature barley kernel were studied by La Berge et al.[104] A total of 14 cationic peroxidase isoenzymes were detected using polyacrylamide slabs for disc electrophoresis at pH 4.75. The actual number of isoenzymes detected on electropherograms of a particular barley cultivar was dependent on the hydrogen donor used for staining the peroxidase isoenzymes. In this respect, 3-amino-ethyl carbazole and *ortho*-dianisidine were superior to guaiacol, catechol, and benzidine as donors for differentiating the isoenzymes. Barley cultivars could be classified into three categories based on varietal differences of enzymes; peroxidase isoenzymes might be useful for identifying positively barley cultivars by fingerprint methods. Phospholipases of cereals were reviewed by Acker.[105]

2. Enzyme Inhibitors

Cereals contain proteins with inhibitor activity against animal α-amylases; this was determined by early research work of Kneen and Sandstedt[106] and later by others.[107,108] Endogenous α-amylase inhibitors in cereals were reported only recently by Warchalewski.[109] Endogenous α-amylase inhibitors were isolated from barley, too.[110-113] It was found that the inhibitor is a low molecular weight protein with an

TABLE 9
Amino Acid Composition of Some α-Amylase and Protease Inhibitors (mol %)

Amino Acid	α-Amylase Inhibitor		Trypsin Inhibitor	
	Wheat[126]	Barley[113]	Barley[127]	Barley Embryo[128]
ASP	7.4	8.9	7.6	7.4
THR	2.5	8.4	5.3	6.8
SER	7.4	5.2	6.1	6.8
GLU	10.7	9.1	11.4	7.4
PRO	8.2	8.0	9.9	12.2
GLY	9.1	10.6	7.6	6.8
ALA	8.2	8.6	8.3	6.1
CYS	8.2	2.5	6.8	12.2
VAL	10.7	7.0	4.6	5.4
MET	2.5	1.4	1.5	2.0
ILE	1.6	3.6	3.8	2.0
LEU	7.4	6.1	7.6	3.4
TYR	3.3	3.3	3.8	2.0
PHE	0	3.6	2.3	2.0
HIS	0	4.8	2.3	0.7
LYS	4.9	3.4	1.5	6.1
ARG	4.9	6.1	7.6	8.1
TRP	3.3	ND	1.5	ND

Note: ND, not determined.

isoelectric point of 7.1 to 7.3. A high amount of basic amino acid residues and cysteine (cystine) content is typical for the majority of these proteins (Table 9).

The inhibitor inhibits endogenous high-pI α-amylase of barley. The inhibitor activity is also detectable in wheat and rye.[112,114] The inhibitor content of barley seeds was found to be highest during early seed development.[115] These inhibitors were also found to have inhibitor activity against subtilisin, a microbial protease.[113,116] N-terminal amino acid sequence studies and similarities in activity conditions suggest that the inhibitors belong to a common family. From a practical point of view the studies of Zawistowska et al.[117] showing that barley α-amylase inhibitor may be successfully used for improving bread-making properties of wheat flour containing barley malt are interesting.

Barley and other cereal grains contain a large number of proteins and peptides inhibiting proteases. Recently a number of amino acid sequences of cereal protease inhibitors have been reported. Some of them are "bifunctional" ("double-headed") in that they also inhibit α-amylase activity. In a review (Reference 19) these proteins were classified into four families: chymotrypsin inhibitors, bifunctional α-amylase/subtilisin inhibitors, bifunctional α-amylase/trypsin inhibitors, and embryo trypsin inhibitors. Barley grain contains all four types of inhibitors. Their quantity is surprisingly high. It has been calculated that trypsin inhibitors may contribute up to 5 to 10% of the water-soluble proteins of barley grain.[118] These inhibitors have been shown to accumulate in the barley endosperm at about the same time as the major storage protein, hordein. They also behave like storage proteins in that the amounts accumulated in the endosperm are markedly increased by increasing nitrogen fertilizer,[119] and they are broken down relatively rapidly during germination.[120] More detailed data about the chemistry and physiology of protease inhibitors are given in a number of reviews.[121-125]

C. Other Proteins

A major group of low molecular weight hydrophobic proteins of barley are called A-hordein; they can be extracted in aqueous alcohol or chloroform-methanol mixtures. They can be partially extracted also with 0.5 *M* sodium chloride and are present in both salt-soluble and hordein fractions extracted according to the Osborne procedure. Using two-dimensional IEF-PAGE Salcedo et al.[129] demonstrated the presence of four major components having molecular weights from 12 to 16 kDa and amino acid composition similar to the CM proteins of wheat. Aragoncillo et al.[130] separated a second group of CM proteins of barley having low mobility and giving a major band with a molecular weight of 18 kDa.

A purothionin analog was isolated from barley by Redman and Fisher[131] and named hordothionin. Later other research workers separated three components of hordothionin, and its amino acid sequence was determined and reported.[132,134] Hordothionin components are highly homologous with purothionins. The lipid complex of hordothionin, called lipohordothionin, was also prepared. Its structure is closely related to that of lipopurothionin. Recently antifungal proteins (e.g., ribosome-inactivating proteins) were detected and studied by several authors.[139-141]

IV. NUTRITIVE (FEEDING) VALUE OF BARLEY PROTEINS

The nutritive value of barley proteins may be generally characterized as being similar to that of other cereal proteins. From the viewpoint of biological value, the low molecular weight storage proteins are of the poorest quality because of their very low lysine content. As for other cereals, the cytoplasmic proteins are richer in essential amino acids than the storage proteins. The better total protein composition of high-lysine mutants is related to a lower content of hordeins and an increased amount of water- and salt-soluble cytoplasmic proteins. The greatest proportion of barley is used for feed and brewing; the importance of barley as food is small. Nevertheless, expanding world requirements for food have stimulated increased use of barley as human food. Today barley consumption occurs in such foodstuff as flour for flat bread, pearled barley, ground and flaked grain for porridge, and malt enrichment for various food products.

A possible new use of barley for food is in the production of protein concentrates[135] (high-protein flours or fractions[136-138]). Use of barley flour and high-protein barley flour in weaning foods and pasta was also reported.[139]

REFERENCES

1. Hoseney, R. C., *Principles of Cereal Science and Technology,* American Association of Cereal Chemists, St. Paul, MN, 1994.
2. Pomeranz, Y., Industrial uses of barley, in *Industrial Uses of Cereal Proteins,* Pomeranz, Y., Ed., American Association of Cereal Chemists, St. Paul, MN, 1973, 371.
3. Anderson, A. J., Effects of fertilizers on barley protein quality and quantity, *Cereal Res. Commun.,* 5, 159, 1977.
4. Anderson, A. J. and Knie, B., N-fertilization and yield response of high lysine and normal barley, *Agron. J.,* 67, 695, 1975.
5. Pomeranz, Y., Robbins, G. S., Gilbertson, J. T., and Boot, G. D., Effects of nitrogen fertilization on lysine, threonine and methionine of hulled and hull-less barley cultivars, *Cereal Chem.,* 54, 1034, 1978.
6. Jenkins, G., Rhodes, A. P., Gill, A. A., and Hanson, P. R., The effect of irrigation and nitrogen supply on the yield and quality of protein in high-lysine barley, *J. Sci. Food Agric.,* 30, 647, 1979.
7. Kirkman, M. A., Shewry, P., and Miflin, B., The effect of nitrogen nutrition on the lysine content and protein composition of barley seeds, *J. Sci. Food Agric.,* 33, 115, 1982.
8. Eppendorf, W., The effect of nitrogen and sulphur on changes in nitrogenous fraction of barley plants at various stages of growth and on yield and amino acid composition of grain, *Plant Soil,* 29, 424, 1968.
9. Tkachuk, A. A. and Irvine, G. N., Amino acid composition of cereal and oilseed meals, *Cereal Chem.,* 46, 206, 1969.
10. Woodham, A. A., The effect of nitrogen fertilization on the amino acid composition and nutritive value of cereals, *Qual. Plant. Plant Foods Hum. Nutr.,* 23, 281, 1973.
11. Rhodes, A. P. and Mathers, J. C., Varietal differences in the amino acid composition of barley grain during development and under varying nitrogen supply, *J. Sci. Food Agric.,* 25, 963, 1974.
12. Rhodes, A. P. and Jenkins, G., The effect of varying nitrogen supply on the protein composition of a high-lysine mutant of barley, *J. Sci. Food Agric.,* 26, 705, 1975.
13. Shewry, P. R., Field, J. M., Kirkman, M. A., Faulks, A. J., and Miflin, B. J., The extraction, solubility, and characterization of two groups of barley storage proteins, *J. Exp. Bot.,* 121, 393, 1980.
14. Brandt, A., Endosperm protein formation during kernel development of wild type and high-lysine barley mutant, *Cereal Chem.,* 53, 890, 1976.
15. Larkins, B. and Hurkman, W. J., Synthesis and deposition of zein in protein bodies of maize endosperm, *Plant Physiol.,* 62, 256, 1978.

16. Adams, C. A., Novelle, L., and Leibenberg, N. V. d. W., Biochemical properties and ultrastructure of protein bodies isolated from selected cereals, *Cereal Chem.,* 53, 1, 1976.
17. Martens, H. and Knudsen, K. E. B., Fractioning barley proteins by computer factor analysis, *Cereal Chem.,* 53, 1, 1976.
18. Cameron-Mills, V., Brandt, A., and Ingversen, J., The molecular biology of barley storage protein synthesis, in *Cereals for Food and Beverages. Recent Progress in Cereal Chemistry,* Inglett, G.E. and Munck. L., Eds., Academic Press, New York, 1980, 335.
19. Shewry, P. R. and Miflin, B. J., Seed storage proteins of economically important cereals, in *Advances in Cereal Science and Technology,* Vol. 7, Pomeranz, Y., Ed., American Association of Cereal Chemists, St. Paul, MN, 1985, 1.
20. Miflin, B. J. and Shewry, P. R., The biology and biochemistry of cereal seed prolamins, in *Seed Protein Improvement in Cereals and Grain Legumes,* Vol. 1, International Atomic Energy Agency, Vienna, 1979, 137.
21. Baxter, E. D. and Wainwright, P. R., Hordein and malting quality, *J. Am. Soc. Brew. Chem.,* 5(37), 8, 1979.
22. Miflin, B. J. and Shewry, P. R., The synthesis of protein in normal and high-lysine barley seeds, in *Recent Advances in the Biochemistry of Cereals,* Laidman, D.L. and Nones, R.G.W., Eds., Academic Press, New York, 1979, 239.
23. Lauriére, M. and Mossé, J., Selective extraction and purification of barley alcohol soluble proteins and their analysis on starch gel electrophoresis, in *Techniques for the Separation of Barley and Maize Proteins,* Miflin, B.J. and Shewry, P.R., Eds., Commission of the European Communities, Kirchberg, Luxembourg, 1977, 49.
24. Shewry, P. R., Ellis, J. R., Pratt, N. M., and Miflin, B. J., Comparison of methods for the extraction and separation of hordein fractions from 29 barley varieties, *J. Sci. Food Agric.,* 29, 433, 1978.
25. Salcedo, G., Sanchez-Monge, R., Argamenteria, A., and Aragoncillò, C., The A-hordein as a group of salt soluble hydrophobic proteins, *Plant Sci. Lett.,* 19, 109, 1980.
26. Miflin, B. J. and Shewry, P. R., An introduction to the extraction and characterization of barley and maize proteins, in *Techniques for the Separation of Barley and Maize Proteins,* Miflin, B.J. and Shewry, P.R., Eds., Commission of the European Communities, Kirchberg, Luxembourg, 1977, 13.
27. Miflin, B. J., Burgess, S. R., and Shewry, P. J., The development of protein bodies in the storage tissues of seeds: subcellular separations of homogenates of barley, maize and wheat endosperms and of pea cotyledons, *J. Exp. Bot.,* 32, 199, 1981.
28. Du Cros, D. L. and Wrigley, C. W., Improved electrophoretic methods for identifying cereal varieties, *J. Sci. Food Agric.,* 30, 785, 1979.
29. Autran, J. C. and Scriban, R., Recherche sur la pureté variétale d'un malt, in Proc. 16th Congr. Eur. Brew. Convent., Amsterdam, 1977, 47.
30. Konarev, V. G., Yakubziner, N. M., Trofimovskaya, A. Y., Gavrilyuk, I. P., Gubareva, N. K., and Chernoburova, A. D., The determination of cultivars of wheat and barley grain by protein formulas (in Russian), *Vestn. Skh. Nauki,* 7, 84, 1976.
31. Gavrilyuk, I. P. and Diaguileva, G. E., Varietal identification of barleys from hordein electrophoretic patterns (in Russian), in *Dokl. V.I.R.,* Konarev, V.G. and Trofimovskaya, A.Y., Eds., V.I.R., Leningrad, 1975 1.
32. McCausland, J. and Wrigley, C. W., Identification of Australian barley cultivars by laboratory methods: gel electrophoresis and gel isoelectric focusing of the endosperm proteins, *Aust. J. Exp. Agric. Anim. Husb.,* 17, 1020, 1977.

33. Mesrob, B. K. and Ivanov, C. P., Comparative fraction composition of hordein from different barley varieties, *C.R. Acad. Bulg. Sci.*, 23, 291, 1970.
34. Neyreneuf, O. and Bourdet, A., Identification of barley varieties, *Bios*, 10, 73, 1979.
35. Scriban, R. and Strobbel, B., Etude chimiotaconomique de l'orge et du malt par electrofocalisation, *C.R. Acad. Sci. Paris Ser. D.*, 287, 841, 1978.
36. Shewry, P. R., Pratt, H. M., and Miflin, B. J., Varietal identification of barley by analysis of hordein polypeptides, *J. Sci. Food Agric.*, 29, 587, 1978.
37. Shewry, P. R., Faulks, A. J., Parmar, S., and Miflin, B. J., Hordein polypeptide pattern in relation to malting quality and the varietal identification of malted barley grain, *J. Inst. Brew.*, 86, 138, 1980.
38. Van Lonkhuysen, H. J. and Marseille, J. P., Identifizierung von Gerstensorten durch Starkegelektrophorese, *Getreide Mehl Brot*, 32, 288, 1978.
39. Bietz, J. A. and Schmalzried, E., Capillary electrophoresis of wheat proteins: optimization and use for variety identification, *Cereal Food World*, 37, 555, 1992.
40. Deichl, A. and Donhauser, S., Die immunchemische Bestimmung der Sortenreinheit und des Vermischungsgrades von Braugerste und Braumalz, *Eur. Brew. Conv. Proc. Congr.*, 20, 611, 1985.
41. Vaag, P. and Munck, L., Immunochemical methods in cereal research and technology, *Cereal Chem.*, 64, 59, 1987.
42. Bietz, J. A., Amino-terminal amino acid sequence of hordein, *Cereal Chem.*, 58, 83, 1981.
43. Shewry, P. R., Pratt, H. M., Charlton, M. J., and Miflin, B. J., Two-dimensional separation of the prolamins of normal and high-lysine barley (*Hordeum vulgare* L.), *J. Exp. Bot.*, 28, 597, 1977.
44. Holder, A. A. and Ingversen, J., Peptide mapping of the major components of in vitro synthesized barley hordein: evidence of structural homology, *Carlsberg Res. Commun.*, 43, 177, 1978.
45. Shewry, P. R., Autran, J. C., Nimmo, C. C., Lew, E. J. L., and Kasarda D. D., N-terminal amino acid sequence homology of storage protein components from barley and a diploid wheat, *Nature (London)*, 286, 520, 1980.
46. Shewry, P. R., Lew, E. J., and Kasarda, D. D., Structural homology of storage proteins coded by the *Hor-1* locus of barley (*Hordcum vulgare* L.), *Planta*, 153, 246, 1981.
47. Shewry, P. R., March, J. F., and Miflin, B. J., N-terminal amino acid sequence of C-hordein, *Phytochemistry*, 19, 2113, 1980.
48. Schmitt, I. M. and Svendsen, I., Amino acid sequences of hordein polypeptides, *Carlsberg Res. Commun.*, 45, 143, 1980.
49. Brandt, A. and Ingversen, J., In vitro synthesis of barley endosperm proteins on wild type and mutant templates, *Carlsberg Res. Commun.*, 41, 311, 1977.
50. Brandt, A. and Ingversen, J., Isolation and translation of hordein messenger RNA-s from wild type and mutant endosperm in barley, *Carlsberg Res. Commun.*, 43, 351, 1978.
51. Forde, B. G., Kreis, M., Bahramian, M. B., Matthews, J. A., Miflin, B. J., Thompson, R. D., Bartels, D., and Flavell, R. B., Molecular cloning and analysis of cDNA sequence from poly A^+ RNA from barley endosperm: identification of B-hordein related clones, *Nucleic Acids Res.*, 9, 6689, 1981.
52. Field, J. M., Shewry, P. R., and Miflin, B. J., Aggregation states of alcohol-soluble storage proteins of barley, rye, wheat and maize, *J. Sci. Food Agric.*, 34, 262, 1983.

53. Faulks, A. J., Shewry, P. R., and Miflin, B. J., The polymorphism and structural homology of storage polypeptides (hordein) coded by Hor-2 locus in barley (*Hordeum vulgare* L.), *Biochem. Genet.,* 19, 841, 1981.
54. Kreis, M., Rahman, S., Forde, B. G., Pywell, J., Shewry, P. J., and Miflin, B. J., Subfamilies of hordein mRNA-s encoded at the Hor-2 locus of barley, *Mol. Gen. Genet.,* 191, 194, 1983.
55. Shewry, P. R., Kreis, P. M., Parmar, S., Lew, E. J., and Kasarda, D. D., Identification of γ-type hordeins in barley, *FEBS Lett.,* 190, 61, 1985.
56. Schmitt, J. M. and Svendsen, I., Amino acid sequences of hordein polypeptides, *Carlsberg Res. Commun.,* 44, 431, 1980.
57. Brandt, A., Montembault, A., Cameron-Mills, V., and Rasrmussen, S. V., Primary structure of a B1 hordein gene from barley, *Carlsberg Res. Commun.,* 50, 333, 1985.
58. Shewry, P. R., Field, J. M., Kirkman, M. A., Faulks, A. J., and Miflin, B. J., The extraction, solubility, and characterization of two groups of barley storage polypeptides, *J. Exp. Bot.,* 31, 393, 1980.
59. Miflin, B. J., Field, J. M., and Shewry, P. R., Cereal storage proteins and their effects on technological properties, in *Seed Proteins,* Daussant, J., Mossé, J., and Vaughan, J., Eds., Academic Press, London, 1983, 255.
60. Bietz, J. A., Huebner, F. R., Sanderson, J. E., and Wall, J. S., Wheat gliadin homology revealed through N-terminal amino acid sequence analysis, *Cereal Chem.,* 54, 1070, 1977.
61. Forde, B. G., Heyworth, A., Pywell, J., and Kreis, M., Nucleotide sequence of a B1 hordein gene and the identification of possible upstream regulatory elements in endosperm storage protein genes from barley wheat and maize, *Nucleic Acids Res.,* 13, 7327, 1985.
62. Forde, B. G., Kreis, M., Williamson, M. S., Fry, R. P., Pywell, J., Shewry, P. R., Brunce, N., and Miflin, B. J., Short tandem repeats shared by B- and C-hordein cDNA-s suggest a common evolutionary origin for two groups of cereal storage protein genes, *EMBO J.,* 4, 9, 1985.
63. Faulks, A., Shewry, P. R., and Miflin, B. J., The polymorphism and structural homology of storage polypeptides (hordein) coded by the Hor-2 locus in barley (*Hordeum vulgare* L.), *Biochem. Genet.,* 19, 841, 1981.
64. Shewry, P. R., Lew, E. J., and Kasarda, D. D., Structural homology of storage proteins coded by *Hor*-1 locus of barley (*Hordeum vulgare* L.), *Planta,* 153, 246, 1981.
65. Tatham, A. S., Shewry, P. R., and Belton, P. S., Structural studies of cereal prolamins, including wheat gluten, in *Advances in Cereal Science and Technology,* Vol. 10, Pomeranz, Y., Ed., American Association of Cereal Chemists, St. Paul, MN, 1990, 1.
66. Kasarda, D. D., Autran, J. C., Lew, E. J., Nimmo, C. C., and Shewry, P. R., N-terminal amino acid sequences of ω-gliadins and ω-secalins: implications for the evolution of prolamin genes, *Biochim. Biophys Acta,* 747, 138, 1983.
67. Field, J. M., Tatham, A. S., Baker, A., and Shewry, P. R., The structure of C-hordein, *FEBS Lett.,* 200, 76, 1986.
68. Landry, J., Moureaux, T., and Huet, J. C., Extractibilité des proteins du grain d'orge, *Bios,* 7(8), 281, 1972.
69. Graveland, A., Extraction of wheat proteins with sodium dodecyl sulphate, *Ann. Technol. Agric.,* 29, 113, 1980.
70. Shewry, P. R. and Miflin, B. J., Genes for the storage proteins of barley, *Qual. Plant Plant Foods Hum. Nutr.,* 31, 251, 1982.

71. Shewry, P. R. and Miflin, B. J., Characterization and synthesis of barley seed proteins, in *Seed Protein: Biochemistry, Genetics, Nutritive Value,* Gottschalk, W. and Müller, H., Eds., Martinus Nijhoff, The Hague, 1983, 143.
72. Shewry, P. R., Finch, R., Parmar, S., Franklin, J., and Miflin, B. J., Chromosomal location of *Hor*-3, a new locus governing storage proteins in barley, *Heredity,* 50, 179, 1983.
73. Kreis, M., Shewry, P. R., Forde, B. G., Rahman, S., Bahramian, M. V., and Miflin, B. J., Molecular analysis of the effects of the mutant lys 3a gene on the expression of Hor loci in developing endosperms of barley (*Hordeum vulgare* L)., *Biochem. Genet.,* 62, 231, 1984.
74. Field, J. M., Shewry, P. R., Miflin, B. J., and March, J. F., The purification and characterization of homologous high molecular weight storage proteins from grain wheat, rye and barley, *Theor. Appl. Genet.,* 62, 329, 1982.
75. Shewry, P. R., Field, J. M., Faulks, A. J., Parmar, S., Miflin, B. J., Dietler, M. D., Lew, E. J., and Kasarda, D. D., Purification and N-terminal amino acid sequence analysis of high molecular weight (HMW) gluten polypeptides of wheat, *Biochim. Biophys. Acta,* 788, 23, 1984.
76. Lundin, H., The proteins of barley and malt, *Wallerstein Lab. Commun.,* 26, 75, 1963.
77. Waldschmidt-Leitz, E. and Hochstrasser, K., Über die Albumine aus Gerste und Weizen. VII. Mitteilung über Samenproteine, *Hoppe-Seylers Z. Physiol. Chem.,* 324, 243, 1961.
78. Ingversen, J. and Koie, B., Lysine-rich proteins in the salt soluble protein fraction of barley, *Phytochemistry,* 12, 73, 1973.
79. Ingversen, J., Koie, B., and Doll, H., Induced seed mutant of barley, *Experientia,* 29, 1151, 1973.
80. Rhodes, A. P. and Gill, A. A., Fractionation and amino acid analysis of the salt-soluble protein fractions of normal and high-lysine barleys, *J. Sci. Food Agric.,* 31, 467, 1981.
81. Miflin, B. J. and Shewry, P. R., The synthesis of proteins in normal and high-lysine barley seeds, in *Recent Advances in the Biochemistry of Cereals,* Laidman, D.L. and Wyn Jones, R.G., Eds., Academic Press, London, 1979, 239.
82. Simmonds, H., Structure, composition and biochemistry of cereal grains, in *Cereals 78: Better Nutrition for the World Millions,* Pomeranz, Y., Ed., American Association of Cereal Chemists, St. Paul, MN, 1978, 105.
83. Wrigley, C. W., Autran, J. C., and Bushuk, W., Identification of cereal varieties by gel electrophoresis of the grain proteins, in *Advances in Cereal Science and Technology,* Vol. 5, Pomeranz, Y., Ed., American Association of Cereal Chemists, St. Paul, MN, 1982, 211.
84. Almgard, G. and Landegren, O., Isoenzymatic variation used for the identification of barley varieties, *Z. Pflanz,* 72, 63, 1974.
85. Matlashewsky, G. J., Urquhart, A. A., Sahasrabudhe, M. R., and Altosaar, I., Lipase activity in oat flour suspensions and soluble extracts, *Cereal Chem.,* 59, 418, 1982.
86. Hill, R. D. and McGregor, A. W., Cereal α-amylases in grain research and technology, in *Advances in Cereal Science and Technology,* Vol. 9, Pomeranz, Y., Ed., American Association of Cereal Chemists, St. Paul, MN, 1988.
87. Kruger, J. E., Lineback, D. R., and Stauffer, C. E., Eds., *Enzymes and Their Role in Cereal Technology,* American Association of Cereal Chemists, St. Paul, MN, 1987.
88. McGregor, E. A. and McGregor, A. W., Studies of cereal α-amylases using cloned DNA, *Crit. Rev. Biotechnol.,* 5, 129, 1987.
89. La Berge, D. E. and Meredith, W. O. S., The β-amylase enzymes of barley and malt. I. Purification of the malt enzymes, *J. Inst. Brew.,* 77, 436, 1971.

90. Allison, M. J. and Swantson, J. S., Relationships between β-amylase polymorphisms in developing, mature and germinating grains of barley, *J. Inst. Brew.*, 80, 285, 1974.
91. McGregor, A. W., La Berge, D. E., and Meredith, W. O. S., Separation of α- and β-amylase enzymes from barley malt by ion exchange chromatography, *Cereal Chem.*, 48, 490, 1971.
92. La Berge, D. E., McGregor, A. W., and Meredith, W. O. S., Changes in α- and β-amylase activities during the maturation of different barley cultivars, *Can. J. Plant Sci.*, 51, 469, 1971.
93. La Berge, D. E. and Marchylo, B. A., Heterogeneity of the β-amylase enzymes of barley, *J. Am. Soc. Brew. Chem.*, 41, 120, 1983.
94. Heygaard, J., Koie, B., Karisson, K. E., and Tallber, A., β-amylase activity — a simple screening test in Hiproly barley breeding, *Hereditas*, 90, 145, 1979.
95. Daussant, J. and Hill, R. D., Combined immunoabsorption and isoelectric focusing of barley and malt amylases in polyacrylamide gels, *Anal. Biochem.*, 93, 261, 1979.
96. Marchylo, B. A. and McGregor, A. W., Separation of barley malt α-amylase by chromatofocusing, *Cereal Chem.*, 60, 311, 1983.
97. Marchylo, B. A. and Kruger, J. E., Methods for purification and separation of cereal enzymes and their multiple forms, in *Enzymes and Their Role in Cereal Technology*, Kruger, J.E., Lineback, D.R., and Stauffer, C.E., Eds., American Association of Cereal Chemists, St. Paul, MN, 1987, 37.
98. McGregor, A. W., Marchylo, B. A., and Kruger, J. E., Multiple α-amylase components in germinated cereal grains by isoelectric focusing and chromatofocusing, *Cereal Chem.*, 65, 326, 1988.
99. Meredith, P. and Pomeranz, Y., Sprouted grain, in *Advances in Cereal Science and Technology*, Vol. 7, Pomeranz, Y., Ed., American Association of Cereal Chemists, St. Paul, MN, 1985, 239.
100. McGregor, A. W., McDougall, F. H., Mayer, C., and Daussant, J., Changes in levels of α-amylase components in barley tissues during germination and early seedling growth, *Plant Physiol.*, 75, 203, 1984.
101. Takano, T. and Takeda, G., Polymorphism for α-amylase in germinating seed and malt of barley varieties detected by isoelectric focusing gel electrophoresis, *Jpn. J. Breed.*, 35, 9, 1985.
102. Burger, W. C., The proteases of barley and malt. Recent research, *Cereal Sci. Today*, 11, 19, 1966.
103. Palmer, G. H., The morphology and physiology of malting of barleys, in *Cereals for Food and Beverages, Recent Progress in Cereal Chemistry*, Inglett, G.E. and Munck, L., Eds., Academic Press, New York, 1980.
104. La Berge, D. E., Kruger, J. E., and Meredith, W. O. S., Peroxidase isozymes in mature barley kernels, *Can. J. Plant Sci.*, 53, 705, 1973.
105. Acker, L., Phospholipases of cereals, in *Advances in Cereal Science and Technology*, Vol. 7, Pomeranz, Y., Ed., American Association of Cereal Chemists, St. Paul, MN, 1985, 175.
106. Kneen, B. and Sandstedt, R. M., An amylase inhibitor from certain cereals, *J. Am. Chem. Soc.*, 65, 247, 1943.
107. Shainkin, R. and Birk, Y. D., α-Amylase inhibitors from wheat: isolation and characterization, *Biochim. Biophys. Acta*, 221, 502, 1970.
108. Silano, V., Pocchjiari, F., and Kasarda, D. D., Physical characterization of α-amylase inhibitors from wheat, *Biochim. Biophys. Acta*, 317, 319, 1973.
109. Warchalewski, J. R., Isolation and purification of native alpha-amylase inhibitors from winter wheat, *Bull. Acad. Pol. Sci. Ser. Sci. Biol.*, 25, 725, 1977.

110. Hejgaard, J., Svendsen, I., and Mundy, J., Barley α-amylase subtilisin inhibitor. N-terminal amino acid sequence and homology with inhibitors of the soybean trypsin inhibitor (Kunitz) family, *Carlsberg Res. Commun.*, 48, 91, 1983.
111. Weselake, R. J., McGregor, A. W., Hill, R. D., and Duckworth, H. W., Purification and characteristics of an endogeneous α-amylase inhibitor from barley kernels, *Plant Physiol.*, 73, 1008, 1983.
112. Weselake, R. J., McGregor, A. W., and Hill, R. D., Endogeneous alpha-amylase inhibitor in various cereals, *Cereal Chem.*, 62, 120, 1985.
113. Mundy, J., Svendsen, I., and Hejgaard, J., Barley α-amylase/subtilisin inhibitors. I Isolation and characterization, *Carlsberg Res. Commun.*, 48, 81, 1983.
114. Törrönen, A., Leisola, M., and Haarasilta, S., Inhibition of rye α-amylase activity by barley α-amylase inhibitor, *Cereal Chem.*, 69, 355, 1992.
115. Robertson, M. and Hill, R. D., Accumulation of an endogenous alpha-amylase inhibitor in barley during grain development, *J. Cereal Sci.*, 9, 237, 1990.
116. Mundy, J., Hejgaard, J., and Svendsen, I., Characterization of a bifunctional wheat inhibitor of endogenous α-amylase and subtilisin, *FEBS Lett.*, 167, 210, 1984.
117. Zawistowska, U., Langstaff, J., and Bushuk, W., Improving effect of a natural alpha-amylase inhibitor on the baking quality of wheat flour containing malted barley flour, *J. Cereal Sci.*, 8, 207, 1988.
118. Mikola, J. and Kirsi, M., Differences between endospermal and embryonal trypsin inhibitors in barley, wheat and rye, *Acta Chem. Scand.*, 26, 787, 1972.
119. Hejgaard, D. J. and Boisen, J., High lysine proteins in Hyproly barley breeding. Identification, nutritional significance and new screening methods, *Hereditas*, 93, 311, 1980.
120. Kirsi, M., Proteinase inhibitors in germinating barley embryos, *Physiol. Plant.*, 29, 141, 1974.
121. Ryan, C. A., Protease inhibitors, in *Herbivores, Their Interaction with Secondary Plant Metabolites*, Rosental, G.A. and Janzen, D.H., Eds., Academic Press, London, 559, 1979.
122. Richardson, M., The protease inhibitors of plants and microorganisms, *Phytochemistry*, 16, 159, 1977.
123. Micola, J., Proteinases, peptidases and inhibitors of endogenous proteinases in germinating seeds, in *Seed Proteins*, Daussant, J., Mossé, J., and Vaughan, J., Eds., Academic Press, London, 1983, 35.
124. Whitaker, J. R., Naturally occurring peptide and protein inhibitors of enzymes, in *Impact of Toxicology on Food Processing*, Ayres, J.C. and Kirschman, J C., Eds., AVI, Westport, CT, 1981, 57.
125. Belitz, H. D. and Weder, J. K. P., Protein inhibitors of hydrolases occurring in foods, in Proc. Int. Conf. EURO FOOD TOX-II, Institute of Toxicology, Zürich, Switzerland, 1987, 92.
126. Buoconore, V., Petrucci, T., and Silano, V., Wheat protein inhibitors of α-amylase, *Phytochemistry*, 16, 811, 1977.
127. Boisen, S., Comparative physicochemical studies on purified trypsin inhibitors from the endosperm of barley, rye and wheat, *Z. Lebensm. Unters. Forsch.*, 176, 434, 1983.
128. Mikola, J. and Suolinna, E. M., Purification and properties of a trypsin inhibitor from barley, *Eur. J. Biochem.*, 9, 555, 1969.
129. Salcedo, G., Sanchez-Monge, R., Argamentaria, A., and Aragoncillo, C., The A-hordeins as a group of salt-soluble hydrophobic proteins, *Plant Sci. Lett.*, 19, 109, 1980.

130. Aragoncillo, C., Sanchez-Monge, R., and Salcedo, G., Two groups of low molecular weight hydrophobic proteins from barley endosperm, *J. Exp. Bot.,* 32, 1279, 1981.
131. Redman, D. G. and Fisher, N., Purothionin analogues from barley flour, *J. Sci. Food Agric.,* 20, 427, 1969.
132. Mak, A. S., Studies of the Primary Structures of Purothionins and Purothionin-Like Proteins from Cereals, Ph.D. thesis, University of Manitoba, Winnipeg, 1975.
133. Ozaki, Y., Wada, K., Hase, T., Matsubara, H., Nakanishi, T., and Yoshizumi, H., Amino acid sequence of a purothionin homolog from barley flour, *J. Biochem.,* 87, 549, 1980.
134. Békés, F. and Lásztity, R., Comparative analysis of the primary structure of grain thionins, *Acta Aliment.,* 10, 357, 1981.
135. Wu, Y. V., Sexson, K. R., and Sanderson, J. E., Barley protein concentrate from high-protein, high-lysine varieties, *J. Food Sci.,* 44, 1580, 1979.
136. Linko, R., Lapvetelainen, A., Lakso, P., and Kallio, H., Protein composition of a high-protein barley flour and barley grain, *Cereal Chem.,* 66, 478, 1989.
137. Sumner, A. K., Gebre-Egziabher, A., Tyler, T. R., and Rossnagel, B., Composition and properties of pearled and fines fractions from hulled and hull-less barley, *Cereal Chem.,* 62, 112, 1985.
138. Vose, J. R. and Youngs, C. G., The fractionation of barley and malted barley flours by air classification, *Cereal Chem.,* 55, 280, 1978.
139. Leah, R., Tommerup, H., Svensen, I., and Mundy, J., Biochemical and molecular characterization of barley seed proteins with antifungal properties, *J. Biol. Chem.,* 266, 1564, 1991.
140. Roberts, W. K. and Selitrennikoff, C. P., Isolation and partial characterization of two antifungal proteins from barley, *Biochim. Biophys. Acta,* 880, 161, 1986.
141. Lagemann, J., Jach, G., Tommerup, H., Mundy, J., and Shell, J., Expression of a barley ribosome inactivating protein leads to increased fungal protein in transgenic tomato plants, *Biotechnology,* 10, 305, 1992.
142. Martin, A. and Sanchez-Monge Laguna, E., Cytology and morphology of the amphiploid *Hordeum chilense* × *Triticum turgidum* conv. *durum, Euphytica,* 31, 262, 1982.
143. Cubero, I. L., Martin, A., Millan, T., Gomez, L., Cabrera, A., and de Haro, A., Tritordeum: a new alloploid of potential importance as a protein source crop, *Crop Sci.,* 26, 1186, 1986.
144. Ballesteros, I., Base Genetica del Contenido Proteico en Tritordeo, Ph.D. Thesis, Universidad de Cordoba, Cordoba, Spain, 1993.
145. McGregor, A. W. and Matsuo, R. R., Starch degradation in endosperm of barley and wheat kernels during initial stages of germination, *Cereal Chem.,* 59, 210, 1982.
146. Gibbons, G. C., On the localization and transport of α-amylase during germination and early seedling growth of *Hordeum vulgare, Carlsberg Res. Commun.,* 44, 353, 1979.
147. Gibbons, G. C., On the sequential determination of α-amylase transport and cell wall breakdown in germinating seeds of *Hordeum vulgare, Carlsberg Res. Commun.,* 45, 177, 1980.
148. Munck, L., Barley for food, feed and industry, in *Cereals: A Renewable Resource, Theory and Practice,* Munck, L., Ed., American Association of Cereal Chemists, St. Paul, MN, 1981, 427.

6 Maize Proteins

I. INTRODUCTION, GENERAL CHARACTERIZATION OF MAIZE PROTEINS

World maize production has increased rapidly in recent decades and has surpassed the 400 million tons/year level; together with wheat and rice it is the cereal produced in the greatest quantity. Every continent produces maize, but North America produces over 50% of the world's total. China is the main producer in Asia; France, Italy, Rumania and Hungary in Europe. Most maize is directly used for feeding. In developed countries over 90% of the maize produced or imported is used for animal feed. Among food uses of maize in these countries, sweet corn (consumed fresh, canned, dehydrated, or frozen), maize-based breakfast cereals (e.g., corn flakes), maize flour-containing mixtures, and popcorn snacks may be mentioned. Maize is widely used directly for human food in some parts of Asia, Africa, Latin America, and Eastern Europe. White maize is generally preferred for food use, although yellow maize is preferred for some products (e.g., polenta). Porridges are traditional foods in Latin American, Asian, and African countries. In Mexico 72% of total maize production is used for human food, mainly in the form of tortillas.

The maize kernel is the largest of all cereals. Kernels are usually flattened due to pressure from adjacent kernels during growth. An average dent maize kernel weighs 250 to 300 mg and measures about 4 mm thick, 8 mm wide, and 12 mm long. Variety and environment influence the shape and size.

Differences in size and shape of kernels are due to genetic background and also to placement on the ear. Kernels at the shank end are large and rounded, and those at the tip end are small and round. Their color may be white to orange, cherry red, red, dark red, brown, or variegated.

As with other cereal grains, the maize kernel has three main morphological parts: pericarp, endosperm, and embryo or germ. The pericarp constitutes about 6% of the whole kernel.[1] The endosperm comprises about 80 to 84% of the kernel. The outer layer of endosperm (aleurone layer) is richer in protein than the starchy endosperm, containing about 85% starch and 10% protein. Two types of starchy endosperm — horny (hard) and floury (soft) — are found beneath the aleurone layer. The horny endosperm is harder and contains more protein. The proportion of germ is the highest among the cereal grains — about 10%. This morphological part of the kernel is the richest in protein.

The five general classes of maize — dent corn, flint corn, sweet corn, popcorn, and flour corn — are based on kernel characteristics. In dent maize varieties the horny endosperm is found on the sides and back of the kernel. The floury endosperm fills the crown (upper part), extends downward to surround the germ, and shrinks as dent maize matures, causing an indentation at the top of the kernel. Flint corn has a rounded crown and the hardest kernels due to the presence of a large horny endosperm. Further details about maize kernel structure may be found in some monographs and review papers.[1-4]

The protein content of the whole kernel varies widely depending on the variety, agronomic conditions, and other factors and ranges from 6 to 18%.[1-5] Generally popcorn and sweet corn have a higher protein content than dent and flint corn. The protein contents of some dent maize hybrids grown in Hungary are summarized in Table 1. As reported,[2] the average protein content of corn purchased on the open market during the period 1980 to 1984 in Illinois, Iowa, and Indiana was 9.5%. Brazilian maize values, ranging from 8.94 to 12.50%, were reported by Mendes.[7] According to a recent publication[72] the average protein content of yellow maize grown in South Africa is 9.8% and that of white maize 9.7%.

TABLE 1
Protein Content of Maize Hybrids Grown in Hungary

		Growing Region				
Maize Hybrid	**Year**	**1**	**2**	**3**	**4**	**Ave.**
SzeTC	1974	10.5	10.2	10.9	9.9	10.5
255	1975	9.9	10.3	9.9	10.0	10.0
KSC	1974	10.1	10.3	10.2	9.5	10.0
360	1975	9.4	9.6	9.7	9.3	9.5
BC-SK	1974	10.9	10.4	9.9	10.3	10.4
22-25	1975	9.7	9.3	9.5	9.6	9.5
Ave.	1974	10.6	10.3	10.3	9.6	10.3
	1975	9.7	9.7	9.7	9.9	9.7

The protein content of the pericarp is the lowest (4 to 6%); the endosperm contains an average of 8 to 9% protein, and the proportion of protein in the embryo is the highest (17 to 20%). Although the concentration of protein is lower in endosperm than in the whole kernel, it contains about 75% of the kernel protein. Protein concentration decreases from the outer regions toward the center of the kernel.

For the extraction of maize proteins the procedure of Osborne is widely used, and on the basis of solubility, albumins, globulins, prolamins (zein), and glutelins may be separated. The proportions of the different fractions vary widely depending on the variety and agronomic conditions. The data published in the literature also vary widely (see Table 2). Nevertheless, it can be stated that the main protein components of the maize kernel are the storage proteins of the endosperm, which are practically identical to zein and corn glutelin.

TABLE 2
Distribution of the Solubility Fractions of Maize Proteins (% of Total Protein)

	Whole Kernel				Endosperm		Embryo	
Fraction	1	2	3	4	1	2	1	2
Albumins	8.0	15.6	10.9	22.0	4.0	7.8	30.0	77.2
Globulins	9.0	10.1	16.2		4.0		30.0	
Zeins	39.0	35.2	38.6	41.0	47.4	50.0	5.0	2.0
Glutelins	40.0	39.1	34.3	31.0	89.0	38.2	23.0	0.6
Residue	—	—	—	6.0	—	4.0	—	20.2
Reference	8	9	10	15	8	15	8	15

The great differences between the data of different authors probably can be connected to the technical difficulties and differences in the extraction of the various fractions (see Chapter 2). Among the extraction procedures used in the investigation of maize proteins, the procedures of Mertz et al.[69] may be mentioned. Landry and Moureaux[11,12] developed a quite different method of extraction and fractionation. After extraction of the salt-soluble proteins and zeins by the classical Osborne method, 2-mercaptoethanol was systematically added to the solvents used for glutelin subgroup extraction. After treatment with β-mercaptoethanol three glutelin subgroups were extracted — with alcohol-water (G1), alkaline buffer solution (G2), and SDS solution (G3). An advantage of the procedure was its exhaustivity. Only about 5% of the total nitrogen remained unextracted. A somewhat different procedure was used by Paulis and Wall.[13,14] After discarding salt-soluble proteins, zeins were extracted by means of an alcoholic solution containing 0.5% sodium acetate. They added a reducing agent to the remaining mixture, and the glutelins were fractionated by dialysis into water-insoluble and water-soluble glutelins.

The amino acid composition of the total protein of the maize kernel is characterized by a low content of lysine and tryptophan (see Table 3).

Since Mertz et al.[19] discovered the high-lysine corn opaque-2, considerable effort has been expended to develop hybrids with high-quality proteins. Unfortunately, different problems such as lower grain yields, higher moisture content, and susceptibility to certain pests hindered the commercial acceptability of the opaque-2 hybrids. Nevertheless, some newer breeding results show that opaque-2 hybrids with higher yield and hard vitreous endosperm may be developed.[20,24] The higher lysine content of the opaque-2 mutants is related to the fact that in these mutants the synthesis of zein (the protein fraction with the lowest lysine content) is suppressed.[21-25] As a result of the lower zein content, the amino acid composition of high-lysine mutants is different from that of normal maize. Some data have been collected in Table 4. The high-lysine mutants have not only a higher lysine content, but also lower glutamic acid and proline contents.

TABLE 3
Amino Acid Composition of the Protein of Maize Kernel (g/100 g Protein)

Amino Acid	Maize Grain[a]	Opaque-2 Grain Endosperm[b]	Normal Grain Endosperm[c]	Total Grain
Lysine	2.6	3.4	2.0	3.0
Histidine	2.8	3.4	2.8	3.1
Arginine	3.8	5.1	3.8	4.5
Aspartic acid + asparagine	8.2	8.5	6.2	7.6
Glutamic acid + glutamine	26.9	19.1	21.3	19.7
Threonine	3.6	3.9	3.5	3.1
Serine	4.8	5.0	5.2	5.8
Tyrosine	4.4	4.7	5.3	4.4
Proline	8.3	9.4	9.7	9.9
Glycine	3.4	4.0	3.2	3.7
Alanine	7.9	7.0	8.1	8.3
Valine	5.3	5.0	4.7	4.2
Methionine	1.8	2.0	2.8	1.9
Isoleucine	3.7	3.9	3.8	3.6
Leucine	13.6	11.6	14.3	12.7
Phenylalanine	5.1	4.7	5.3	4.9
Tryptophan	0.7	ND	ND	1.2
Cystine	1.1	2.4	1.8	—

Note: ND, not determined.

[a] From Baudet et al.[16]
[b] From Mertz et al.[17]
[c] From El Kady.[18]

The amount of zein, the major maize endosperm storage protein, is also reduced in seeds with the homozygous sugary-1 *(su)* mutation, the gene for common sweet maize.[26-28] When used as a feed for poultry, maize supplemented with soybean meal is deficient in methionine. This fact stimulated the search for maize variants with increased endosperm methionine concentrations. The biochemical basis and some initial results of these investigations are reviewed by Phillips and McLure.[29]

II. STORAGE PROTEINS OF MAIZE

A. Low Molecular Weight Storage Proteins (Zeins)

According to Osborne's classification *zein* is the alcohol-soluble protein of maize endosperm. The name *native zein,* or zein-I, is also used, making the difference

TABLE 4
Amino Acid Compositions of Some High-Lysine Maize Mutants

	Mutant				
Amino Acid	**Oh43 O_2[a]**	**W22[a]**	**O_2[b]**	**bt_2[b]**	**su_2[b]**
Lysine	3.5	3.8	3.7	3.3	3.0
Tryptophan	0.8	0.7	0.8	0.7	0.6
Leucine	12.1	12.5	9.8	11.8	12.1
Isoleucine	4.3	4.3	3.2	3.9	5.0
Threonine	4.4	4.4	3.6	3.9	3.4
Methionine	2.7	3.2	1.2	1.4	1.4
Cystine	2.1	1.9	2.1	1.5	1.5
Phenylalanine	6.0	5.2	4.0	4.9	4.2
Tyrosine	5.2	4.9	—	—	—
Valine	5.9	6.7	5.8	5.6	5.1
Histidine	3.4	4.1	3.6	2.6	2.7
Arginine	5.1	5.2	5.7	4.2	4.0
Glycine	4.9	5.2	—	—	—
Alanine	8.2	7.9	—	—	—
Serine	5.4	5.6	—	—	—
Aspartic acid	9.5	9.4	—	—	—
Glutamic acid	23.6	25.5	—	—	—
Proline	9.8	11.0	—	—	—

[a] From Misra et al.[31]
[b] From Sysoyev.[32]

between protein extracted with ethanol (or propanol) and the protein fraction solubilized using ethanol + β-mercaptoethanol (or some other disulfide bond reducing agent) this is also called *total zein*. When the residue obtained after sequential extraction (according to the procedure of Osborne) of albumins, globulins, and zein is treated with ethanol + reducing agent, some portion of the glutelins may be extracted. Several authors call this protein fraction *zein-II* or *alcohol-soluble reduced glutelin* (ASG). A review concerning the nomenclature of zeins is given by Wilson.[30]

In the framework of this chapter the properties of the protein fraction extracted with ethanol (without a reducing agent) will be discussed. Early work on zein was reviewed by Mossé.[33] More recent reviews were published by Wall and Paulis,[34] Mossé and Landry,[35] Wilson,[30] and Tatham et al.[36]

Zein is also soluble in other alcohols. Isopropanol may especially be used successfully.[37] Glacial acetic acid, phenol, and some other organic solvents (e.g., diethylene glycol) are also suitable, but these are not widely applied. For the preparation of relatively pure zein an extraction with an isopropanol/water mixture free of salt and reducing agents is recommended.[35]

After washing the extract with petroleum ether, zein is salted out, chromatographed on Sephadex LH-20, and lyophilized from a solution of aqueous tertiary butyl alcohol.

The heterogeneity of zein was detected even in early investigations using solvent fractionation procedures. On the basis of the differences in solubility, two zein components were isolated: α-zein, soluble in 95% ethanol, and β-zein, soluble in 60% ethanol.[38] Significant differences in amino acid composition were observed between α- and β-zeins[38] (see Table 5). α-Zein contains less histidine, arginine, proline, and methionine than β-zein.

TABLE 5
Amino Acid Composition of Zein Preparations (g/100 g Protein)[39]

Amino Acid	Total	Zein α	Zein β
Lysine	0.1	0.0	0.2
Histidine	2.6	1.8	3.3
Ammonia	4.4	5.1	3.9
Arginine	3.1	2.6	3.6
Aspartic acid	4.2	4.4	3.9
Threonine	2.6	2.2	2.7
Serine	4.5	4.4	4.6
Glutamic acid	24.2	23.1	24.8
Proline	8.9	7.1	10.1
Glycine	1.3	0.9	1.8
Alanine	8.4	7.9	8.0
Valine	3.4	3.1	3.5
Methionine	1.3	0.5	2.4
Isoleucine	3.5	3.2	3.4
Leucine	17.7	17.0	17.0
Tyrosine	4.3	3.3	4.9
Phenylalanine	6.0	5.6	5.7

The crude zein as well as purified preparations showed heterogeneity when fractionated on Sephadex G-100 and G-200 columns. As reported by Mossé and Landry,[35] gel filtration chromatography of crude and purified samples of zein preparations performed on Sephadex G-200 columns in 8 *M* urea at pH 3.5 yielded two major peaks.

Characteristic elution profiles of the zeins extracted from two maize hybrids are shown in Figure 1.[44] The separation achieved by Sephadex columns is relatively poor. A more effective separation may be assured with ion-exchange chromatography on phosphocellulose and sulfopropyl Sephadex.[45,46] Whole zein (extracted with 60%

isopropanol) was dissolved in a lactate-ethylene glycol-isopropanol buffer (pH 3.8) containing mercaptoethanol, loaded on phosphocellulose columns, and eluted by a gradient of NaCl in the same buffer. It was reported that the elution profile had 12 overlapping peaks. An additional fractionation by gel electrophoresis showed the heterogeneity of all peaks. The reduced and alkylated α-zein was also fractionated on sulfopropyl Sephadex columns. The elution profile obtained had about 10 peaks.

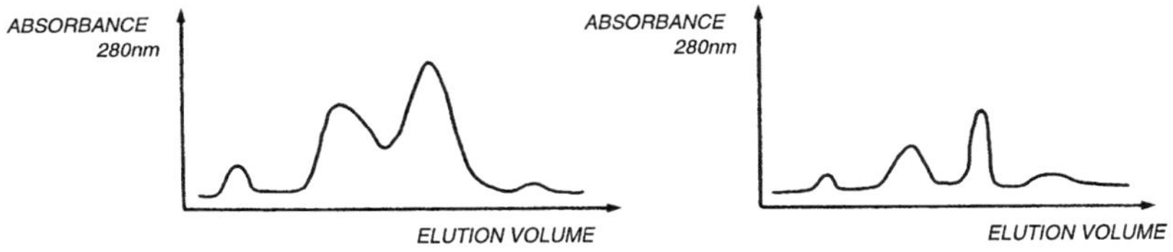

FIGURE 1 Elution profiles of the zeins of two maize hybrids. (From El Kady, A. and Lásztity, R., *Gabonaipar,* 29, 94, 1982. With permission.)

A very effective separation may be realized by using an HPLC (RP-HPLC) technique[47,48] (Figure 2).

The fractionation of zein components by gel electrophoresis is one of the most effective separation procedures. SDS-PAGE of the zein fraction extracted with aqueous alcohol (but without a reducing agent) shows two major bands and some minor ones with low mobilities. Molecular weights varying from 19,000 to 22,000 for the faster, major band and from 22,000 to 26,000 for the slower band have been determined by SDS-PAGE. The common practice of naming the bands by apparent molecular masses can lead to confusion because different laboratories have applied overlapping estimates of molecular mass to the polypeptides of the two bands. Therefore Wilson[30] proposed the name A-zein for the larger, slower-moving zein and B-zein for the smaller, faster-moving ones. In the recent literature[36] the nomenclature of Argos et al.[49] is recommended and the two major zein components are named Z19 and Z22. The low-mobility minor bands have higher molecular weights. If zein is treated with reducing agents before electrophoresis only the two major bands may be observed. This fact suggests that higher molecular weight bands contain aggregates composed of A and B monomers linked by disulfide bonds.

This suggestion may be confirmed, e.g., by the results reported by Mossé and Landry.[35] They resolved the purified zein from a hybrid maize in several bands using SDS-PAGE. Along with the major bands, with apparent molecular weights of about 22 and 24 kDa, slow-moving bands with a molecular weight of around 45 kDa were also observed. When the sample was pretreated with 2-mercaptoethanol, slow-moving bands in the 45-kDa region disappeared and the relative intensity of the 22 to 24-kDa bands increased. The apparent sizes of the low-mobility component suggest that this is a dimer composed of A or B monomers linked by disulfide bonds. The presence of trimers and sometimes even larger oligomers is also possible.[30,50]

Both major bands are in fact mixtures of related compounds. They could be separated by isoelectric focusing (IEF) or — more effectively — by two-dimensional gel electrophoresis (IEF/SDS-PAGE).

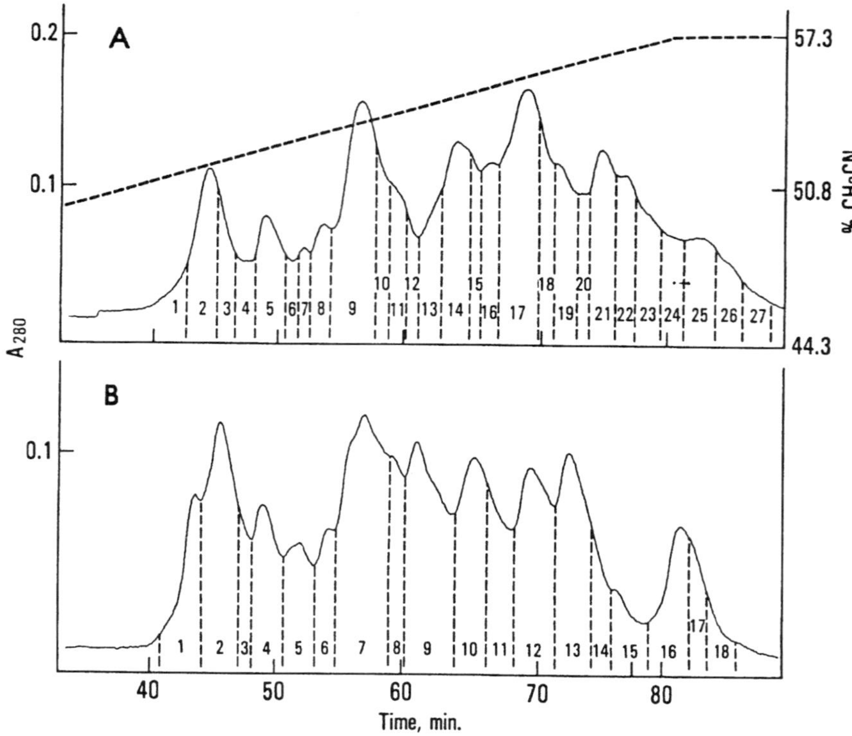

FIGURE 2 Reversed phase high-performance liquid chromatography of (A) native and (B) reduced and alkylated zein, dissolved in 8 *M* urea, on SynChropak RP-P(C_{16}) using a linear gradient from 42.3 to 57.3% CH_3CN (+0.1% CF_3COOH). (From Paulis, J.W. and Bietz, J.A., *Cereal Chem.,* 65, 215, 1988. With permission.)

Research workers[51-53] separated 25 individual polypeptides from the zein preparations. Wilson et al.,[54] using two-dimensional separation (first isoelectric focusing, then SDS-PAGE), fractionated zein into 22 different polypeptide spots. A minor protein fraction named reduced soluble protein was extracted from either the salt-soluble fraction or the total zein fraction, depending on which solvent contained a reducing agent. The reduced soluble protein has a unique amino acid composition with much more proline, histidine, cysteine, glycine, and valine and less aspartate, alanine, glutamic acid, and leucine than zein. This protein is also low in lysine (see Table 6).

Summarizing the results of the electrophoretic investigations, it can be stated that the reduced and alkylated zein may be separated into up to 25 to 30 components belonging to two major groups having molecular weights of about 22 and 24 kDa, respectively. The large number of bands obtained by different electrophoretic techniques, the similarities and differences in amino acid composition of different zein preparations, and the fairly simple molecular size distribution of zein led some authors[53,55] to consider reasons for the observed heterogeneity. They concluded that

TABLE 6
Amino Acid Composition of Reduced Soluble (Rs) Protein of Maize and Zein (μmol/100 μg)

Amino Acid	RS Protein[a] 1	RS Protein[a] 2	Zein[b]	Zein[c]
Lysine	0.4	0.1	0.1	0.5
Histidine	7.0	8.0	0.9	0.9
Arginine	2.2	2.9	1.0	2.4
Aspartic acid	0.7	0.2	5.1	5.5
Threonine	4.3	1.7	2.9	2.4
Serine	4.3	0.2	6.0	6.3
Glutamic acid	16.5	18.5	20.7	25.7
Proline	23.4	28.1	10.8	10.2
Glycine	7.8	8.1	2.2	1.7
Alanine	5.3	6.2	13.7	10.9
PE (cysteine)	3.7	—	0.3	—
Valine	6.4	9.1	4.4	2.1
Methionine	0.5	0.2	0.8	1.8
Isoleucine	2.9	2.3	4.0	3.5
Leucine	9.5	11.9	19.2	17.3
Tyrosine	3.1	0.9	3.2	3.1
Phenylalaninc	2.0	1.4	4.9	5.3
Tryptophan	—	—	—	0.6

[a] From Wilson et al.[54]
[b] From Sodek and Wilson.[55]
[c] From El Kady.[18]

spot mutations in genes for zein synthesis, deriving from a common ancestral gene, were primarily responsible for the observed heterogeneity of zein. It was supposed that some *in vivo* cellular deamidation was also possible. An almost total lack of selective pressure against diversification of genes controlling zein synthesis must exist, similar to the mutations to which are attributed the heterogeneity and homology of wheat gliadin. In addition, it was also supposed that the two major zein subunit classes must be homologous. The more recent results on the molecular biology of zeins will be discussed later in this chapter.

Concerning the zein group component with low electrophoretic mobility it may be stated that some components consisting of monomers linked by disulfide bonds are present.

The minor high molecular weight bands extracted with ethanol and appearing on the electropherogram of zein are also mixtures of different aggregates of AA, AB, and BB, for example.

The amino acid compositions of the Z19 (A-zein) and Z22 (B-zein) groups of polypeptides are both characterized by a relatively low content of proline (9 to 10 mol%), but high glutamate plus glutamine (20 mol%), leucine (18 to 20 mol%), and alanine (12 to 24 mol%). Tryptophan is absent (Table 7).

TABLE 7
Amino Acid Composition of Zein (Extracted Without Reducing Agent) and the Two Major Groups (A [Z19] or B [Z 22]) of Zein Polypeptides (mol%)

Amino Acid	Zein (A+B)	A-Zein	B-Zein	Z22[a]	Z19[b]
ASP	5.1	5.7	5.7	0.00	0.0–0.1
THR	3.0	3.1	3.1	3–4	2–3
SER	6.3	6.4	7.4	7–8	7–8
GLU	21.4	21.4	20.7	0.5–1	0.4
PRO	10.7	8.7	10.0	8–9	9–10
GLY	2.2	2.5	2.9	1–2	1–2
ALA	13.3	13.6	13.2	14–15	13–15
CYS	1.0	0.8	0.4	0.5	1
VAL	3.6	5.6	3.2	6–7	2–3
MET	0.9	1.3	0.4	2	0–0.5
ILE	3.8	3.7	3.6	3–5	4–5
LEU	18.7	18.4	18.7	17–19	17–20
TYR	3.5	2.7	3.2	3–4	3
PHE	5.2	3.7	5.3	3–4	5–6
HIS	1.0	1.1	1.1	1–2	0.5–1
LYS	0.1	0.2	0.4	0	0
ARG	1.2	1.1	1.1	1–2	1–2
TRP	ND	0.0	0.0	0.0	0.0
ASN	ND	ND	ND	5–6	4–5
GLN	ND	ND	ND	20–22	19–21
Reference	56	57	57	58	59–62

[a] Range of values.
[b] Recalculated from residue/mol.

Bietz[63] separated zein into 16 or more peaks by RP-HPLC, using acetonitrile as the major solvent. When individual fractions were run on IEF gels, additional heterogeneity was found. Separation was largely on the basis of surface hydrophobicity, providing another characteristic of proteins that can be used in classification.

The rapid development of genetics and nucleic acid research led to new ways to investigate maize proteins: the isolation of mRNAs coding for zein polypeptides and the *in vitro* translation of these mRNAs. Isolation, purification, and *in vitro* translation of zein mRNAs were realized by Burr et al.,[64] Viotti et al.,[65] Wienand and Feix,[66] and Larkins et al.[67] Duplex DNAs were synthesized enzymatically using purified zein mRNAs as the template material, and restriction endonuclease fractions of maize DNA were investigated.[68,70] The results of these investigations confirmed that zein is a multigene family composed of sequences with limited heterogeneity.[70] Although zein is being synthesized in large amounts in the endosperm at mid-development, no rearrangements or amplifications of genomic endosperm sequences seem to be implicated.

When duplex DNAs were synthesized enzymatically using purified zein mRNAs as template material and inserted into a bacterial plasmid vector, recombinant clones were obtained containing zein sequences hybridized specifically to mRNAs encoding polypeptides in either the light or the heavy zein class.[70] The clones might be divided into two heavy class subgroups and at least three light class subgroups. The protein sequence of a representative of zeins has been derived from the nucleotide sequence of a zein cDNA clone by Geraghty et al.[59] The first published complete amino acid sequence of a plant storage protein is shown in Figure 3.

The possible differences in quality between the storage proteins of normal and high-lysine maize were also investigated.[71,75,78] The view that high-lysine maize endosperm contains lower amounts of zein because of decreased zein biosynthesis is widely accepted. The reduced zein content of high-lysine mutants was reported by many research workers. A screening method based on the determination of zein content was proposed by Esen.[45] A summary of the earlier research work was given in the review by Wall and Paulis.[34] Earlier electrophoretic investigations could distinguish no qualitative differences in the electrophoretic patterns of near isogenic normal and high-lysine endosperm zeins, although quantitative differences in some bands occurred. On the basis of more recent investigations it was reported that patterns obtained by the isoelectric focusing of zeins from an O_2 mutant exhibited fewer of the more alkaline components than the isogenic normal zein. It was also found that opaque-2 zein has less of the high molecular weight component separated by SDS-PAGE than zein from isogenic normal maize. Some results of the investigation of the zeins of the high-lysine mutants opaque-2 and floury-2 were published by Paulis.[71] It was stated that SDS-PAGE and PAGE confirmed that the whole zeins from the endosperms of the near isogenic normal opaque-2 and floury-2 maizes are qualitatively similar to the zein patterns from normal endosperm, but some quantitative differences may occur. Native zeins from all mutant endosperms also lacked protein migrating at 22-kDa molecular weight and contained 20,000-mol wt subunits, but had a smaller proportion of 24-kDa subunits than did normal zein.

Since the first complete amino acid sequence of a zein polypeptide was reported by Geraghty et al.,[59] as a result of the work of several research groups today the majority of structural genes coding for zein polypeptides are now known, and based on known DNA sequences; the amino acid sequences of several individual polypeptides have also been determined.

The structural genes of zeins appear to be located on three different chromosomes.[15,36,50,85] Seven genes coding for Z19 polypeptides are present in the region

```
   MET ALA ALA LYS ILE PHE CYS LEU LEU MET LEU LEU GLY LEU SER
CA ATG GCA GCC AAA ATA TTT TGC CTC CTT ATG CTC CTT GGT CTT TCT

   ALA SER ALA ALA THR ALA THR ILE PHE PRO GLN CYS SER GLN ALA
   GCA AGT GCT GCT ACG GCG ACC ATT TTC CCG CAA TGC TCA CAA GCT

   PRO ILE ALA SER LEU LEU PRO PRO TYR LEU SER PRO ALA VAL SER
   CCT ATA GCT TCC CTT CTT CCC CCG TAC CTC TCA CCA GCG GTG TCT

   SER VAL CYS GLU ASN PRO ILE LEU GLN PRO TYR ARG ILE GLN GLN
   TCG GTA TGT GAA AAC CCA ATT CTT CAA CCC TAC AGG ATC CAA CAG

   ALA ILE ALA ALA GLY ILE LEU PRO LEU SER PRO LEU PHE LEU GLN
   GCA ATC GCA GCT GGC ATC TTA CCT TTA TCA CCC TTG TTC CTC CAA

   GLN SER SER ALA LEU LEU GLN GLN LEU PRO LEU VAL HIS LEU LEU
   CAA TCA TCA GCC CTA TTA CAG CAG TTA CCT TTG GTG CAT TTA TTG

   ALA GLN ASN ILE ARG ALA GLN GLN LEU GLN GLN LEU VAL LEU ALA
   GCA CAA AAC ATC AGG GCA CAA CAA CTA CAA CAA CTT GTG CTA GCA

   ASN LEU ALA ALA TYR SER GLN GLN GLN GLN PHE LEU PRO PHE ASN
   AAC CTT GCT GCC TAC TCT CAG CAA CAG CAG TTT CTT CCA TTC AAC

   GLN LEU ALA ALA LEU ASN SER ALA SER TYR LEU GLN GLN GLN GLN
   CAA CTA GCT GCA TTG AAC TCT GCT TCT TAT TTG CAA CAA CAA CAA

   LEU PRO PHE SER GLN LEU PRO ALA ALA TYR PRO GLN GLN PHE LEU
   CTA CCA TTC AGC CAG CTA CCT GCT GCC TAC CCC CAG CAA TTT CTT

   ALA ALA LEU ASN SER PRO GLU ASN GLN LEU PRO ALA TYR LEU GLN
   GCA GCA TTG AAC TCT CCA TTC AAC CAA CTG CCT GCT TAT TTA CAG

   GLN GLN GLN LEU LEU PRO PHE SER GLN LEU ALA GLY VAL SER PRO
   CAG CAA CAA CTA CTA CCA TTC AGC CAG CTA GCT GGT GTG AGC CCT

   ALA THR PHE LEU THR GLN PRO GLN LEU LEU PRO PHE TYR GLN HYS
   GCT ACC TTC TTG ACA CAA CCA CAG TTG TTG CCG TTC TAC CAG CAC

   ALA ALA PRO ASN ALA GLY THR LEU LEU GLN LEU GLN GLN LEU LEU
   GCT GCG CCT AAC GCT GGC ACC CTC TTA CAA CTG CAA CAA TTG CTG

   PRO PHE ASN GLN LEU ALA LEU THR ASN LEU ALA ALA PHE TYR GLN
   CCA TTC AAC CAA CTT GCT TTG ACA AAC CTA GCA GCG TTC TAC CAA

   GLN PRO ILE ILE GLY GLY ALA LEU PHE STOP
   CAA CCC ATC ATT GGT GGT GCC CTC TTT TAG ATT TCT TAT GAG TTA

   TAG TTC AAT AAT AAA GTT TTT TGT CTG ATG TTT GTG GCT TCC CAG
   AAA TAA GAA AGT ACA TTT CTA GAT TCT (polyA)
```

FIGURE 3 The nucleotide sequence of a zein cDNA and the deduced amino acid sequence. (From Geraghty, D., Peifer, M.A., Rubinstein, J., and Messing, J., *Nucl. Acids Res.,* 9, 5163, 1981. With permission.)

of about 30 crossover units on the short arm of chromosome 7, and nine genes coding for Z22 polypeptides and three coding for Z19 polypeptides are scattered on both arms of chromosome 4. Structural genes of zeins were found on chromosome 10, too.[79,80] Estimates of the number of genes for zein range up to 100, though not all would be present in any one inbred strain.[81] The suggestion has been made that different numbers of copies of each gene are present, possibly leading to variable levels of the different polypeptides. Heidecker and Messing[82] recognized four subfamilies of genes for Z19 and Z22 zeins, based on the hybridization of their messenger RNAs with cloned DNAs. Two subfamilies encode predominantly Z19 zeins and one encodes predominantly Z22 zeins. The fourth encodes mostly Z19 zeins, but also some Z22 components. Recently the genetic basis of the regulation of synthesis of individual polypeptides influencing their ratios has also been studied.[83,84]

Determination of the nucleotide sequences of cDNA clones allowed the amino acid sequences of the encoded proteins to be deduced. The Z19 cDNA and genomic DNA clones encode proteins with 210 to 220 amino acid residues, and the Z22 clones encode proteins with 240 to 245 residues.[59,60,62,86,89] The Z19 and Z22 zeins have similar amino acid sequences. The consensus sequences of three domains of zein polypeptides are shown in Figure 4, based on data of Larkins[86] and Messing.[87]

AMINO TERMINAL SEQUENCE (36)

SER—ILE—PHE—PRO—GLN—CYS—SER—GLN
PRO—LEU—LEU—SER—ALA—ILE—PRO—ALA
PRO—TYR—LEU—PRO—PRO—VAL—MET—SER
LEU—ALA—PRO—ASN—GLU—CYS—VAL—SER
GLN—PRO—TYR—ARG

REPEATING SEQUENCE (9×20)

GLN—GLN—LEU—LEU—PRO—PHE—ASN
SER—ASN—ALA—ALA—ALA—LEU—GLN
PRO—ALA—TYR—LEU—GLN—GLN

CARBOXY TERMINAL SEQUENCE (10 or 29)

GLN—GLN—GLN—LEU—LEU—PRO—TYR—ASN—ARG
SER—LEU—VAL—PRO—ASN—MET—LEU—SER—PHE
ARG—GLN—GLN—PRO—ILE—ILE—GLY—GLY—ALA
PHE—LEU

FIGURE 4 Consensus sequence of the three domains in the Z19 zeins.[36,86,87]

The sequences have nonrepetitive domains at the N- and C-termini, with a central repetitive domain. The Z19 zeins have nine repeated blocks of about 20 amino acids, and the Z22 zeins have either 10 or 9, depending on how the sequence is interpreted. This repeat motif is longer than that in the prolamins of wheat, rye, and barley. The structural organization of typical Z19 and Z22 zeins is shown in Figure 5, based on data of Messing[88] and Prat et al.[89] The N-terminal domains in the Z19 and Z22 clones are clearly homologous, and the first 10 residues appear to be the most conserved, with only two differences between the two sequences. The remaining part of the N-terminal domain is less conserved. The central part of the zein polypeptide consists of tandem repeats of a sequence of about 20 residues. The main size difference between these two groups is due to an insertion of 19 residues in the C-terminal region of the Z22 zein. This results in an increase in the size of the C-terminal domain from 10 to 29 residues. Apart from the position of the glutamine residues, the first two repeats bear little structural relationship to the succeeding seven. The N-terminus contains almost all of the charged residues and one (Z22 zeins) or two (Z19 zeins) cysteine residues.

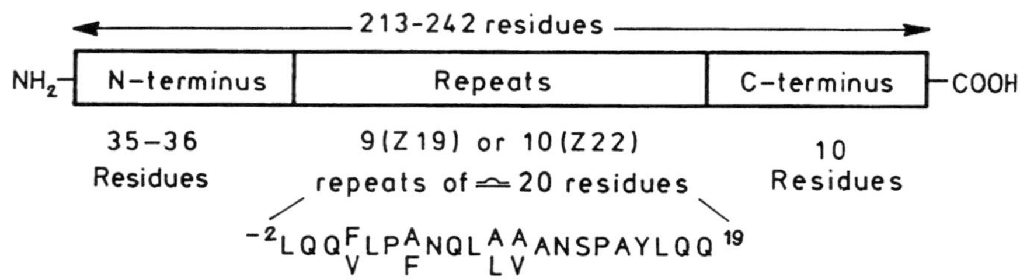

FIGURE 5 Typical structural organization of Z19 and Z22 zeins.[36]

The early conformational studies of zein (reviewed by Tatham et al.[36]) agreed that zeins are asymmetric molecules, approximating prolate ellipsoids or rods. More recent studies[90] using optical rotatory dispersion (ORD) and circular dichroism (CD) techniques suggest that the average α-helical portion amounts to about 45% of the zein molecule. The proportion of β-sheets is about 15%, and the remainder of the molecule is aperiodic.

Argos et al.[49] have proposed an interesting model for the molecular conformation of zeins (Figure 6). This structural model is based on the presence of nine homologous repeat units in Z19 and Z22. The additional blocks of residues in the Z22 zeins show sufficient homology with the repeating units to be considered a 10th repeat by other workers.[88] Their consensus sequence for the repeat units in the Z19 and Z22 zeins is shown in Figure 7.

This sequence is flanked by glutamine residues and has alternating blocks of polar residues (underlined) and hydrophobic residues. The authors suggested, based on the hydration potential, polarity, and secondary structure properties of the residues, that each of these repeat units forms an α-helix, with positions -2, -1, and 19 constituting turn regions. When these units are displayed as an α-helical wheel, three

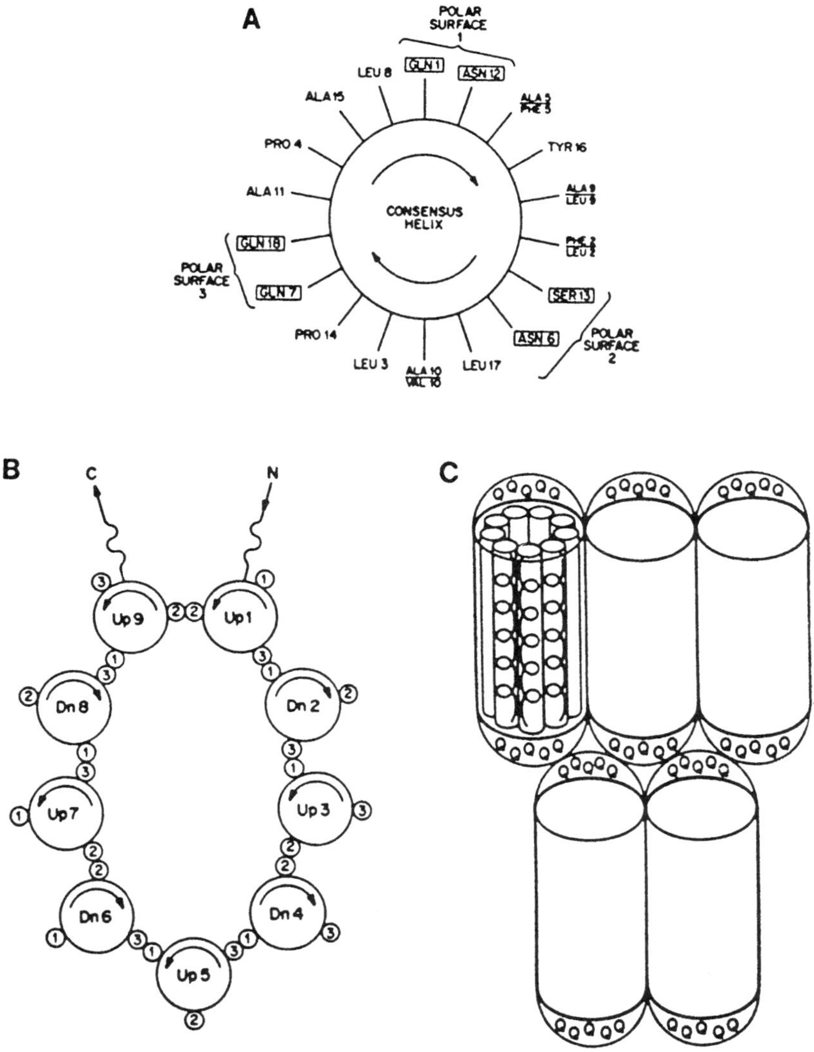

FIGURE 6 The structural model for zein. (A) Helical wheel representation of the consensus repetitive sequences of the Z19 and Z22 zeins. The three polar regions are indicated by brackets. (B) A possible nine-helix zein protein with the helical axis orthogonal to the plane of the figure. The hydrogen bonding polar segments (shown as small circles) are numbered as in helical wheel shown in part A. "Up" and "Dn" indicate directions of the antiparallel helices. (C) Possible model for arrangement of zein proteins within and between planes, with hydrogen bonding between glutamine residues in the turn regions between the helices. (From Argos, P., Pedersen, K., Marks, M.D., and Larkins, B.A., *J. Biol. Chem.,* 257, 988, 1982. With permission.)

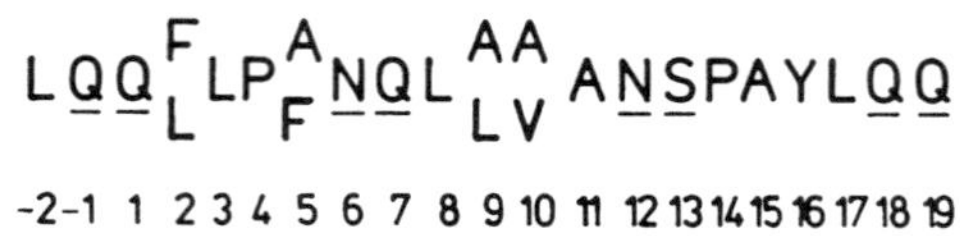

FIGURE 7 Consensus sequence for the 18 repeat units present in the Z19 and Z22 components.[49]

polar segments are revealed, corresponding to residues 1 and 12, 7 and 18, and 6 and 13, as shown in Figure 6A.

Argos et al.[49] further suggest that the nine helices are arranged in an antiparallel ring, stabilized by intramolecular hydrogen bonds involving residues on two of the three polar segments (Figure 6B). This arrangement would leave the third polar segment free to form intermolecular hydrogen bonds with other zein molecules in the same planes (Figure 6C). The model predicts that the protein molecule would be only slight asymmetric, which is not consistent with the results of earlier investigations.

B. High Molecular Weight Storage Proteins (Maize glutelins)

1. Extraction and Separation

The alkali-soluble portion of the maize endosperm proteins (to be extracted from residue remaining after solubilization of water-, salt-, and alcohol-soluble proteins according to Osborne's procedure) is not as precisely defined as the zein fraction. In the widest sense the glutelin fraction contains all the endosperm proteins remaining after the extraction of the salt- and alcohol-soluble proteins. In this definition the glutelin fraction is composed not only of storage proteins, but also of some structural proteins (membrane proteins, complex proteins, and cell wall proteins). The extraction of proteins with alkaline solutions may cause degradation of the proteins. First of all, cystine and arginine may be degraded, and the glutamine side chains may be partially deamidated. Alternative solvents and extraction procedures causing no degradation were also investigated, but each of the investigated solvents removed only small amounts of the glutelin proteins. Because of the difficulties in the extraction of glutelin proteins, methods based on the addition of reducing agents (for splitting the disulfide bonds) have recently been widely used. The procedures of Landry and Moureaux[11,12] and Mertz et al.[69] are described in the previous section of this chapter. To prevent further reoxidation of the thiol groups and the formation of new disulfide bonds, most of the reduced glutelin peptides are alkylated. Detergent solutions containing reducing agents (2-mercaptoethanol, sulfite) dissolve practically all of the proteins of maize. The reduced glutelin proteins may be effectively solubilized by SDS solutions. A procedure using reducing agent-containing solvents[54] is shown in Figure 8. The native glutelin may be separated by gel filtration chromatography into several components using Sepharose columns. In Figure 9 some elution profiles of different glutelin preparations are shown. The separation is in general relatively poor.

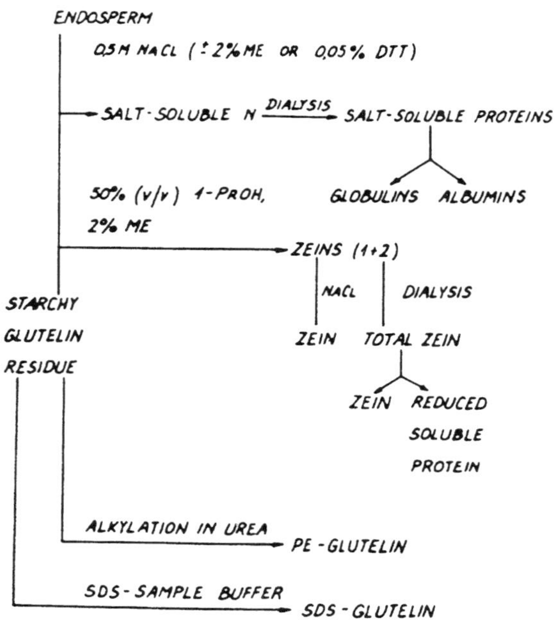

FIGURE 8 A combined procedure for extraction of maize proteins using reducing agent-containing solvents. ME = mercaptoethanol; DTT = dithiothreitol. (From Wilson, C.M., Shewry, P.R., and Miflin, B.J., *Cereal Chem.,* 58, 275, 1981. With permission.)

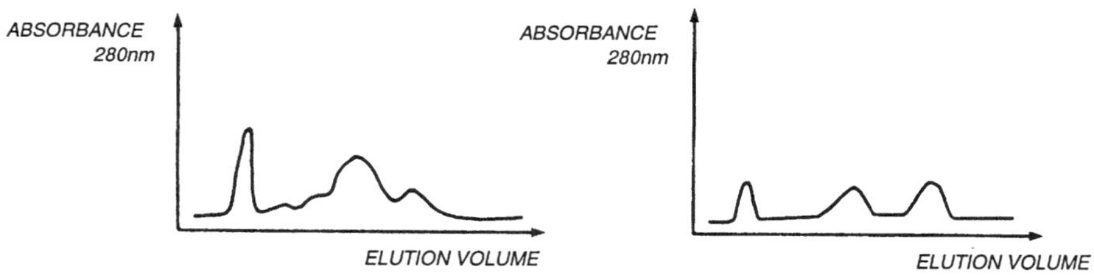

FIGURE 9 Characteristic elution profiles of the glutelins of two maize hybrids on Sepharose 4B columns. (From El Kady, A. and Lásztity, R., *Gabonaipar,* 29, 94, 1982. With permission.)

The reduced (and alkylated) glutelins may be separated in different ways. In the Landry-Moureaux procedure[11,12] three fractions (G_1, G_2, and G_3 glutelins) were separated on the basis of different solubility (G_1 being soluble in alcohol containing 2-mercaptoethanol, G_2 being soluble in pH 10 buffer with 2-mercaptoethanol, and G_3 being soluble in pH 10 buffer containing 2-mercaptoethanol and SDS). The term alcohol-soluble reduced glutelin (ASG) is also used, with a subsequent division into water-soluble and water-insoluble components.[14] The reduced glutelins may be separated by gel filtration chromatography. Using Sephadex G-200 columns and 6 *M* guanidine hydrochloride, six components (A, B, C, D, E, and F) were separated by Paulis and Wall.[92] Based on the elution values of reduced and alkylated proteins of known molecular weight, the molecular weights of the reduced glutelin fractions were >70, 70, 53, 38, 25, and 17.5 kDa. Esen et al.[93] fractionated the alcohol-soluble reduced maize glutelins on phosphocellulose columns. Eight different fractions were obtained having molecular weights ranging from 20 to 30 kDa.

Recently RP-HPLC has also been used for separation of reduced glutelins[63,94] and for variety identification.[95,98]

As is the case with other cereal proteins, the best separation of the subunits of maize glutelin may be achieved by gel electrophoresis.[96,97,99] The electrophoretic studies of glutelin subunits revealed the presence of a number of other types of polypeptides in addition to Z19 and Z22. The whole reduced glutelin consists of at least 20 components ranging in molecular weight from 11 to 120 kDa. Some of bands are very similar to those of the native zeins. Comparison of the electrophoretic patterns of glutelin polypeptides and those of salt-soluble proteins also revealed a similarity of several bands.[54] These observations raised several questions, including the following:

1. Are they specific glutelin polypeptides, and if so, are these polypeptides homologous?
2. Are some zein polypeptides included in the macromolecules of maize glutelin?
2. Are part of the polypeptides separated from reduced glutelin identical to the polypeptides obtained by PAGE of salt-soluble proteins?

2. Amino Acid Composition and Structure of High Molecular Weight Storage Proteins (Glutelins) of Maize

The amino acid compositions of some glutelin preparations and of some subfractions of the glutelins are shown in Tables 8 and 9. In comparison with zein the glutelin has higher lysine, arginine, histidine, and tryptophan contents, but lower quantities of glutamic acid. The amino acid composition of ASG is similar to that of zein, but amounts of histidine, arginine, proline, glycine, and methionine are higher in ASG, whereas those of leucine, isoleucine, aspartic acid, and phenylalanine are higher in zein. The proline-rich fractions obtained from alcohol-soluble glutenin have an interesting amino acid composition.

Concerning the molecular structure of maize glutelin it may be stated that these proteins consist of different polypeptides which have diverse properties and which are linked by disulfide bonds. This view is widely accepted by research workers. Based on the physical properties of the proteins before and after disulfide cleavage, three types of disulfide bonds were postulated:[30] intramolecular bonds, intermolecular bonds that link proteins into linear-soluble polymers of limited size, and intermolecular bonds that cross-link proteins extensively in three dimensions so as to render the proteins insoluble.

TABLE 8
Amino Acid Compositions of the Glutelin Preparations and Alcohol-Soluble Glutelin (ASG)

	Glutelin		ASG	
Amino Acid	Alkylated Reduced[a]	Native Unreduced[b]	Ethanol Insoluble[a]	Ethanol Soluble[a]
Lysine	3.7	3.0	5.4	0.1
Histidine	4.0	2.5	3.6	4.3
Arginine	5.6	4.1	6.9	3.1
Aspartic acid	6.2	7.1	8.5	2.4
Threonine	3.7	3.4	4.2	3.1
Serine	4.4	5.9	5.1	3.8
Glutamic acid	18.6	20.0	16.5	21.0
Proline	11.0	10.9	7.3	18.6
Glycine	3.8	4.5	4.7	2.6
Alanine	5.4	6.2	5.6	5.6
Half cystine	3.7	3.4	2.4	4.2
Valine	5.0	5.1	5.8	3.9
Methionine	4.7	2.4	3.4	7.0
Isoleucine	3.6	3.2	4.4	2.2
Leucine	10.6	12.0	9.5	12.0
Tyrosine	5.7	4.6	5.2	5.7
Phenylalanine	4.9	4.9	5.2	3.2
Tryptophan	—	0.8	—	—

[a] From Paulis and Wall.[92]
[b] From El Kady.[18]

Although the consensus of the researchers is that the improved amino acid composition of high-lysine maize mutants is due to shifts in protein class distribution rather than to changes in the amino acid composition of the individual proteins, some investigators have reported differences in the amino acid composition of glutelins from normal and high-lysine maize.[100-102] The differences in amino acid composition may be explained by differences in distribution of glutelin polypeptides: e.g., the higher lysine content of O_2 mutants is probably associated with a higher amount of lysine-rich polypeptides. The gel electrophoresis investigations of different mutants show very similar electrophoretic patterns, but quantitative differences have been observed between several bands.[103,104] On the basis of all these studies it can be stated that in high-lysine mutants not only the distribution of the macrofractions is changed (the zein content is lower and the salt-soluble and glutelin contents are higher), but also the composition (polypeptide distribution) of the glutelin is changed. The O_2, fl_2, and other genes may function not only to suppress zein biosynthesis, but also to decrease the proportion of some polypeptides of lysine content in the glutelin fraction.

TABLE 9
Amino Acid Composition of Some Glutelin Subfractions (g/100 g Proteins)

Amino Acid	Proline-Rich Fractions from ASG[a]		Glutelin Subfractions Extracted by the Landry-Moureaux Method[b]		
	1	2	G1	G2	G3
ASP	0.5	0.2	4.5	2.3	9.0
THR	4.1	4.1	2.8	3.9	4.3
SER	3.8	3.6	5.0	4.1	5.0
GLU	16.4	15.9	23.8	24.2	14.9
PRO	25.6	25.0	19.6	20.4	12.1
GLY	6.9	6.6	3.6	7.0	7.9
ALA	5.6	5.1	9.8	5.7	8.2
VAL	7.0	7.2	3.4	6.6	7.1
CYS	6.5	6.2	—	0.2	—
MET	0.7	0.9	7.2	1.2	3.0
ILE	1.9	2.0	4.1	3.1	6.0
LEU	9.4	9.4	16.3	10.2	9.8
TYR	2.2	2.2	6.7	4.1	4.0
PHE	1.1	1.5	6.1	3.0	5.7
TRP	—	—	—	—	—
LYS	0.1	0.1	0.1	1.2	6.0
HIS	5.5	6.0	1.4	8.5	3.5
ARG	2.6	3.2	2.3	4.6	7.7

Note: ASG = alcohol-soluble glutenin.

[a] From Esen et al[93]

[b] From Mossé and Landry[35]

The structure of maize glutelin has not been studied as intensively as that of zein. It is generally accepted that glutelin is a macromolecule composed of different polypeptides (subunits) linked together by disulfide bonds. Based on solubility the subunits may be classified into the following groups: (1) water-soluble (and alcohol-soluble) polypeptides (alcohol-soluble glutelin [ASG], also known as water-soluble ASG [WSASG]; G-2 glutelin, prolamin-like proteins; proline-rich or γ-zein; reduced soluble protein [RSP]); (2) alcohol-soluble polypeptides (known also as C-zeins and D-zeins); and (3) alkali-soluble (insoluble residue) subunits. The classification of glutelin subunits mentioned above clearly shows the difficulties — particularly in the case of maize proteins — in this field, which resulted in a considerable amount of disputes and confusion. Nowadays minimally four systems are used: the classical Osborne nomenclature, the system proposed by Wilson,[30] Landry-Moureaux nomenclature,[11,12] and the classification proposed by Esen.[105] Further, more detailed knowledge of the maize endosperm proteins is needed in order to find an internationally agreed upon and more accurate classification.

Of the polypeptides obtained after reduction of glutelin, the water-soluble proteins have been investigated the most thoroughly. In the following part of this chapter the name reduced soluble glutelin (RSG) will be used. As revealed by gel electrophoresis the major, most characteristic component of RSG is a polypeptide with an apparent molecular weight of 28 kDa named RSG-1. This component has been studied at the molecular level by several researchers.[30,88,89,106-108] Although charge variants of RSG-1 have been isolated, the protein is probably a single species.[107,108] It consists of about 200 amino acid residues and contains a high amount of cysteine (7 mol%). A short N-terminal sequence of 11 residues is followed by a repetitive domain consisting of eight highly conserved hexapeptides with the sequence Pro–Pro–Pro–Val–His–Leu. The rest of the molecule, including the C-terminal domain, is nonrepetitive. Some sulfur-rich and HMW prolamins of wheat, rye, and barley showed sequence homology with certain parts of RSG-1. The polar nature of the repetitive domain may be responsible for the solubility of RSG-1 in water when in the reduced state, while the high content of cysteine facilitates the formation of alcohol-insoluble and water-insoluble aggregates. The RSG fraction mainly contains components with a molecular weight of 28 kDa, but smaller amounts of components with slower mobilities (M_r = 58,000) are also present (RSG-2). Vitale et al.[106] purified the two fractions and compared their amino acid compositions (Table 10). The 28-kDa fraction (RSG-1) contained relatively little glutamate + glutamine (about 16 mol%), but was high in proline and cysteine (about 21 mol% and 7 mol%, respectively). Lysine was absent, but about 8 mol% histidine was present. The amino acid composition of RSG-2 was distinctly different, with 34 mol% glutamate + glutamine, but only 4.7 mol% proline. Less cysteine (4.4 mol%) but more histidine (11 mol%) was present. The total content of basic amino acids was about 15 mol%. The compositions of both groups of polypeptides were different from those of the major zein polypeptides (Z19 and Z22).

The localization of RSG proteins in the maize endosperm was also studied.[94,103,104] It was found that they are distributed at the periphery of protein bodies. Changes in the major polypeptide groups among different genotypes were found; e.g., QPM (Quality Protein Maize) varieties, which combine high levels of lysine and tryptophan with high yields, traditional appearance, and conventional kernel hardness, were also shown to contain relatively high amounts of RSG (γ-zein) in the endosperm. γ-Zein was found in very small amounts in the endosperm of opaque-2 and floury-2 genotypes, which have a very soft endosperm texture. Considering the location of γ-zein at the periphery of protein bodies,[113] its high cysteine content, and the fact that this protein requires a reducing agent for extraction, it is possible that γ-zein is involved in disulfide interactions that influence kernel hardness. Recent investigations by Dombrink-Kurtzman and Bietz[104] of zein composition in the hard and soft endosperm portions of maize suggest that the question of hardness or softness is of a more complex nature. These researchers mentioned above, investigating endosperm proteins extracted with alcohol containing a reducing

TABLE 10
Amino Acid Compositions of Some Types of Maize Glutelin Components (mol%)

Amino Acid	RSG-1	RSG-2	RSG (Glutelin-2)	RSG-1
ASP	0.3	4.3	0.3	0.5
THR	4.5	2.5	4.5	4.3
SER	4.2	7.3	4.2	4.3
GLU	16.3	33.6	16.3	16.0
PRO	21.2	4.7	21.2	24.9
CYS	7.3	4.4	7.3	5.5
GLY	6.8	4.9	6.8	7.3
ALA	5.1	3.5	5.2	5.7
VAL	8.3	5.1	8.4	7.5
MET	0.4	1.3	0.4	0.8
ILE	1.6	2.2	1.6	2.0
LEU	9.0	4.7	9.0	10.0
TYR	2.5	3.5	2.5	2.1
PHE	1.1	1.9	1.2	1.3
HIS	8.2	11.0	8.2	7.2
LYS	0	2.6	0	0.2
ARG	2.5	2.1	2.5	2.7
Reference	106	106	106[a]	Average data from 106, 109–112

Note: RSG = reduced soluble glutelin.

[a] Mean values of two fractions, recalculated from Vitale et al.[106] by Tatham et al.[36]

agent using the RP-HPLC technique, have found that the main differences involve the quantity of α-zeins (Z19 + Z22).

γ-Zein (RSG) content is even lower in the hard-texture endosperm parts (which were separated by hand dissection of individual kernels). A typical RP-HPLC chromatogram is shown in Figure 2, and some data about distribution of alcohol-soluble polypeptide fractions in different maize hybrids are summarized in Table 8.

The alcohol-soluble fraction of polypeptides obtained after reduction of maize glutelin contains some other protein components, too. The presence of two proteins with molecular weights of about 15 to 17 kDa and 9 to 11 kDa has been reported by Gianazza et al.[114] The names Z15 and Z10[36,50] are used, as are zein-C and zein-D.[30] The amino acid compositions of these components differ from those of the major group of polypeptides in that they contain more methionine and more cysteine.[115]

The 9- to 11-kDa components (Z10-zein, D-zein) also have a high methionine content (over 10%), a high glycine content, and a moderate leucine content.[116] C-zein does not seem to form aggregates in protein bodies.[106] These proteins are much more likely to form intermolecular disulfide bonds, due to the high number of cysteine residues, than are the Z19- and Z22-zeins.

III. CYTOPLASMIC (METABOLICALLY ACTIVE) PROTEINS OF MAIZE

A. Albumins and Globulins

Metabolically active proteins include a lot of components which are soluble in water and/or salt solutions. The proteins in this group include enzymes, nucleoproteins, glycoproteins, membrane proteins, etc. The problem of the solubility of the proteins belonging to this group was reviewed by Wall and Paulis.[34] In general, three procedures are used for the extraction of albumins and globulins: the classic procedure of Osborne, the method of Mertz et al.,[69] and the procedure of Landry and Moureaux.[11,12]

The separation of the cytoplasmic proteins into subfractions has been widely studied. The fractionation on the basis of selective solubility used in earlier research work has now been replaced by gel chromatography and electrophoresis methods, and the role of the HPLC technique is also steadily growing.

The heterogeneity of the water-soluble albumins was investigated by gel filtration chromatography on Sephadex G-100 columns.[117] Five different peaks were observed. The distribution of the peaks depends on the solvent chosen. Urea increases the proportion of the peaks, and alkaline buffers give better separation than acidic ones. The presence of a reducing agent does not influence the elution profile. These findings support the suggestion that albumins contain only intramolecular disulfide bonds. Some characteristic elution profiles of albumins separated on Sephadex G-200 columns are shown in Figure 10.[44] Halasi et al.[118] reported on the separation of albumins and globulins of maize using gel chromatography. More than ten subfractions were separated with molecular weights ranging from 16 to about 400 kDa, and extreme heterogeneity of both fractions was shown. The presence of some high molecular weight components probably indicated that the preparations also contained some proteins not belonging to the albumin and globulin fractions. Ion exchange chromatography with carboxymethyl cellulose (CMC)[119] and DEAE-cellulose[120] has also been effectively used for the separation into subfractions.

At this time the most widely used technique for the separation of the components of metabolically active proteins is gel electrophoresis. Both starch gels and polyacrylamide gels are used, as is isoelectric focusing. Using this technique both albumin and globulin fractions may be separated into about 20 different components. Results of gel electrophoresis investigations of the albumins and globulins of maize have been published by many research workers.[54,120-122] All of the reported results confirm the heterogeneity of the water- and salt-soluble fractions. There are some indications that at least some bands of the soluble proteins are probably identical to the bands of reduced glutelin.[34] The possibility that mutant and normal endosperm of corn (*Zea mais* L.) differ predictably in the electrophoretic banding patterns of their soluble endosperm proteins was examined by Wilson[122] using polyacrylamide gel electrophoresis. The system for designating the bands obtained is illustrated by a scan of a long gel in Figure 11. The bands were classified into three groups (A, B, and C). The major band in the upper region was called A′. The next major band below A′ was B_1, the first of the seven bands in the B region. The fastest-moving major band found for all genotypes was labeled C. The reproducibility of banding patterns was quite good. No differences were noted between the PAGE patterns of hetero- and homozygous normal endosperms. The B_2 and B_3 band intensities were characteristic for normal inbred strains. In comparison with the patterns for 50-day-old endosperms, those of younger endosperms often differed somewhat in relative band intensity. In the gels of fully mature endosperm the A′ band was greatly reduced.

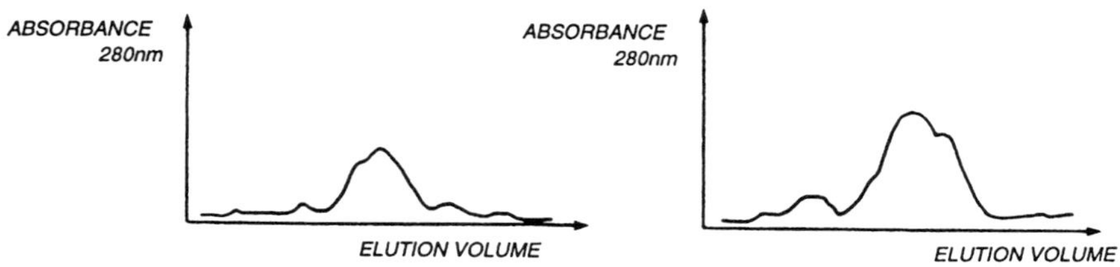

FIGURE 10 Characteristic elution profiles of the albumins of two maize hybrids on Sephadex G-150 columns. (From El Kady, A. and Lásztity, R., *Gabonaipar*, 29, 94, 1982. With permission.)

The banding patterns for the opaque-2 endosperms consistently differed from those of the corresponding normal endosperms in only one minor respect. The B_6-B_7 band pair of the opaque-2 sample became less distinct. The banding patterns of the homozygous floury-2 versions of the five sets of inbred strains did show a major characteristic difference from the patterns of normal endosperms: the B_1 band decreased in intensity.

The amino acid compositions of the soluble proteins differ from those of the storage proteins of maize and are characterized by higher amounts of essential amino acids and lower concentrations of glutamic acid. Some data concerning amino acid compositions of albumins and globulins are summarized in Tables 11 and 12. As is seen, the amino acid compositions of the albumins and globulins are similar and only slight differences occur. Albumins are richer than globulins in aspartic acid, proline, glycine, and alanine, but poorer in glutamic acid and arginine.

SDS-PAGE patterns of endosperm globulins differ from those of albumins in that they have fewer bands, with several bands being present in relatively large amounts.[30] Small changes in pattern were induced by the O_2 mutation, and some differences are apparent between inbred strains.

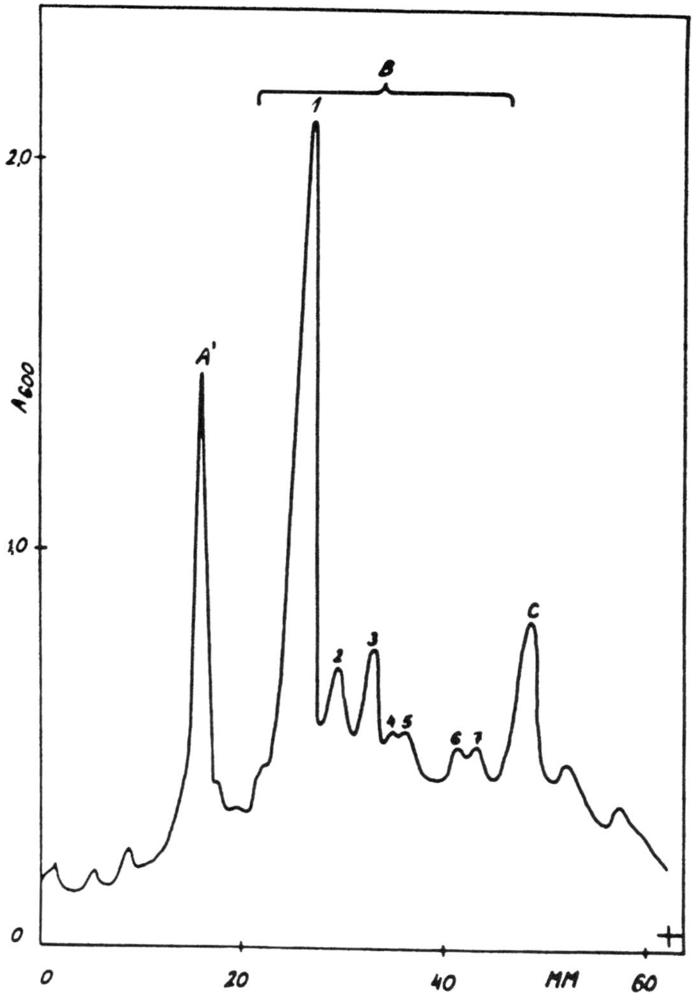

FIGURE 11 Designation of protein bands after polyacrylamide gel electrophoresis of an endosperm extract from maize. A′ = sucrose synthetase; B1 = the major marker protein in the B region; C = the major marker band for the fast-moving proteins; B2-7 = minor bands in the middle region. (From Wilson, C.M., *Cereal Chem.*, 58, 401, 1981. With permission.)

B. Enzymes and Enzyme Inhibitors

The maize kernel, like other cereal grains, contains a lot of enzymes. From a practical technological view the amylases, proteases, lipoxidases, and other redox enzymes are the most important. The amylases of corn have not been investigated as thoroughly as those of barley and wheat. Their activity varies widely. Investigations at the Hungarian Grain Research Laboratory[9] showed activity ranging from 60 to 1000 as measured by the Hagberg method. Amylase activity of sound maize kernel is low; however, the α-amylase activity increases rapidly during germination of

TABLE 11
Amino Acid Composition of the Albumins of Maize (g/100 g Protein)

Amino Acid	Endosperm Albumin[a]	Maize Albumin[b]	Germ Albumin[a]	Albumin + Globulin[c]	Germ Protein Isolate
Lysine	5.6	6.9	6.4	5.2	5.9
Histidine	2.2	3.4	2.5	2.0	3.4
Arginine	6.7	8.5	6.9	5.4	9.0
Aspartic acid	8.4	8.4	8.2	8.4	8.4
Threonine	4.5	4.8	4.8	5.0	4.1
Serine	4.2	4.2	4.3	5.6	4.9
Glutamic acid	11.1	14.3	12.6	12.0	13.6
Proline	4.3	7.8	2.6	7.1	6.1
Glycine	5.3	6.4	4.7	10.7	5.6
Alanine	6.0	6.6	6.0	10.7	5.6
Valine	5.0	5.5	5.0	7.0	6.1
Methionine	1.3	1.7	1.0	1.2	1.7
Cysteine	—	—	—	0.7	2.0
Isoleucine	3.2	4.0	2.7	4.3	4.0
Leucine	5.6	6.9	5.1	8.7	8.3
Tyrosine	3.1	4.0	2.8	2.6	2.8
Phenylalanine	3.1	3.6	4.1	3.4	3.9
Tryptophan	—	3.1	—	—	—

[a] From Paulis and Wall.[127]
[b] From El Kady.[18]
[c] From Sodek and Wilson.[55]

maize. The status of research on cereal α-amylases is the subject of a review by Hill and McGregor.[123] The study of amylases in germinating maize is less advanced than in other cereals. Polymorphism for α-amylase in germinating maize was revealed even in early investigations. In a recent study McGregor et al.,[124] using a combination of IEF and chromatofocusing, separated α-amylases of several germinating grains. Grains were classified into two groups: those that contain both a high- (>5.8) and a low-pI (<5.5) component (barley, wheat, rye, and triticale) and those with only low-pI components (oats, maize, millet, sorghum, and rice). However, maize had intermediate-pI (5.5 to 6.0) amylases as well as low-pI components and did not strictly fit either classification.

Warner et al.[125] found eight or nine identifiable IEF bands having α-amylase activity (amylases were fractionated by affinity chromatography, anion exchange chromatography, and chromatofocusing). At least three groups of α-amylases were found, with pI ranges of 5.2 to 5.7, 4.6 to 4.8, and 4.0 to 4.2. Differences were found in starch-degrading activity of these groups.

Proteases (peptidases) are present in practically all parts of the maize kernel. Acidic proteases of maize were described by Polnik.[126] Heterogeneity of the protease

TABLE 12
Amino Acid Composition of the Globulins of Maize (g/100 g Protein)

Amino Acid	Endosperm Globulin[a]	Maize Globulin[b]	Germ Globulin[a]	Salt-Soluble Protein[c]
Lysine	5.3	6.6	4.7	7.2
Histidine	3.4	4.1	2.9	3.5
Arginine	11.2	11.1	9.8	10.8
Aspartic acid	6.7	9.5	6.1	9.2
Threonine	2.8	5.1	2.7	3.9
Serine	4.6	5.3	4.3	5.1
Glutamic acid	14.7	15.4	12.4	15.0
Proline	3.2	5.8	3.7	8.6
Glycine	4.2	6.8	4.0	8.1
Alanine	4.3	4.4	4.1	7.7
Valine	4.9	6.0	4.4	8.8
Methionine	0.9	2.1	0.7	2.4
Cystine	—	—	—	1.9
Isoleucine	2.6	2.7	2.5	5.2
Leucine	5.1	4.6	5.0	6.6
Tyrosine	2.8	2.6	2.5	3.8
Phenylalanine	4.1	3.4	4.0	5.1
Tryptophan	—	4.4	—	—

[a] From Paulis and Wall.[127]
[b] From E1 Kady.[18]
[c] From Mossé, and Landry.[35]

preparation was revealed and the presence of more enzymes, probably isoenzymes, was suggested.

An endopeptidase was found by Melville and Scandalios[128] in all parts of the maize kernel except the pericarp and the starchy endosperm. The endopeptidase has trypsin-like activity and exists in the form of genetic variants or isoenzymes distinguished by their electrophoretic mobility. Maize contains appreciable levels of trypsin inhibitors.[50,128] The inhibitors are similar in molecular size and properties to the inhibitors found in other cereals. A trypsin inhibitor was characterized and sequenced by Mahonney et al.[139]

The peroxidases of normal and high-lysine maize were thoroughly investigated by Russian research workers.[129] In Figure 12 the peroxidase spectra of normal and opaque-2 maize are demonstrated. The germs are the richest in peroxidase isoenzymes. Significant differences were observed between normal and opaque-2 maize.

The lipases and lipoxygenases of maize are relatively poorly investigated. A recent review of these enzymes has been published by Gardner.[160] Their importance in storage of maize needs further investigation.

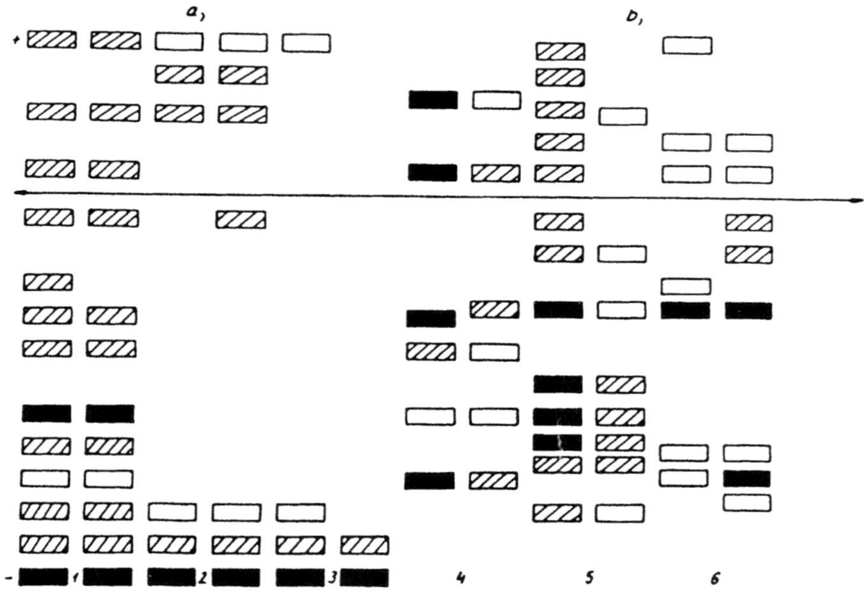

FIGURE 12 Electropherograms of the peroxidases of the embryo, endosperm, and bran; a = opaque-2; b = normal. (1) Germ (mature kernel). (2) Endosperm (mature kernel). (3) Bran (mature kernel). (4) Germ (immature kernel). (5) Endosperm (immature kernel). (6) Bran (immature kernel). Boxes represent electrophoretic bands of different intensity. (From Skolenko, V.V., in *Biochimitcheskoje Issledovnye v Processe Selekeciji Kukuruzy,* Kovarskyi, A.E., Ed., Izdanija Stiinga, Kishinev, 1973, 167. With permission.)

Sucrose synthase has been investigated by several research workers.[30,130,131] This enzyme may be separated easily by PAGE. The molecular weight of sucrose synthase was estimated to be about 365 kDa. This enzyme makes up about 2.8% of the soluble endosperm protein, as estimated from the purification experiments of Su and Preiss.[130] Chourey and Nelson[131] report that the shrunken (sh) mutation is specific for a deficiency in sucrose synthase.

Ribonuclease was isolated from maize seed and characterized by Wilson.[132] Ribonuclease activity of normal and opaque-2 mutant maize was also investigated, including genetic control of ribonuclease activity.[133,134]

In addition to the α- and β-amylases that degrade polysaccharides, Chiba and Shimomura[135] have described a very active α-glucosidase in maize.

C. Other Proteins

Van Etten et al.[136] found that in the pericarps of maize kernels hydroxyproline was present. Later, Boundy et al.[137] established that the hydroxyproline of maize pericarp was a component of a carbohydrate-protein complex. Lamport and Miller[138] demonstrated that the hydroxyproline in maize pericarp was attached through its hydroxyl group via glycosidic linkage to arabinose residues of hemicelluloses.

Several unusual proteins can be extracted from maize seeds with 0.5 *M* sulfuric acid. These are thought to be similar in chemical composition to wheat purothionins, but are different in structure[140] and do not have the toxic properties of wheat and barley thionins. Six different proteins in the extract are all high in basic amino acids and cysteine.

The growing interest in the use of cereal germs (germ protein concentrates and isolates) in food production has stimulated research on maize germ proteins. The distribution of N among the various classical protein fractions of the germ is quite different than that in the endosperm. Albumins and globulins are the main fractions. Landry and Moureaux[141] present a complete picture of the germ protein fractions, with comparisons to similar fractions from the endosperm. Small amounts of zein, identified by alcohol extractability and amino acid composition, were found. The major protein fractions all consisted of many proteins. Cross and Adams[142] compared the SDS-PAGE patterns of albumins and globulins from several inbred strains and a hybrid. A large number of bands were observed. A few differences were apparent among different inbreds, with bands from both parents appearing in the hybrid. SDS-PAGE of the globulins revealed fewer bands, with some being predominant. Several bands appear to be characteristic of certain inbred strains and possibly could be used for inbred identification.

More recently, Tömösközi et al.[143,144] and Lásztity et al.[145] investigated the fraction distribution, amino acid composition, and functional properties of different germ proteins, including maize germ proteins. Although some losses of cysteine and lysine content occur during isolation of proteins, the isolates have good nutritive value and high *in vitro* digestibility. Some advances in supercritical extraction of oils relating to functional properties of protein preparation were observed.

Zeamatin, an antifungal protein with membrane-permeabilizing activity, was isolated from maize by Roberts and Selitrennikoff,[73] and a ribosome-inactivating protein was studied by Bass et al.[74]

IV. PROTEIN CONCENTRATES AND NUTRITIVE VALUE OF MAIZE PROTEINS

The germ of maize is potentially a copious source of protein for human use. It can be used directly or in defatted form in the baking industry or in the form of protein preparations (protein concentrates), as well as for protein enrichment or protein substitution in different food products.

The demand for low-cost vegetable protein supplements to increase the nutritional value of cereals and other foods encouraged research into improved products from maize germ. The chemical and nutritional problems of the cereal germs used in bakery products were recently reviewed by Tsen.[146]

Defatted maize germ protein has considerable potential for use as a protein supplement in a variety of foods. A good maize germ protein source can be obtained by drying maize germ meal at low temperatures and extracting the oil using solvents. Recently, successful use of supercritical fluid extraction was also reported.[145,146] Functional properties of maize germ proteins have been intensively studied by several researchers.[144-148]

Current industrial dry-milling processes using a complex system of grinding, sieving, aspiration, and flotation provide the possibility of producing germ preparations and protein-enriched flours. The air classification process — generally used as a means of producing high-protein fractions from cereal flours — results in maize flour fractions with moderately increased protein contents. The goal of the wet-milling process is separation of highly pure starch from protein and other constituents of maize. However, important feeds and other products are derived in large quantities from protein-rich by-products. An essential initial step in the wet-milling process is steeping the maize in 0.1 to 0.2% SO_2 solution. The effect of this treatment, plus increased proteolytic activity, is an increase in the amount of soluble proteins and N-containing compounds being collected in the steep waters. Condensed fermented maize extracts contain 24.8% protein.[37] The maize germ meal produced in the wet-milling process contains more than 20% protein. One of the most valuable products of wet milling is the gluten meal, containing about 60% protein. The protein is mainly composed of zein and maize glutelin; consequently it is low in lysine and tryptophan, but relatively rich in sulfur-containing amino acids. The feed gluten meal has a strong odor and flavor and a tendency to develop rancidity due to the high content of unsaturated fatty acids. To upgrade the gluten meal for human use it is necessary to extract the oil, pigments, and typical flavor. A process resulting in maize protein concentrate suitable for human consumption is described by Sternberg et al.[150] It was also reported that this protein concentrate has good water-binding capacity and also fat-emulsifying properties. The essential amino acid contents of the different products of the wet-milling process are summarized in Table 13.

For quite some time the zein of maize has been one of the industrially produced proteins. The world production is estimated to be 500 tons/year. In the current production process the zein is extracted at 60°C using 88% isopropyl alcohol containing 0.25% sodium hydroxide. After clarification the solution is chilled to –15°C to precipitate zein. The normal commercial product contains 3 to 4% oil and about 500 mg/kg xanthophyll.

The possibility of improving the nutritional quality of zein by using the plastein reaction was investigated by Arai et al.[151] This reaction permits, after hydrolysis of the zein, the introduction of essential amino acids into the polypeptide chain. During the plastein reaction not only are new essential amino acids incorporated, but a condensation of the peptides also occurs. Zein is currently used primarily as a coating agent in pharmaceutical or food applications. For nuts, zein coatings retard rancidity; for candies, they restrict moisture access and provide a glaze.

Recently potential use of water-soluble zein (produced by enzymatic modification) as a food ingredient was reported.[152]

TABLE 13
Essential Amino Acid Content of Some Products of the Wet-Milling Process of Gluten

Amino Acid	Condensed Fermented Maize Extracts[a]	Maize Germ Meal[a]	Maize Gluten Protein Concentrate[b]	Maize Gluten Feed[a]	Soya Concentrate[b]
Lysine	3.4	4.2	1.7	2.9	6.3
Methionine + cystine	5.2	4.5	5.4	4.3	2.8
Threonine	3.7	5.0	3.6	4.1	4.3
Leucine	8.2	8.0	15.4	8.6	7.9
Isoleucine	2.8	3.3	3.6	2.9	4.6
Phenylalanine + tyrosine	5.4	7.1	11.1	6.2	8.9
Valine	4.7	5.5	4.7	4.8	4.8
Tryptophan	0.2	0.8	0.7	0.4	1.5

[a] From Reiners et al.[37]
[b] From Sternberg et al.[150]

Fermentation of the cereal grains to make alcohol produces a protein-rich material (spent grain stillage) after the alcohol is distilled. Most of the spent grain stillage is recovered in different forms as a dried feed ingredient.[153] Distiller's dried grains with solubles (CDDGS) are a dried base of still material (whole stillage). When this is screened, the part that remains on top (on-screen residue) is pressed and dried; it is then known as distiller's dried grains. The part passing through the screen (off-screen material) is concentrated in an evaporator and drum-dried; it is called distiller's dried soluble.[153] The eventual increase in use of alcohol as fuel enhanced the investigations connected with more effective use of these protein-containing by-products.[153-156]

Some data about the amino acid composition of some products are collected in Table 14.

Protein-rich residue from ethanolic fermentation of high-lysine, dent, waxy, and white corn varieties potentially may be used in human foods, as reported by Wu.[157]

The nutritive value of total maize protein, and especially of zein, is relatively low because of the poor lysine and tryptophan contents of these proteins. The biological value of maize proteins, calculated on the basis of different chemical indexes, varies between 30 and 47 (see Table 15). Nevertheless, maize proteins may be well supplemented with proteins containing more lysine and tryptophan and which are poor in sulfur-containing amino acids. Casein or proteins of legumes, including soya, are suitable for these purposes. Also, a combination of wheat and maize flours may be advantageous.[127] The germ proteins, and also germ protein isolates, have a more convenient amino acid composition and a higher biological value. The high-lysine mutants also have a higher biological value.

TABLE 14
Amino Acid Composition of Corn Distiller's Grains and Soluble Fractions[153]

		Base of Still		Residue	
Amino Acid	CDDGS	Supernatant	Residue	On Screen	Off Screen
Aspartic acid	6.4	7.9	6.4	6.6	6.7
Threonine	4.0	5.1	4.1	4.1	3.7
Serine	5.3	5.5	5.5	5.3	4.9
Glutamic acid	20.1	22.5	20.7	19.1	18.8
Proline	10.2	15.4	9.8	9.2	8.9
Glycine	4.3	6.9	4.0	4.1	3.5
Alanine	8.0	8.4	8.3	8.1	8.1
Valine	5.4	5.8	5.3	5.6	5.1
Cystine	0.9	1.5	1.5	2.0	1.5
Methionine	2.5	1.6	2.1	2.1	2.1
Isoleucine	5.3	4.3	4.2	4.1	4.2
Leucine	15.1	8.6	14.2	13.5	13.6
Tyrosine	5.5	2.5	4.7	4.3	4.7
Phenylalanine	5.2	4.4	6.2	5.6	6.2
Lysine	3.1	3.4	3.1	3.2	2.5
Histidine	2.6	2.8	2.7	3.0	2.4
Arginine	4.2	3.1	5.2	5.0	4.3

TABLE 15
Biological Value of Mixtures of Maize and Wheat Flours[158]

	Biological Value				
Product	Mitchell Index	Korpáczy Index	FAO/WHO Index	Morup-Olesen Index	Limiting Amino Acid
Maize flour	41,134	39,642	47,650	31,093	Tryptophan
Wheat flour	48,640	45,552	46,444	60,781	Lysine
Wheat flour + 20% maize flour	48,334	45,056	47,082	61,156	Lysine
Wheat flour + 40% maize flour	47,136	43,567	47,198	65,021	Lysine

REFERENCES

1. Pomeranz, Y. and Bechtel, D. E., Structure of cereal grains as related to end use properties, in *Cereals '78: Better Nutrition for the World Millions,* Pomeranz, Y., Ed., American Association of Cereal Chemists, St. Paul, MN, 1978, 85.
2. Watson, S. A., Structure and composition, in *Corn: Chemistry and Technology,* Watson, S.A. and Ramstad, E., Eds., American Association of Cereal Chemists, St. Paul, MN, 1991, 53.
3. Hoseney, R. C., *Principles of Cereal Science and Technology,* 2nd ed., American Association of Cereal Chemists, St. Paul, MN, 1994.
4. Salunkhe, D. K., Chavan, J. K., and Kadam, S. S., *Postharvest Biotechnology of Cereals,* CRC Press, Boca Raton, FL, 1985.
5. Jegorov, G. A., *Technologija Pererabotki Serna,* Kolos, Moscow, 1977.
6. Gabonatermesztési Kutató Intézet, Kukoricahibridek Minõsége 1974-ben és 1975-ben, Szeged, Hungary, 1977.
7. Mendes, D. D., Estudio Quimico Comparativo las Variedades des Milho Cultivades en Diversas Regiones do Pais, Boletin Technico No. 4, Centro de Technologia Agricola e Alimentar, Rio de Janeiro, 1972.
8. Reiners, R., Wall, J. S., and Inglett, G. E., Corn proteins: potential for their industrial use, paper presented at the 58th Annu. Meet. Am. Assoc. Cereal Chemists, St. Louis, MO, 1973.
9. Grain Research Laboratory, Budapest, Hungary, unpublished data.
10. Hecksch-Hajdú, É., Kukoricafehérjék, Vizsgálata, Ph.D. thesis, Technical University of Budapest, Budapest, Hungary, 1978.
11. Landry, J. and Moureaux, T., Heterogenité des glutelines du grain du mais. Extraction selective et composition en acides aminées des trois fractions isolées, *Bull. Soc. Chim. Biol.,* 52, 1021, 1970.
12. Moureaux, T. and Landry, J., Extraction sélective des protéines du grain de mais et en particulier de la fraction "glutelines", *C.R. Acad. Sci. Ser. D.,* 266, 2302, 1968.
13. Paulis, J. W. and Wall, J. S., Comparison of the protein composition of selected corns and their wild relatives teosinte and tripsacum, *J. Agric. Food Chem.,* 52, 265, 1977.
14. Paulis, J. W. and Wall, J. S., Fractionation and characterization of alcohol-soluble reduced corn endosperm glutelin proteins, *Cereal Chem.,* 54, 1223, 1977.
15. Watson, S. A. and Ramstad, P. E., *Corn: Chemistry and Technology,* American Association of Cereal Chemists, St. Paul, MN, 1991.
16. Baudet, T., Mossé, J., Landry, J., and Moureaux, T., Étude sur les protéines de mais. I. Composition en acides aminées des fractions du grain, *Ann. Physiol. Veg.,* 8, 321, 1966.
17. Mertz, E. T., Nelson, O. E., Bates, L. S., and Viron, O. N., Better protein quality in maize, *Adv. Chem.,* 57, 228, 1966.
18. El Kady, A., Investigation of the Maize Proteins and Their Biological Value, Ph.D. thesis, Technical University of Budapest, Budapest, Hungary, 1982.
19. Mertz, E., Nelson, O., and Bates, L. S., Mutant gene that changes composition and increases lysine content of maize endosperm, *Science,* 154, 279, 1964.
20. Vasal, S. K., Villegas, E., Bjarnason, M., Gelau, B., and Goerzt, P., Genetic modifiers and breeding strategies for developing hard opaque-2 materials, in *Improvement of Quality Traits of Maize for Grain and Silage Use,* Pollmer, W.G. and Phipps, P.H., Eds., Martinus Nijhoff, The Hague, 1980, 37.

21. Mertz, E. T., *Quality Protein Maize,* American Association of Cereal Chemists, St. Paul, MN, 1992.
22. Wall, J. S. and Bietz, J. A., Differences in corn endosperm proteins in developing seeds of normal and opaque-2 corn, *Cereal Chem.,* 64, 275, 1987.
23. Vasal, S. K., Use of genetic modifier to obtain normal type kernels with the opaque-2 gene, in *High Quality Protein Maize,* Dowden, Hutchinson, Ross, Stroudsburg, PA, 1975, 197.
24. Ortega, E. I. and Bates, L. S., Biochemical and agronomic studies in two modified hard-endosperm opaque-2 maize (*Zea mays* L.) populations, *Cereal Chem.,* 60, 107, 1983.
25. Gevers, H. O., Progress in the implementation of high lysine maize in South Africa, in *Cereal Science and Technology: Impact on a Changing Africa,* Taylor, J.R.N., Randall, P.G., and Viljoen, J.H., Eds., CSIR, Pretoria, 1993, 53.
26. Paulis, W., Wall, J. S., and Sanderson, J., Origin of high methionine content in sugary-1 corn endosperm, *Cereal Chem.,* 55, 705, 1978.
27. Wilson, C. M., Sprague, G. F., and Nelsen, T. C., Linkages among zein genes determined by isoelectric focusing, *Theor. Appl. Genet.,* 77, 217, 1989.
28. Wilson, C. M., Zeins in sweet corn (sugary-1), *Cereal Chem.,* 69, 113, 1992.
29. Phillips, R. L. and McLure, R. A., Elevated protein-bound methionins in seeds of a maize line resistant to lysine plus threonine, *Cereal Chem.,* 62, 213, 1985.
30. Wilson, C. M., Proteins of the kernel, in *Corn: Chemistry and Technology,* Watson, A. and Ramstad, P.E., Eds., American Association of Cereal Chemists, St. Paul, MN, 1991, 273.
31. Misra, P. S., Jambunathan, R., Mertz, E. T., Glover, D. V., Barbose, H. M., and McWhirter, K. S., Endosperm protein synthesis in maize mutants with increased lysine content, *Science,* 176, 1425, 1972.
32. Sysoyev, A. F., O razlitchijach aminokyslotnogo sostava mutantov opak-2 i floury-2 i obychnych form kukuruzy, *Trudy Vasnil.,* Kolos, Moscow, 1971.
33. Mossé, J., Monographie sur une protéine du mais: la zeine (preparation, composition, propriétés physiochimiques, technologiques et physiologiques), *Ann. Physiol. Veg.,* 3, 105, 1961.
34. Wall, J. S. and Paulis, J. W., Corn and sorghum grain proteins, in *Advances in Cereal Science and Technology,* Vol. 2, Pomeranz, Y., Ed., American Association of Cereal Chemists, St. Paul, MN, 1977.
35. Mossé, J. and Landry, J., Recent research on major maize proteins: zeins and glutelins, in *Cereals for Food and Beverages, Recent Progress in Cereal Chemistry,* Inglett, G.E. and Munck, L., Eds., Academic Press, New York, 1980, 255.
36. Tatham, A. S., Shewry, P. R., and Belton, P. S., Structural studies of cereal prolamins, including wheat gluten, in *Advances in Cereal Science and Technology,* Vol. 10, Pomeranz, Y., Ed., American Association of Cereal Chemists, St. Paul, MN, 1990, 1.
37. Reiners, R. A., Wall, J. S., and Inglett, G. E., Corn proteins: potential for their industrial use, in *Industrial Uses of Cereals,* Pomeranz, Y., Ed., American Association of Cereal Chemists, St. Paul, MN, 1973, 235.
38. Turner, J. E., Boundy, J. A., and Dimler, R. J., Zein: a heterogeneous protein containing disulphide linked aggregates, *Cereal Chem.,* 42, 452, 1965.
39. Paulis, J. W., Disulfide structures of zein proteins from corn endosperm, *Cereal Chem.,* 58, 542, 1981.

40. Landry, J., Franctionnement de la zeine par chromatographie sur Sephadex, *C.R. Acad. Sci.,* 261, 275, 1965.
41. Ganchev, K. D., Ivanov, C. P., and Drenska, A. I., Studies on the heterogeneity of zein and its fractions by disc electrophoresis, *Dokl. Bolg. Akad. Nauk,* 29, 689, 1976.
42. Ganchev, K. D., Stoyanova, R. Z., and Ivanov, C. P., Characterization of A_1, B_1, C^a and C^b fractions isolated by gel chromatography of zein, *Dolk. Bol. Akad. Nauk,* 25, 633, 1972.
43. Fraij, B. and Melcher, V., Proteins of the zein extracts of corn, *Plant Physiol.,* 61, 40, 1978.
44. El Kady, A. and Lásztity, R., Kukoricafehérjék vizsgálata. III. A fehérjék gélkromatográfiás frakcionálása, *Gabonaipar,* 29, 94, 1982.
45. Esen, A., Fractionation of zein by ion-exchange chromatography on phosphocellulose, *Cereal Chem.,* 57, 75, 1980.
46. Esen, A., Chromatography of zein on phosphocellulose and sulfopropyl Sephadex, *Cereal Chem.,* 59, 272, 1982.
47. Bietz, J. A., High performance liquid chromatography: how proteins look in cereals, *Cereal Chem.,* 62, 201, 1985.
48. Paulis, J. W., Bietz, J. A., Lambert, R. J., and Villegas, E. M., Identification of modified high-lysine maize genotypes by reversed-phase high-performance liquid chromatography, *Cereal Chem.,* 68, 361, 1991.
49. Argos, P., Pedersen, K., Marks, M. D., and Larkins, B. A., A structural model for maize zein proteins, *J. Biol. Chem.,* 257, 998, 1982.
50. Shewry, P. R. and Miflin, B. J., Seed storage proteins of economically important cereals, in *Advances in Cereal Science and Technology,* Vol. 7, Pomeranz, Y., Ed., American Association of Cereal Chemists, St. Paul, MN, 1985, 1.
51. Alexandrescu, V., Chihaia, C., and Cosmin., O., Zein specificity in inbred lines of maize, *Rev. Roum. Biochim.,* 13, 169, 1976.
52. Gentinetta, E., Maggiore, T., Salamini, F., Lorenzoni, C., Pioli, F., and Soave, C., Protein studies in 46 opaque-2 strains with modified endosperm texture, *Maydica,* 20, 145, 1975.
53. Vitale, A., Soave, C., and Galante, E., Peptide mapping of IEF zein components of maize, *Plant Sci. Lett.,* 18, 57, 1980.
54. Wilson, C. M., Shewry, P. R., and Miflin, B. J., Maize endosperm proteins compared by sodium dodecyl sulphate gel electrophoresis and isoelectric focusing, *Cereal Chem.,* 58, 275, 1981.
55. Sodek, L. and Wilson, C. M., Amino acid composition of proteins isolated from normal, opaque-2 and floury-2 corn endosperm by a modified Osborne procedure, *J. Agric. Food Chem.,* 19, 1144, 1971.
56. Wilson, C. M., Seed protein fractions of maize, sorghum, and related cereals, in *Seed Proteins: Biochemistry, Genetics, Nutritive Value,* Gottshalk, W. and Muller, H. P., Eds., Martinus Nijhoff/Junk, The Hague, 1983, 271.
57. Abe, M., Arai, S., Kato, H., and Fujimaki, M., Electrophoretical analysis of zein and isolation of its components, *Agric. Biol. Chem.,* 45, 1467, 1981.
58. Marks, M. D. and Larkins, B. A., Analysis of sequence microheterogeneity among zein messenger RNAs, *J. Biol. Chem.,* 257, 9976, 1982.
59. Geraghty, D. E., Peifer, M. A., Rubinstein, T., and Messing, J., The primary structure of a plant storage protein: zein, *Nucleic Acids Res.,* 9, 5163, 1981.

60. Geraghty, D. E., Messing, J., and Rubinstein, I., Sequence analysis and comparison of cDNAs of the zein multigene family, *EMBO J.*, 1, 1329, 1982.
61. Hu, N. T., Peifer, M. A., Heidecker, H., Messing, J., and Rubinstein, I., Primary structure of a genomic zein sequence of maize, *EMBO J.*, 1, 1337, 1982.
62. Pedersen, K., Devereux, J., Wilson, D. R., Sheldon, E., and Larkins, B. A., Cloning and sequence analysis reveal structural variation among related zein genes in maize, *Cell,* 29, 1015, 1982.
63. Bietz, J. A., Separation of cereal proteins by reversed phase high-performance liquid chromatography, *J. Chromatogr.*, 255, 219, 1983.
64. Burr, B., Burr F. A., Rubinstein, I., and Simon, M. N., Purification and translation of zein messenger RNA from maize endosperm protein bodies, *Proc. Natl. Acad. Sci. U.S.A.*, 75, 696, 1978.
65. Viotti, A., Sala, B., Morotta, R., Alberi, P., Balducci, C., and Soave, C., Genes and mRNAs coding for zein polypeptides in *Zea mays, Eur. J. Biochem.*, 102, 213, 1979.
66. Wienand, V. and Feix, G., Electrophoretic fractionation and translation in vitro of poly(rA)-containing RNA from maize endosperm, *Eur. J. Biochem.*, 92, 605, 1979.
67. Larkins, B. A., Jones, R. A., and Tsai, Y., Isolation and in vitro translation of zein messenger ribonucleic acid, *Biochemistry,* 15, 5506, 1976.
68. Wienand, V., Langridge, P., and Feix, G., Isolation and characterization of a genomic sequence of maize coding for a zein gene, *Mol. Gen. Genet.*, 182, 440, 1981.
69. Mertz, E. T., Bressani, R., and Lloyd, M. E., Studies on corn proteins. I. A new method of extraction, *Cereal Chem.*, 55, 146, 1968.
70. Burr, B., Burr, F. A., St. John, T. P., Thomas, M., and Davis, R. W., Zein storage gene family of maize. An assessment of heterogeneity with cloned messenger RNA sequences, *J. Mol. Biol.*, 154, 33, 1982.
71. Paulis, J. W., Disulphide structures of zein from corn endosperm, *Cereal Chem.*, 58, 542, 1981.
72. Cownie, P. I., The maize giant in a changing Africa and its challenge for cereal science and technology, in *Cereal Science and Technology: Impact on a Changing Africa,* Taylor, J.R.N., Randall, P.G., and Viljoen, J.H., Eds., CSIR, Pretoria, 1993, 31.
73. Roberts, W. K. and Selitrennikoff, C. P., Zeamatin, an antifungal protein from maize with membrane permeabilising activity, *J. Gen. Microbiol.*, 136, 1771, 1990.
74. Bass, H. W., Webster, C., Brian, G. R. O., Roberts, J. K. M., and Boston, R. S., A maize ribosome inactivating protein is controlled by the transcription activator opaque-2, *Plant Cell,* 4, 225, 1992.
75. Geetha, K. B., Lending, C. R., Lopez, M. A., Wallace, J. C., and Larkins, B. A., Opaque-2 modifiers increase γ-zein synthesis and utter its spatial distribution in maize endosperm, *Plant Cell,* 3, 1207, 1991.
76. Wallace, J. C., Lopes, M. A., Paliva, E., and Larkins, B. A., New methods for extraction and quantitation of zeins reveal a high content of γ-zein in modified opaque-2 maize, *Plant Physiol.*, 92, 191, 1990.
77. Wilson, C. M., Multiple zeins from maize endosperms characterized by reversed-phase high-performance liquid chromatography, *Plant Physiol.*, 95, 777, 1991.
78. Misra, P. S. and Mertz, E. T., Studies on corn proteins. X. Polypeptide molecular weight distribution in Landry-Moureaux fractions of normal and mutant endosperms, *Cereal Chem.*, 53, 705, 1976.
79. Viotti, A., Pogna, N. E., Balducci, C., and Durante, M., Chromosomal localization of zein genes by in situ hybridization of *Zea mays, Mol. Gen. Genet.*, 178, 35, 1980.

80. Viotti, A., Abildsten, G., Pogna, N. E., Sala, E., and Pirotta, V., Multiplicity and diversity of cloned zein cDNA sequences and their chromosomal location, *EMBO J.*, 1, 53, 1982.
81. Soave, C. and Salamini, F., Organization and regulation of zein genes in maize endosperm, *Philos. Trans. R. Soc. London Ser. B.*, 304, 341, 1984.
82. Heidecker, G. and Messing, J., Structural analysis of plant genes, *Annu. Rev. Plant Physiol.*, 37, 439, 1986.
83. Giovinazzo, G., Manzocchi, L. A., Bianchi, M. W., Coraggio, I., and Viotta, A., Functional analysis of the regulatory region of a zein gene in transiently transformed protoplasts, *Plant Mol. Biol.*, 19, 257, 1992.
84. Mass, C., Laufs, J., Grant, S., Korfhage, C., and Werr, W., The combination of a novel stimulatory element in the first exon of the maize Shrunken-1 gene with the following intron 1 enhances reporter gene expression up to 1000-fold, *Plant Mol. Biol.*, 16, 199, 1991.
85. Rubinstein, Z. and Geraghty, D. E., The genetic organization of zein, in *Advances in Cereal Science and Technology,* Vol. 8, Pomeranz, Y., Ed., American Association of Cereal Chemists, St. Paul, MN, 1986, 297.
86. Larkins, B. A., Genetic engineering of seed storage proteins, in *Genetic Engineering of Plants,* Kosuge, T., Meredith, D.P., and Hollaender, A., Eds., Plenum Press, New York, 1983, 93.
87. Messing, J., The manipulation of zein genes to improve the nutritional value of corn, *Trends Biotechnol.*, 1, 1, 1983.
88. Messing, J., The genes encoding seed storage proteins in higher plants, *Genet. Eng.*, 6, 1, 1987.
89. Prat, S., Perez-Grau, L., and Puigomenech, P., Multiple variability in the sequence of a family of maize endosperm proteins, *Gene,* 52, 41, 1987.
90. Wu, Y., Paulis, J. W., Sexson, K. R., and Wall, J. S., Conformation of corn zein and glutelin fractions with unusual amino acid sequence, *Cereal Chem.*, 60, 342, 1983.
91. Nielsen, H. C., Paulis, J. W., James, C., and Wall, J. S., Extraction and structure studies on corn glutelin proteins, *Cereal Chem.*, 47, 501, 1970.
92. Paulis, J. W. and Wall, J. S., Fractionation and properties of alkylated-reduced corn glutelin proteins, *Biochim. Biophys. Acta,* 251, 57, 1971.
93. Esen, A., Bietz, J. A., Paulis, J. W., and Wall, J. S., Fractionation of alcohol-soluble reduced corn glutelins on phosphocellulose and partial characterization of two proline-rich fractions, *Cereal Chem.*, 58, 534, 1981.
94. Paulis, J. W. and Bietz, J. A., Characterization of zeins fractionated by reversed-phase high-performance liquid chromatography, *Cereal Chem.*, 65, 215, 1988.
95. Bietz, J. A., Identification of maize inbreds and hybrids by reversed-phase high-performance liquid chromatography, *Cereal Foods World,* 30, 562, 1985.
96. Paulis, J. W., Bietz, J. A., and Wall, J. S., Corn protein subunits: molecular weights determined by sodium dodecyl sulfate-polyacrylamide gel electrophoresis, *J. Agric. Food Chem.*, 23, 197, 1975.
97. Wilson, C. M., Shewry, P. R., and Miflin, B. J., Maize endosperm proteins compared by sodium dodecyl sulfate gel electrophoresis and isoelectric focusing, *Cereal Chem.*, 58, 275, 1981.
98. Paulis, J. S., Bietz, J. A., Lambert, R. J., and Villegas, E. M., Identification of modified high-lysine maize genotypes by reversed-phase high-performance liquid chromatography, *Cereal Chem.*, 68, 361, 1991.

99. Wall, J. S. and Bietz, J. A., Differences in corn endosperm proteins in developing seeds of normal and opaque-2 corn, *Cereal Chem.,* 64, 275, 1987.
100. Jimenez, J. R., Protein fractionation studies of high lysine corn, in *Proc. High-Lysine Corn Conf.,* Mertz, E. T. and Nelson, O. T., Eds., Corn Refiner's Association, Washington, D.C., 1966, 74.
101. Paulis, J. W., James, C., and Wall, J. S., Comparison of glutelin proteins in normal and high lysine corn endosperm, *J. Agric. Food Chem.,* 17, 1301, 1969.
102. Paskarj, S. I., Nekotorye zakonomernosty biochimitcheskoj izmentchivosty nabljudayemye pri selekciji kukuruzy na katchestvo, in *Biochimitcheskoje Issledovnye v Processe Selekciji Kukuruzy,* Kovarskyi, A.D., Ed., Stiinga, Kisinev, 1975, 53.
103. Paiva, E., Kriz, A. L., Peixoto, M. J. V. V., Wallace, J. C., and Larkins, B. A., Quantitation and distribution of γ-zein in the endosperm of maize kernels, *Cereal Chem.,* 68, 276, 1991.
104. Dombrink-Kurtzman, M. A. and Bietz, J. A., Zein composition in hard and soft endosperm of maize, *Cereal Chem.,* 70, 105, 1993.
105. Esen, A., A proposed nomenclature for the alcohol soluble proteins (zeins) of maize (*Zea mays* L.), *J. Cereal Sci.,* 5, 117, 1987.
106. Vitale, A., Smaniotto, E., Longhi, R., and Galante, E., Reduced soluble proteins associated with maize protein endosperm bodies, *J. Exp. Bot.,* 33, 439, 1982.
107. Prat, S., Cortadas, J., Puigdomenech, P., and Palau J., Nucleic acid (cDNA) and amino acid sequences of the maize endosperm protein glutelin-2, *Nucleic Acids Res.,* 13, 149, 1985.
108. Esen, A., Bietz, J. A., Paulis, J. W., and Wall, J. S., Tandem repeats in the N-terminal sequence of a proline-rich protein from corn endosperm, *Nature (London),* 296, 678, 1982.
109. Esen, A., Bietz, J. A., Paulis, J. W., and Wall, J. S., Fractionation of alcohol soluble reduced corn glutelins on phosphocellulose and partial characterization of two proline rich fractions, *Cereal Chem.,* 58, 534, 1981.
110. Landry, J., Paulis, J. W., and Fey, D. A., Relationship between alcohol-soluble proteins extracted from maize by different methods, *J. Agric. Food Chem.,* 31, 1317, 1983.
111. Paulis, J. W. and Wall, J. S., Fractionation and characterization of alcohol-soluble reduced corn endosperm glutelin proteins, *Cereal Chem.,* 54, 1223, 1977.
112. Wilson, C. M., Shewry, P. R., and Miflin, B. J., Maize endosperm proteins compared by sodium dodecyl sulphate gel electrophoresis and isoelectric focusing, *Cereal Chem.,* 46, 253, 1981.
113. Lending, C. R. and Larkins, B. A., Changes in the zein composition of protein bodies during maize endosperm development, *Plant Cell,* 1, 1011, 1989.
114. Gianazza, A., Viglienghi, V., Righett, P. C., Salamini, F., and Soave, C., Amino acid composition of zein molecular components, *Phytochemistry,* 16, 315, 1977.
115. Pedersen, K., Argos, P., Naravana, S. V. L., and Larkins, B. A., Sequence analysis and characterization of a maize gene encoding a high-sulfur zein protein of M_r 15000, *J. Biol. Chem.,* 261, 6279, 1986.
116. Philips, R. L. and McLure, B. A., Elevated protein-bound methionine in seeds of maize resistant to lysine plus threonine, *Cereal Chem.,* 62, 213, 1985.
117. Moureaux, T., Baudet, J., and Mossé, J., Fractionnement des albumines du mais par chromatographie sur Sephadex, *C.R. Acad. Sci. Ser. D.,* 266, 1710, 1966.
118. Halasi, R., Adamov, I., and Medakovic, S., Uticaj Djubrenja na Sastav Odnos i Molekulsku Masu Frakcije Proteina u Hibridu Kukuruza NSSC-6666, Res. Rep., University of Novi Sad, Novi Sad, Yugoslavia, 1980.

119. Moureaux, T. and Sallantin, M., Fractionnement des albumines du grain de mais par chromatographie sur carboxymethylcellulose, *C.R. Acad. Sci. Ser. D.,* 264, 1619, 1967.
120. Artemie, V., Medeleanu, M., and Cretu-Arindt, V., Chromatographie on DEAE-cellulose of albumins and globulins from maize, *An. Stiinte. Univ. Al. I. Cuza Iasi Sect.* 1c, 20, 217, 1974.
121. Paulis, J. W., Bietz, J. A., and Wall, J. S., Corn protein subunits. Molecular weights determined by sodium dodecyl sulphate-polyacrylamide gel electrophoresis, *J. Agric. Food Chem.,* 23, 197, 1975.
122. Wilson, C. M., Variations in soluble endosperm proteins of corn (*Zea mays* L.) inbreds as detected by disc gel electrophoresis, *Cereal Chem.,* 58, 401, 1981.
123. Hill, R. D. and McGregor, A. W., Cereal α-amylases in grain research and technology, in *Advances in Cereal Science and Technology,* Vol. 9, Pomeranz, Y., Ed., American Association of Cereal Chemists, St. Paul, MN, 1988, 217.
124. McGregor, A. W., Marchylo, B. A., and Krueger, J. E., Multiple α-amylase components in germinated cereal grains determined by isoelectric focusing and chromatofocusing, *Cereal Chem.,* 65, 326, 1988.
125. Warner, D. A., Grove, M. J., and Knutson, C. A., Isolation and characterization of α-amylases from endosperm of germinating maize, *Cereal Chem.,* 8, 383, 1991.
126. Polnik, I., Kukorica Proteázok Vizsgálata, Ph.D. thesis, Technical University of Budapest, Budapest, Hungary, 1979.
127. Paulis, J. W. and Wall, J. S., Albumins and globulins in extracts of corn grain parts, *Cereal Chem.,* 46, 263, 1969.
128. Melville, J. C. and Scandalios, J. G., Maize endopeptidase: genetic control, chemical characterization and relationship to an endogenous trypsin inhibitor, *Biochem. Genet.,* 7, 15, 1972.
129. Skolenko, V. V., Nekotorye izofermentnye systemy v razlitchnych organach kukuruzy, in *Biochimitcheskie Issledovanya v Processe Selekciji Kukuruzy,* Kovarskij, A.E., Ed., Izdanija Stiinga, Kishinev, 1973, 167.
130. Su, J. C. and Preiss, J., Purification and properties of sucrose synthase from maize kernels, *Plant Physiol.,* 61, 389, 1978.
131. Chourey, P. S. and Nelson, O. E., The enzymatic deficiency conditioned by the shrunken-1 mutations in maize, *Biochem. Genet.,* 14, 1041, 1976.
132. Wilson, C. M., Purification of a corn ribonuclease, *J. Biol. Chem.,* 242, 2260, 1967.
133. Wilson, C. M. and Alexander, D. E., Ribonuclease activity in normal and opaque-2 mutant endosperm of maize, *Science,* 155, 1575, 1967.
134. Wilson, C. M., Plant nucleases. IV. Genetic control of ribonuclease activity in corn endosperm, *Biochem. Genet.,* 9, 53, 1973.
135. Chiba, S. and Shimomura, T., Purification and some properties of flint corn α-glucosidase, *Agric. Biol. Chem.,* 39, 1033, 1975.
136. Van Etten, C. H., Miller, R. W., Earle, F. R., Wolff, I. A., and Jones, Q., Hydroxyproline content of seed meals, *J. Agric. Food Chem.,* 9, 433, 1961.
137. Boundy, A., Wall, J. S., Turner, J. E., Woychik, J. H., and Dimler, R. J., A mucopolysaccharide containing hydroxyproline from corn pericarp, *J. Biol Chem.,* 242, 2410, 1967.
138. Lamport, D. T. A. and Miller, D. H., Hydroxyproline arabinosides in the plant kingdom, *Plant Physiol.,* 48, 454, 1971.
139. Mahonney, W. C., Hermodson, M. A., Jones, B., Powers, D. D., Corfman, R. S., and Reeck, G. R., Amino acid sequence and secondary structural analysis of the corn inhibitor of trypsin and activated Hageman factor, *J. Biol. Chem.,* 259, 8412, 1984.

140. Jones, B. L. and Cooper, D. B., Purification and characterization of corn (*Zea mais* L.) protein similar to purothionins, *J. Agric. Food Chem.*, 28, 90, 1980.
141. Landry, J. and Moureaux, T., Distribution and amino acid composition of protein group located in different parts of maize grain, *J. Agric. Food Chem.*, 28, 1186, 1980.
142. Cross, J. W. and Adams, W. R., Differences in the embryo specific globulins among maize inbred lines and their hybrids, *Crop Sci.*, 23, 1160, 1983.
143. Tömösközi, S., Simándi, B., Borsiczky, E., and Nagy, J., Effect of supercritical extraction on properties of oils and protein products, in *Proc. World Conf. Oilseed Technology and Utilization,* Applewhite, T.H., Ed., AOAC Press, Champaign, IL, 1993, 438.
144. Tömösközi, S., Pungor, A., Lásztity, R., and Stefan, P., Functional properties of some new plant protein isolates, *J. Food Phys.*, 55, 5, 1991.
145. Lásztity, R., Tömösközi, S., Nagy, J., and Pungor, A., The surface properties and other functional parameters of cereal germ proteins, in *Food Proteins: Structure and Functionality,* Schwenke, K.D. and Mothes, R., Eds., VCH, Weinheim, 1993, 310.
146. Tsen, C. C., Cereal germs used in bakery products: chemistry and nutrition, in *Cereals for Food and Beverages, Recent Progress in Cereal Chemistry,* Inglett, G.E. and Munck, L., Eds., Academic Press, New York, 1980, 245.
147. Zayas, J. F. and Lin, C. S., Emulsifying properties of corn germ proteins, *Cereal Chem.*, 66, 263, 1989.
148. Zayas, J. F. and Lin, C. S., Water retention of two types of hexane-defatted corn germ proteins and soy protein flour, *Cereal Chem.*, 66, 51, 1989.
149. Stringfellow, A. C., Brekke, O. L., Pfeifer, V. F., Burbridge, L. H., and Griffin, E. L., Fractionation of defatted wheat- and corn-germ flours by air classification, *Cereal Chem.*, 54, 415, 1976.
150. Sternberg, M., Phillips, R. D., and Daley, L. H., Maize protein concentrate, in *Cereals for Food and Beverages. Recent Progress in Cereal Chemistry,* Inglett, G.E. and Munck, L., Eds., Academic Press, New York, 1980, 275.
151. Arai, S., Yamasita, M., and Fujimaki, M., Plastein reaction and its applications, *Cereal Food World,* 20, 107, 1975.
152. Mannheim, A. and Cheryan, M., Water-soluble zein by enzymatic modification in organic solvents, *Cereal Chem.*, 70, 115, 1993.
153. Wu, Y. V., Sexson, K. R., and Wall, J. S., Protein-rich residue from corn alcohol distillation: fractionation and characterization, *Cereal Chem.*, 58, 343, 1981.
154. Satterlee, L. D., Vavak, D. M., Abdul-Kadir, R., and Kendrick, J. R., The chemical, functional and nutritional characterization of protein concentrates from distillers grains, *Cereal Chem.*, 53, 739, 1976.
155. Chen, M. C., Beeson, W. M., Perry, T. W., and Mohler, M. T., The effects of varying levels of processed distillers solubles and distiller grains with solubles on nitrogen and energy metabolism of beef steers, *J. Anim. Sci.*, 44, 859, 1977.
156. Thong, L. A., Jensen, A. H., Harmon, B. G., and Cornelius, S. G., Distillers dried grains with solubles as a supplemental protein source in diets for gestating swine, *J. Anim. Sci.*, 46, 674, 1978.
157. Wu, Y. V., Protein-rich residue from ethanolic fermentation of high lysine, dent, waxy and white corn varieties, *Cereal Chem.*, 66, 506, 1989.
158. Hussein, M., Plant Proteins and Their Role in the Solving of Protein Problems in Arab Republic of Egypt, Ph.D. thesis, Technical University of Budapest, Budapest, Hungary, 1979.

159. Kulakova, E. V., Vainerman, E. S., and Rogoshin, S. V., Contribution to the investigation of corn germ. I. Corn germ is a valuable source of protein, *Nahrung,* 26, 451, 1982.
160. Gardner, H. W., Lipoxygenase pathway in cereals, in *Advances in Cereal Science and Technology,* Vol. 9, Pomeranz, Y., Ed., American Association of Cereal Chemists, St. Paul, MN, 1988, 161.

7 Sorghum Proteins

I. INTRODUCTION, GENERAL CHARACTERIZATION OF SORGHUM PROTEINS

Grain sorghum is one of the major crops grown for human consumption in arid and semiarid regions of Africa and Asia. In the developed countries, sorghum is grown mainly for animal feed. Asia, northern Central America, and Africa contribute most of the world production of sorghum. India, China, Nigeria, Sudan, and South Africa are the major sorghum-producing countries.

A great variety of sorghum types are known; however, the more simplified classification, based on single grain and glume relationship and panicle type, presented by Harlan and De Wet[1] is widely used. In this classification, sorghum has been divided into two major races: *Sorghum bicolor* subsp. *bicolor* (cultivated) and *Sorghum bicolor* subsp. *arundinaceum* (spontaneous). In India, depending on the growing period during the year, it is classified as kharif (June sowing) or rabi (October sowing) sorghum. Among cultivated races *S. bicolor guinea, S. gaudatum, S. kafir,* and *S. durra* are the most important. The fact that new plants are being developed continuously through hybridization means that the botanical classification may not be universally applicable.[2]

Sorghum cultivars vary considerably with respect to pericarp color (white, yellow, red, brown), kernel size and shape, hardness of endosperm (corneous and floury), and condensed tannin content (low- and high-tannin sorghum). Generally, brown varieties have a high tannin content. Although condensed tannins reduce the nutritive value, this variety is widely grown due to its high resistance to ravaging pests in the field and its protective effect against birds ("birdproof" sorghum). In recent times the utilization of sorghum for beer production has increased, and particularly the red and white sorghums are classified into groups of malting and nonmalting varieties.

The kernel of the sorghum plant is generally spherical (weight 20 to 30 mg) and may be divided into three morphological parts: seed coat, germ, and endosperm. The seed coat constitutes about 4.3 to 7.9% of the dry weight and is composed of the pericarp and testa. The pericarp contains pigments which migrate to the endosperm and affect the quality of milled sorghum. The testa layer, immediately below the pericarp and around the aleurone, contains tannins. Tannins in grain sorghum have been shown to offer resistance against bird attacks. The embryo contributes about 7.8 to 12.1% of the dry weight of the kernel. The germ of some sorghum cultivars is more deeply embedded inside the endosperm and is difficult to remove.[4] The largest part of the grain, the endosperm (81.1 to 84.6% of the dry weight of the kernel), consists of the aleurone layer and peripheral, corneous, intermediate, and floury portions. The relative proportion of corneous to floury endosperm within the sorghum kernel is referred to as endosperm texture. Kernels with almost corneous or entirely floury endosperm have been identified. The corneous endosperm is responsible for greater hardness, less breakage during pearling, easy removal of the bran, greater resistance to pest infestation during storage, and higher yields during milling as compared to the floury type.

On the basis of chemical composition, sorghum endosperm is classified as waxy (100% amylopectin in starch), normal (75% amylopectin + 25% amylose), high lysine, sugary, or yellow.[5] The chemical composition of sorghum is similar to that of other cereals and has been reviewed by several authors.[5-8,95]

In the last decade a great deal of progress has been made in research on sorghum. This progress is connected with a lot of factors — the growing interest in use of sorghum for production of different varieties of food and for beer production, breeding of new high-lysine varieties, and development of new industrial technologies for sorghum processing. As a result our knowledge about sorghum proteins has increased significantly.

The average protein content of sorghum is 11 to 12%. There is considerable variation in the protein content depending on the variety, agricultural technique, and other factors. In his review paper Rooney[9] reported that the protein content varied from 8.7 to 16.8%. Surveys of the world collection of sorghums showed even greater variability in protein: 4.7 to 17.0%.[6,11] A range from about 6 to 25% was reported in the review paper of Hoseney et al.[6]

The protein distribution between different morphological parts of the sorghum grain is uneven, as is the case with other cereals. The embryo is richest in protein content (up to 20%). The protein content of the endosperm is lower; however, the outer layers of the endosperm are richer in proteins. The pericarp has the lowest protein content. More than 80% of the total protein of the sorghum grain is located in the endosperm as it is the largest part of the grain. The greatest part of the sorghum grain protein is concentrated in subcellular organelles and particulates, as in many other cereals. The protein-rich bodies and protein matrix present in the sorghum endosperm were investigated by several authors[12,13] using light scanning and transmission electron microscopy. Scanning electron micrographs of sections of sorghum endosperm tissue destarched by treatment with α-amylase indicated that the roughly spherical bodies 2 to 4 μm in diameter are larger than those of corn. The internal structure of the protein bodies and the protein matrix in which they are embedded were explored by transmission electron microscopy of the sections. The observations indicated a lamellar structure in the protein bodies. Treatment with hot 60% alcohol dissolved most of the protein bodies, but left the matrix. This observation supports the view that protein bodies are composed mainly of prolamins and that the matrix contains glutelins.

The cells of the aleurone layer are rich in protein and also contain protein bodies. Based on solubility it can be stated that the proteins forming protein bodies of the aleurone layer belong to the globulin solubility group. Protein bodies were also isolated from the parenchymal tissue of the germ scutellum.[14] The isolated bodies resembled those of the aleurone layer in appearance and composition. It was reported[15] that protein bodies exhibited some enzymatic activity. Protease, α- and β-glucosidase, pyrophosphatase, and ribonuclease activities were detected. The existence of a dense, high-protein layer of endosperm cells just beneath the aleurone cells has been well documented in sorghum grains.[16]

Differences in protein content were observed between vitreous and opaque endosperms in the same variety.[17] The average protein content of the opaque part of endosperm was 6.1% and that of vitreous endosperm was 10.8%.

The fractionation of the sorghum proteins based on the Osborne procedure was used widely in the investigation of sorghum proteins. The original procedure was modified by Virupaksha and Sastry.[11] After the extraction of the albumins and globulins, the prolamin of sorghum (kafirin) was extracted with 60% ethyl alcohol at a higher temperature. Finally, the glutelins were solubilized using 0.4% sodium hydroxide. The aqueous *tert*-butyl alcohol, as was reported,[18] may be used successfully for the extraction of kafirin.

The procedure of Landry and Moureaux[19] — as reported by Jambunathan and Mertz[20] — was successfully used for the extraction of sorghum proteins. The Landry-Moureaux procedure reduces disulfide bonds and changes the native state of the endosperm proteins. Solvents containing a reducing agent (dithiothreitol) were also used by Wu and Wall.[21] The quantities of the protein solubility fractions are shown in Table 1.

TABLE 1
Protein Solubility Fractions of Sorghum Grain (% of Total Protein)

Albumin	Globulin	Kafirin	Glutelin	Ref.
1.3–7.7	2.0–9.3	32.6–58.8	19.0–37.4	11
16.0	16.0	48.0	25	21
3.0	3.0	37.0	35.0	18
23.4	11.6	51.8	18.9	22
12.2–17.2	—	30.9–43.5	36.2–43.6	8, 23

As seen in Table 1, great differences exist between the reported data. This is partly due to differences in the fractionation procedure and is particularly related to the great number of cultivated sorghum varieties.

After discovery of high-lysine maize in 1964, plant breeders were searching for mutants similar to opaque-2 maize among the other economically important cereal grains. The first naturally occurring mutant from Ethiopia was identified by Munck et al.[24] In 1973 Singh and Axtell[25a] reported the discovery of two lines of Ethiopian origin (IS 11167 and IS 11758) that were high in lysine and protein. These two varieties were found among 62 floury endosperm sorghums selected from the world collection of 9000 entries. Inheritance studies have suggested that the increased lysine content is controlled by a single recessive gene which increases lysine, arginine, aspartic acid, glycine, and tryptophan and decreases glutamic acid, proline, alanine, and leucine. Another high-lysine sorghum, P-721 opaque, was produced by chemical mutagen treatment of normal grain.[26] Unfortunately, the high-lysine mutants had some disadvantageous properties such as lower yield and digestibility, high tannin content, and reduced hardness of endosperm. Axtell and Ejeta[25] have increased yields of the P-721 mutant from 67% to 99% by selective breeding. The improved grain was more vitreous than the original soft-endosperm P-721. Ejeta and Axtell[26a] have extended their studies on breeding high-lysine sorghum for increased kernel hardness. In their studies a varying degree of kernel modification continued to arise from one generation to the next, even when well developed, completely modified kernels were planted. Further work is needed in this area. A review of recent efforts to improve sorghum quality has recently been published by Mertz et al.[27]

Early studies on high-lysine protein sorghum revealed a reduced amount of prolamins (kafirins).[28] High-lysine sorghum endosperm was found to contain fewer and smaller protein bodies. More recent investigations have confirmed the view that changes in protein composition are characterized by quantitative shifts in major protein fractions rather than by qualitative changes in protein fractions.[29] The enhanced lysine content of opaque mutants results primarily from an increase in relatively lysine-rich glutelins and a decrease in lysine-deficient prolamins.

The protein and lysine levels in developing kernels of normal and high-lysine sorghum were also studied by several research workers.[29-32] Seed weight and volume increased steadily over a 45-day period after half-bloom for normal sorghum, but plateaued a week earlier for opaque mutants. Normal endosperm protein declined 0.7% during seed maturation while that of opaque mutants increased 1.2%. Albumins and globulins (determined by the Landry-Moureaux procedure) differed little among lines. Prolamin accumulation in opaque mutants plateaued 2 weeks earlier than in normal sorghum, whereas glutelin increased more rapidly in opaque than in normal endosperm.[29] The highest endosperm protein and lysine content of all genotypes is found during the late dough stage (31 days after flowering).[31] This finding suggests that there is a nutritional basis for the tradition of Ethiopian farmers to consume high-lysine varieties exclusively at the milk dough and late dough stages of grain development.

Hard-endosperm kernels develop faster and have a higher concentration of protein bodies in the outer endosperm than the soft-endosperm kernels.[33] Differences have also been observed in the distribution of kafirin subfractions.[32,96]

Several studies have investigated the amino acid composition of normal sorghum genotypes and high-lysine sorghum mutants. Most of this work has been reviewed by Wall and Paulis,[7] Hoseney et al.,[6] and Chung and Pomeranz.[34] The amino acid composition of sorghum protein is similar to that of maize. Sorghum protein is usually high in glutamic acid, leucine, alanine, proline, and aspartic acid. The lysine content is relatively low except in high-lysine mutants. The gross amino acid composition — as with other cereals — is dependent on the total protein content.

Glutamic acid, alanine, and leucine are highly positively correlated with the protein content. Conversely, lysine and glycine are highly negatively correlated with the protein content.

A study with sorghum using grain samples covering a wide range of N content and employing amino acid analysis conditions of the highest possibly accuracy was undertaken by Mossé et al.[35] The 12 grain samples analyzed corresponded to seven *Sorghum bicolor* (L.) Moench genotypes from field-grown sorghums. One cultivar (Monitor) was grown under different conditions in six locations. The total nitrogen content ranged from 1.5 to 3 g/100 g grain (Table 2). Amino acid composition was determined from six different hydrolysates per sample. It was found that the amino acid levels in grain increased linearly as a function of N, with correlation coefficients close to 1 for most amino acids regardless of sorghum genotype or phenotype. As a result, the amino acid composition of any grain sample of normal sorghum can be predicted from its N content. Amino acids in grain protein changed as hyperbolic functions of N, which increased for alanine, leucine, isoleucine, phenylalanine, and glutamine + glutamic acid, remained constant for serine, tyrosine, tryptophan, and asparagine + aspartic acid, and decreased for the other amino acids. The nitrogen-to-protein conversion factor remained practically constant and close to 5.81 within the N range investigated. The results also showed that the composition of storage proteins accumulated in sorghum grain remained constant, with the rate of deposition of prolamins being roughly 1.5 times that of glutelins. The effect of changes in amino acid composition on the variation of the limiting amino acid score (in percent, according to a report of FAO 1973) is shown in Figure 1 as published by Baudet et al.[36] High-lysine mutants of sorghum have elevated contents of lysine (2.7 to 3.3%) and tryptophan (1.0 to 1.3%).[37]

II. STORAGE PROTEINS

A. Low Molecular Weight Storage Proteins (Kafirins)

The low molecular weight storage protein of sorghum named kafirin is in many aspects similar to zein of maize. Kafirin is generally extracted using hot 70% aqueous ethanol or with 60% *tert*-butyl alcohol. It is also soluble in 6 *M* guanidine hydrochloride and 8 *M* urea as well as in dimethyl sulfoxide, methyl formamide, and 50% acetic acid.[38,39] In the framework of this chapter kafirin is defined as the protein fraction extracted with 70% aqueous ethanol not containing a reducing agent.

The alcohol-soluble fraction is a mixture of different proteins which may be separated by different techniques. Using flour extraction with 30% (v/v) *tert*-butanol only one portion of kafirin can be solubilized, it is called β-kafirin. From the residue the α-kafirin can be extracted with 90% (v/v) *tert*-butyl alcohol.[40-42] By chromatography on Sephadex G-100 columns two main fractions were separated, with molecular weights of >100 kDa and 4 to 30 kDa.[43,44] Early research using PAGE revealed several polypeptide bands.[39,43,44] The electrophoretic patterns of reduced and alkylated

TABLE 2
Amino Acid Composition of Sorghum Samples (g/16 g Nitrogen)

	Variety[a]											
Component	**1**	**2**	**3**	**4**	**5**	**6**	**7**	**8**	**9**	**10**	**11**	**12**
N[b]	1.51	1.67	1.74	1.86	1.86	1.88	2.06	2.25	2.34	2.66	2.86	2.97
Glycine	3.4	3.15	3.05	3.05	3.1	2.9	2.85	2.8	3.0	2.75	2.55	2.5
Alanine	9.1	9.2	9.2	9.4	9.5	9.1	9.6	9.5	9.3	9.8	9.7	10.0
Valine	5.2	5.5	5.3	5.6	5.6	5.2	5.6	5.3	5.3	5.3	5.2	5.1
Leucine	12.7	13.9	13.6	13.8	14.2	13.6	14.4	13.8	14.3	14.2	14.1	14.7
Isoleucine	4.1	4.3	4.2	4.3	4.4	4.1	4.3	4.2	4.2	4.4	4.3	4.4
Serine	4.7	4.6	4.5	4.6	4.7	4.5	4.5	4.7	4.6	4.7	4.5	4.5
Threonine	3.35	3.25	3.15	3.3	3.3	3.2	3.15	3.2	3.2	3.2	3.1	3.0
Tyrosine	3.9	4.2	4.1	4.2	4.3	3.9	4.3	3.9	4.0	4.0	4.0	4.1
Phenylalanine	5.2	5.5	5.4	5.5	5.5	5.2	5.4	5.5	5.3	5.5	5.6	5.7
Tryptophan	1.08	1.03	1.00	1.01	1.11	0.84	1.00	1.05	1.05	1.02	1.00	1.00
Proline	8.1	8.8	8.5	8.6	8.9	8.2	8.9	8.3	8.1	8.4	8.3	8.4
Methionine	2.00	1.65	1.55	1.60	1.70	1.35	1.55	1.35	1.65	1.60	1.40	1.40
Half cystine	2.15	1.90	1.70	1.75	1.90	1.75	1.65	1.85	1.90	1.60	1.45	1.50
Lysine	2.5	2.3	2.3	2.3	2.3	2.1	2.15	2.05	2.3	1.95	1.95	1.65
Histidine	2.3	2.2	2.15	2.25	2.3	2.2	2.15	2.3	2.1	2.05	2.0	2.0
Arginine	4.1	4.0	4.0	4.0	4.1	3.8	3.8	3.7	4.2	3.7	3.7	3.1
Asx[c]	6.7	7.0	7.0	7.0	6.9	6.7	7.0	7.7	7.3	7.3	7.1	6.7
Glx[c]	20.3	21.0	20.8	21.4	21.7	20.8	22.0	22.4	21.2	22.6	22.3	22.9
Amide NH_3	2.45	2.7	2.7	2.75	2.7	2.5	2.85	2.85	2.65	2.95	2.85	3.05
R[d]	92.9	95.3	94.0	95.7	97.3	91.1	96.1	95.6	94.1	96.0	94.2	94.6

[a] 1, BIL 1; 2 to 7, Monitor; 8, SA 10015; 9, F30R; 10, IS 2926; 11, lowar Man Majra; 12, B 4359.
[b] N = grain nitrogen content (g/100 g dry matter).
[c] Asx and Glx were evaluated in grams of aspartic acid and glutamic acid, respectively.
[d] Percentage of nitrogen recovered by amino acid analysis.

From Mossé, J. Huet, J. C., and Baudet, J., *Cereal Chem.*, 65, 271 , 1988. With permission.

kafirin were similar to those of unreduced kafirin. The conclusion was made on the basis of these results that the disulfide bonds of low molecular weight storage proteins of sorghum are predominantly intramolecular. More recent investigations using IEF and SDS-PAGE confirmed the heterogeneity of kafirin and also of subfractions α- and β-kafirin.[40,45] Good separation was achieved also with reversed-phase high-performance liquid chromatography (RP-HPLC).[45]

In Figure 2 RP-HPLC patterns of kafirins (and alcohol-soluble reduced glutelins) published by Sastry et al.[45] are shown. The separation indicates that kafirins from the same genotypes contain mostly the same protein components, but with quantitative differences in amounts. Grains of different inbred strains usually contain some different kafirin proteins. The hybrids contain proteins inherited from both parents,

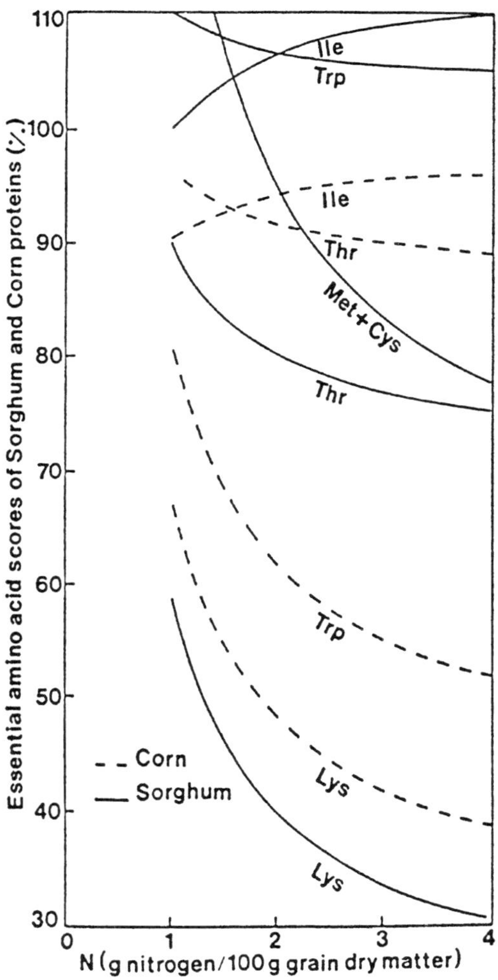

FIGURE 1 Variation of limiting amino acid score (%) in sorghum and corn as a function of grain nitrogen content (N), isoleucine (Ile), tryptophan (Trp), threonine (Thr), methionine plus cysteine (Met + Cys), and lysine (Lys). Essential amino acid scores are from FAO 1973. (From Mossé, J., Huet, C., and Baudet, J., *Cereal Chem.,* 65, 271, 1988. With permission.)

with those from the female predominating. Representatives of the different sorghum races vary in their component alcohol-soluble proteins, with those most widely removed from the geographical center of origin showing the greatest differences. Taylor and Schussler[47] reported that the patterns of kafirins revealed by PAGE in an acidic buffer varied with the sorghum cultivar. Recently enzyme-linked immunosorbent assay (ELISA) was also successfully used to quantitate the relative proportions of α-, β-, and γ-kafirin[46] (γ-kafirin = alcohol-soluble subunits of reduced glutelin[41]).

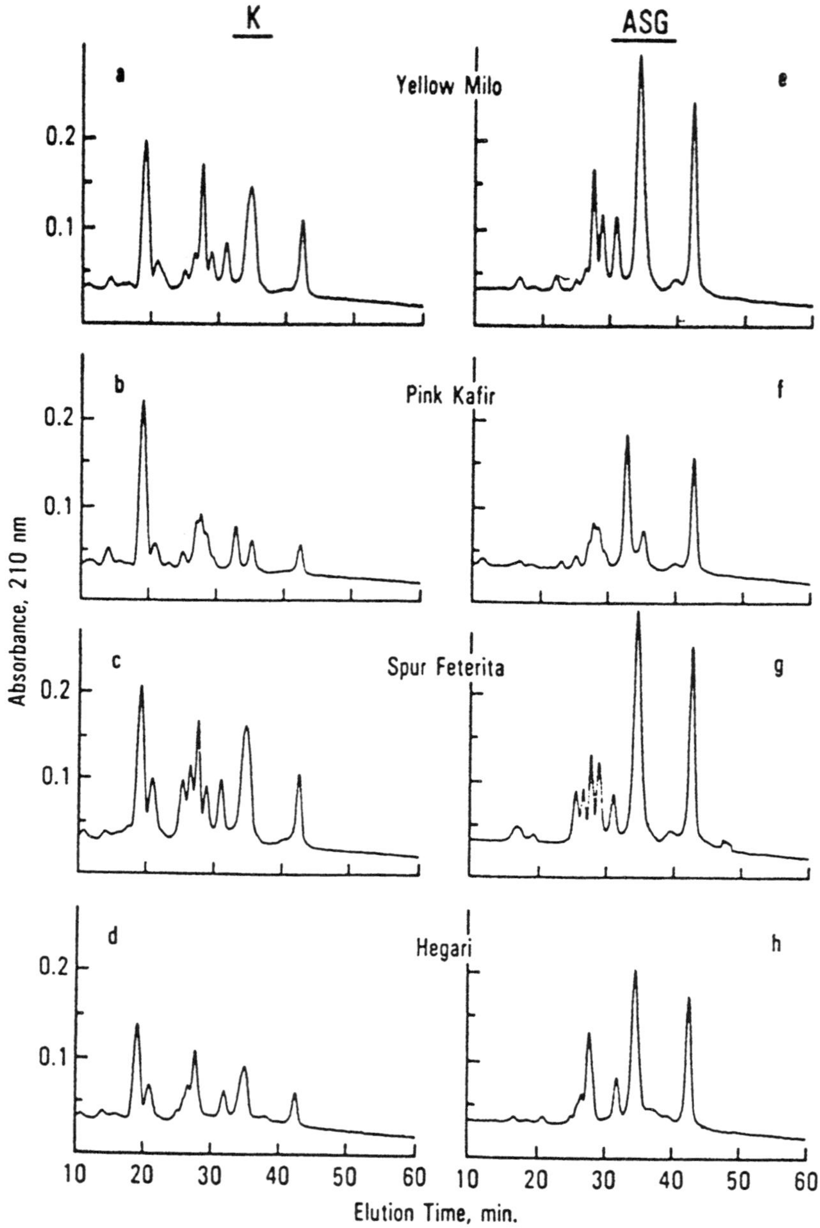

FIGURE 2 Reversed-phase high-performance liquid chromatography (RP-HPLC) elution patterns of kafirins (K) and alcohol-soluble reduced glutelins (ASG) extracted from Standard Yellow Milo (a and e), Pink Kafir (b and f), Spur Feterita (c and g), and Hegari (d and h) sorghum grains. (From Sastry, L.V.S., Paulis, J.E., Bietz, J.A., and Wall, J.S., *Cereal Chem.*, 63, 420, 1986. With permission.)

Correlations were found between kafirin content and distribution and sorghum grain hardness.[46,48,49]

Opaque endosperm contained a significantly lower amount of kafirin than vitreous endosperm. The vitreous endosperm of a hard sorghum variety (Mshimba) contained 80 to 84% α-kafirin, 7 to 8% β-kafirin, and 9 to 12% γ-kafirin. Opaque endosperm contained 66 to 71% α-kafirin, 10 to 13% β-kafirin, and 19 to 21% γ-kafirin.[46] The electrophoretic spectra (SDS-PAGE) of kafirin extracted with alcohol (without a reducing agent) showed three characteristic bands with molecular weights of 28, 22, and 19 kDa.[40,46,50] SDS-PAGE of isolated α-kafirin gave two bands of M_r 28,000 (α_1-kafirin) and M_r 22,000 (α_2-kafirin). The β-kafirin fraction contained a single band of M_r 19,000. γ-Kafirin (the alcohol-soluble subunit of glutelin) also contained a single band of M_r 27,000 as noted by Mazhar et al.[40] Immunochemical studies by these authors showed that α-kafirin antibody reacted with both the M_r 28,000 and M_r 22,000 bands, in addition to that of M_r 50,000. The β-kafirin antibody reacted with the M_r 19,000 band, and the γ-kafirin antibody reacted with only a single band of M_r 27,000. Since there is very little difference in the M_rs of the α_1- and γ-kafirins, the cross-reactivity was also checked by dot-blot ELISA. The antibodies raised against α-kafirin did not cross-react with the γ-kafirin antigen, and vice versa, on dot blots. Similar results were obtained by Watterson et al.,[46] who reported that the α-kafirin serum reacted specifically with M_r 25,000 and 23,000 bands. Anti-β-kafirin serum reacted specifically with the M_r 20,000 band, and anti-γ-kafirin serum reacted with the M_r 28,000 band. It was found that kafirins are immunologically related not only to zeins, but also to prolamins from tropical millets.

The significant progress in investigation of maize proteins and the high degree of similarity between maize and sorghum proteins stimulated research on the finer structure and genetic basis of sorghum proteins. As a result of these investigations our knowledge about sorghum prolamins has increased significantly in the last decade. In a pioneering study by Bietz[51] it was demonstrated by N-terminal amino acid analysis of kafirins isolated from 60% *tert*-butanol extracts of sorghum that different kafirins have a high degree of homology and thus must constitute a family of closely related proteins coded by a multigene system. It was suggested that allelic genes coding for the synthesis of kafirins might show some significant differences among most of the genotypes investigated in this study.[52]

In review papers on cereal prolamins[52,53] the authors expressed the view that the major kafirin components are similar to those of Z19 and Z22 zeins. Proteins related to minor low-M_r zeins and to soluble glutelin subunits are present in kafirin fractions extracted in the presence of a reducing agent.[52]

Electrophoretic analysis of translation products of polyadenylated RNA isolated from mid-maturation sorghum seed in the presence of [^{35}S]-methionine, [^{3}H]-leucine, or [^{3}H]-valine revealed two major proteins of 24 kDa and 21 kDa.[50] These products were not detected when [^{3}H]-lysine was supplied as the radioactive substrate. The molecular weight values were approximately 2 kDa larger than those obtained for native kafirin, consistent with the presence of a signal sequence on each molecular species. Sequence analysis of two cDNA clones (pSK8 and pSKR2) from sorghum seed mRNA revealed them to be highly homologous with each other and to the 22-kDa zeins from maize, suggesting that they represented kafirin (K22) cDNAs. Compared with pSKR2, pSK8 had an insertion of 24 nucleotides and a deletion of 24 nucleotides, so that the coding regions were nearly identical in length. All three sequences had a 21-amino-acid signal sequence (consensus: MATKIESLLMLLA-LSASAATA). N-terminal analysis of the 22-kDa kafirin by Bietz[51] revealed the following amino acid sequence:

F I P C   P I   I
H_2N-   I Q SLA   AIA QFLPAL-
VY A Y   QN   A

This sequence closely matches the amino acid sequence deduced from the cDNA data,[50] starting at amino acid position 22, and provides confirmation that the first 21 amino acids encoded by cDNA clones represent a signal peptide in precursor kafirin that is cleared during maturation to yield the form found in mature seed endosperm.

As mentioned in Chapter 6, a structural model has been proposed by Argos et al.[54] for the 22- and 19-kDa zeins, based on the nine homologous repeat units in their primary structure[55] and on their circular dichroism (CD) spectra.[54] The deduced amino acid sequence of kafirin showed eight copies of a repetitive amino acid block in the C-terminal domain with the consensus sequence

F A P
LL LN LALANPAAYLQQQQ
I P Q

The sequence is highly homologous with corresponding zein sequences published by Spena et al.[55,56] and Geraghty et al.[57] Genetic analysis indicated the presence of less than 20 copies of kafirin genes encoding the 22- and 19-kDa kafirin proteins. As transformation and regeneration of cereal crops are now becoming feasible, the lower genomic copy number of kafirin genes (about 20) relative to zeins (over 100) may indicate that a low number of modified kafirin gene sequences (e.g., high lysine) will have a more pronounced effect on sorghum grain quality than on that of maize.

The determinations of amino acid composition of kafirin showed that, like zein, sorghum prolamins are rich in glutamic acid (glutamine) and nonpolar amino acids (e.g, leucine, alanine). They contain practically no lysine. Unfortunately no data were published about tryptophan content (Table 3.).

B. High Molecular Weight Storage Proteins (Glutelins)

The high molecular weight storage protein of sorghum (sorghum glutelin) may be extracted with dilute sodium hydroxide. To avoid destruction caused by the use of alkali hydroxides as extractants, other solvents were also studied. The urea and SDA-urea solvent solutions are not as effective as sodium hydroxide. If solvents

TABLE 3
Amino Acid Composition of Kafirin (g/l00 g Protein)

Amino Acid	1[a]	2[b]	3[c]	4[d]
LYS	0.1	0.15	Trace	0.2
ARG	0.9	1.50	1.1	1.8
HIS	1.0	1.05	1.2	2.2
ASX	10.6	6.2	5.1	5.2
GLX	25.9	26.0	22.0	22.0
THR	2.6	2.3	2.7	2.8
SER	4.1	4.0	5.0	3.9
TYR	5.5	4.8	3.8	4.9
PRO	10.0	10.0	9.9	9.8
GLY	1.1	1.45	2.3	1.7
ALA	12.4	10.6	15.6	10.6
VAL	5.0	4.3	4.8	4.8
MET	1.0	1.05	1.4	2.4
CYS	0.4	0.9	1.2	0.5
ILE	4.8	4.2	3.5	4.3
LEU	19.2	17.8	16.1	14.7
PHE	6.4	6.2	4.3	5.8
TRP	ND	ND	ND	ND

Note: ND, not determined.

[a] From Jones and Beckwith.[18]
[b] From Mossé et al.[35]
[c] From Bright and Shewry.[59]
[d] From Taylor and Schüssler.[58]

containing reducing agents are used the solubility increases. The alkylated-reduced protein is 85 to 89% soluble in 6 *M* guanidine hydrochloride.[60] The sequential extraction procedure of Landry and Moureaux[19] is also used, producing different glutelin fractions. The reduction of the disulfide bonds also results in the decrease of the average molecular weight. These facts confirm the hypothesis that high molecular weight storage protein contains a lot of subunits (polypeptides) which are linked together with intermolecular disulfide bonds.

The subunits of sorghum glutelin may be separated by common techniques used in the study of other cereal proteins. One portion of the subunits is soluble in aqueous ethanol and water. This fraction is named alcohol-soluble reduced glutelin (ASG) or reduced soluble protein (RSP). The name γ-kafirin is also used.[41,42,46] Phosphocellulose chromatography of sorghum RSP produced three peaks;[61] however, the majority of the protein was present in the third fraction. SDS-PAGE of RSP and the fractions obtained by phosphocellulose chromatography showed that the first fraction consisted of bands of 28 and 17 kDa, the second fraction had bands of 28, 16, and 14 kDa, and the third fraction had a major band of 28 and a lesser band of 15 kDa. The third fraction contained the major components of RSP. Using RP-HPLC and IEF Sastry et al.[45] studied the alcohol-soluble subunits of sorghum glutelin. Both separation techniques confirmed the heterogeneity of the subunits. The IEF patterns of the ASGs had most bands in common with the kafirins of the same cultivar, but ASG bands with pI near 8 appeared to be more prominent than the corresponding kafirin bands. These differences may reflect variations in the extractability of the proteins, variations in their tendencies to form intermolecular disulfide cross-linkages, as well as differences in composition between ASG and kafirins.

Comparison of adjacent patterns of kafirin and ASG obtained by RP-HPLC has indicated that the kafirin and ASG patterns of the same inbred strain may contain some of the same polypeptide units, but there are considerable quantitative differences.

Two-dimensional electrophoresis (SDS-PAGE-IEF) showed that the single bands of sorghum RSP contained multiple isomers with different pI values.[62] SDS-PAGE of RSP by Evans et al.[63] showed a major band of 28 kDa and a minor one of about 49 kDa.

Protein bodies from natural sorghum grain were extracted with aqueous alcohol plus reducing agent by Taylor et al.[64] TEM studies revealed that cross-linked kafirin was located within the protein bodies. Electrophoresis demonstrated great similarity between kafirin and cross-linked kafirin.

The amino acid composition of total sorghum glutelin is characterized by high contents of glutamic acid + glutamine, leucine, proline, and alanine. Lysine content is relatively low, but is higher than that of alcohol-soluble unreduced kafirin (Table 4). The water-soluble fraction of reduced sorghum glutelin (RSP) has a high proline content and also a high amount of cysteine.

Our knowledge about the fine structure of sorghum glutelin subunits is relatively poor. The N-terminal amino acid sequence of sorghum RSP was recently studied by Taylor et al.[61] The N-terminal primary structure of the heterogeneous sorghum RSP showed no polymorphism, and 10 of the first 11 residues were identical to the corresponding sequence of maize RSP (Figure 3). The sorghum homologue also appeared to contain the repeating hexapeptide Pro–Pro–Pro–Val–His–Leu found in maize RSP.

III. CYTOPLASMIC (METABOLICALLY ACTIVE) PROTEINS

A. Enzymes and Enzyme Inhibitors

Like other cereal grains, sorghum contains various enzymes. From a practical point of view the amylases, proteases, and some redox enzymes are the most important. To date little research has been done in the field of sorghum enzymes. Results of such investigations are reviewed in a book edited by Krueger et al.,[66] a review paper of Hill and McGregor,[67] and an article by McGregor et al.[68]

TABLE 4
Amino Acid Composition of Sorghum Glutelin (g/100 g Protein)

		Reduced Glutelin[b]				
Amino Acid	Alkali Soluble[a]	Alcohol Soluble	Buffer Soluble	Detergent Soluble	Glutelin (Buffer + SDS)[c]	RSP[d]
Lysine	2.1	0.15	2.53	4.55	3.4	0.5
Histidine	2.0	1.7	6.0	2.7	3.2	8.1
Arginine	3.6	—	—	—	—	3.0
Aspartic acid	6.2[e]	—	—	—	—	0.7
Glutamic acid	18.7[e]	—	—	—	—	15.7
Threonine	3.5	2.78	5.4	4.13	4.0	4.7
Serine	4.4	—	—	—	—	4.2
Tyrosine	3.1	—	—	—	2.9	—
Proline	10.9	—	—	—	—	28.8
Glycine	2.4	—	—	—	—	5.3
Alanine	9.1	—	—	—	—	5.1
Valine	5.1	5.0	5.1	5.53	5.4	6.1
Methionine	1.4	1.45	1.38	1.73	1.6	1.3
Isoleucine	4.3	4.7	3.05	4.5	3.6	2.9
Leucine	14.9	20.6	8.03	14.88	9.2	8.3
Phenylalanine	5.5	6.88	4.25	6.35	5.1	3.2
Tryptophan	ND	ND	ND	ND	ND	ND
Cystine	1.2	—	—	—	—	6.7

Note: ND, not determined.

[a] From Jones and Beckwith.[18]
[b] From Jambunathan and Mertz.[65]
[c] From Neucere and Sumrell.[22]
[d] From Evans et al.[63]
[e] Aspartic acid and glutamic acid are used interchangably with asparagine and glutamine, respectively.

The growing interest in using sorghum as a raw material for beer production in some sorghum-growing countries has stimulated research connected with germination of sorghum and diastatic activity of sorghum malt.[69-72] McGregor et al.,[68] studying α-amylases of different germinated cereal grains, stated that wheat and rye contained multiple forms of α-amylase that could be divided into low-pI (<5.5) and high-pI (>5.8) groups. However, only low-pI α-amylase components were found in germinated oats, maize, millet, sorghum, and rice. A chromatogram of α-amylases of sorghum separated by chromatofocusing is shown in Figure 4.

Although natural enzyme inhibitors of sorghum have not yet been studied in detail, it has been suggested that they also may occur in sorghum grain.[73]

Adams and Novellie[14] reported that positive results were obtained with protein bodies and spherosomes from whole grain, embryo, and aleurone tissue in tests for protease, α- and β-glucosidase, pyrophosphatase, and ribonuclease activity.

	1 5 10
Sorghum	H-Thr-[Leu]-Thr-Ser-Gly-Gly-Cys-Gly-Cys-Gln-
Maize	H-Thr-His-Thr-Ser-Gly-Gly-Cys-Gly-Cys-Gln-
	15 20
Sorghum	Pro-[Pro-His-Leu-Pro]-Pro-Pro-Pro-Val-His-Leu-
Maize	Pro- — — — — -Pro-Pro-Pro-Val-His-Leu-
	25
Sorghum	Pro-Pro-Pro-Val-[His]-Leu-Pro
Maize	Pro-Pro-Pro-Val- His -Leu-Pro

FIGURE 3 N-terminal amino acid sequence of RSP from sorghum cv. Barnard red aligned with that of maize homologue. Boxed residues within brackets signify uncertainty in identification. The four deletions (–) in the maize sequence were introduced to allow alignment for maximum homology. Numbering follows that of the sorghum RSP sequence. (From Taylor, R.N., Von Benecke, R., and Carlsson, F.H.H., *J. Cereal Sci.,* 9, 169, 1989. With permission.)

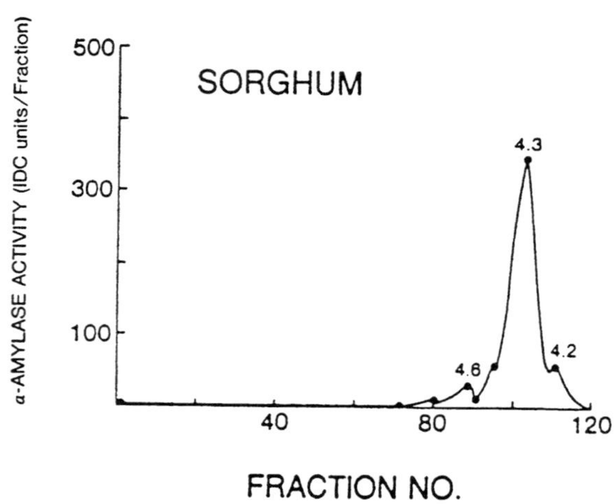

FIGURE 4 Separation of α-amylases of sorghum by chromatofocusing on a pH 4.0 to 6.2 gradient. (From MacGregor, A.W., Marchylo, B.A., and Kruger, J.E., *Cereal Chem.,* 65, 326, 1988. With permission.)

B. Albumins and Globulins

The water- and salt-soluble proteins of sorghum are heterogeneous. High tannin content in whole grain sorghum decreases the quantity of extracted proteins, probably because of the tannin-protein reactions. Jambunathan and Mertz[65] found that the proportion of albumins and globulins extracted from the total protein was much greater than from the high-tannin grains. Subfractions of albumins and globulins may be prepared by partial precipitation, gel filtration chromatography, and gel electrophoresis. The varietal differences have been relatively few, and to date gel electrophoresis has not been used for variety identification. In high-lysine sorghum the levels of albumins and globulins are higher than in grains of normal sorghum.[8,64,74] The albumin and globulin fractions have generally better nutritive value than the storage proteins. Some of the reported data are summarized in Tables 5 and 6.

TABLE 5
Amino Acid Compositions of the Albumins of Sorghum Grain (g/100 g Protein)

	Albumin			
Amino Acid	Endosperm[a]	Whole Grain[b]	Whole Sorghum Grain[c]	Maize[d]
Lysine	6.3	6.5	2.8	5.6
Histidine	2.9	3.8	2.3	2.2
Arginine	6.9	—	4.5	6.7
Aspartic acid	10.4	—	7.7	8.4
Threonine	6.0	4.6	3.3	4.5
Serine	4.8	—	4.2	4.2
Glutamic acid	14.2	—	22.8	11.1
Proline	6.0	—	7.7	4.3
Glycine	7.0	—	3.3	5.3
Alanine	7.4	—	9.2	6.0
Valine	6.0	5.7	5.1	5.0
Methionine	2.0	1.5	1.7	1.3
Isoleucine	4.3	3.4	4.0	3.2
Leucine	7.5	6.6	13.2	5.6
Tyrosine	3.7	—	4.3	3.1
Phenylalanine	3.9	4.9	5.1	3.1
Tryptophan	ND	ND	1.3	ND
Cystine	ND	ND	1.3	ND

Note: ND, not determined.

[a] From Jones and Beckwith.[18]
[b] From Neucere and Sumrell.[22]
[c] From Jambunathan and Mertz.[65]
[d] From Paulis and Wall.[75]

C. Other Proteins

Sorghum also contains complex proteins in first-line glyco- and lipoproteins. To date no investigations have been reported in this field. Recently three antifungal proteins were isolated from sorghum grain endosperm,[93] and their effect on fungal mycelium was studied.[94]

TABLE 6
Amino Acid Compositions of Globulins of the Sorghum Grain (g/100 g Protein)

	Globulin			
Amino Acid	**Endosperm**[a]	**5 *M* NaCl**[b]	**1% NaCl**[c]	**Salt Soluble**[d]
Lysine	4.7	4.5	3.36	5.1
Histidine	2.5	3.9	1.45	2.2
Arginine	10.8	—	—	8.6
Aspartic acid	7.9	—	—	11.3
Threonine	4.6	4.3	4.87	3.4
Serine	5.7	—	—	4.0
Glutamic acid	13.7	—	—	12.8
Proline	4.5	—	—	4.0
Glycine	6.4	—	—	4.4
Alanine	6.0	—	—	4.9
Valine	5.3	4.8	6.46	4.4
Methionine	1.4	1.3	2.24	1.1
Isoleucine	3.5	3.1	3.45	2.7
Leucine	6.4	6.3	6.72	4.8
Tyrosine	3.3	—	—	2.5
Phenylalanine	4.1	5.2	4.77	2.7
Tryptophan	ND	ND	ND	ND
Cystine	ND	ND	ND	1.6

Note: ND, not determined.

[a] From Jones and Beckwith.[18]
[b] From Virupaksha and Sastry.[11]
[c] From Neucere and Sumrell.[22]
[d] From Jambunathan and Mertz.[65]

IV. NUTRITIVE VALUE OF SORGHUM PROTEINS AND PROTEIN CONCENTRATES

Sorghum proteins are low in lysine; therefore, their biological value is relatively low. The digestibility ranged from 71 to 76% as reported by Hari and Conrad.[76] Sorghum varieties with varying kernel structure were analyzed for availability of protein by Hahn et al.[77] It was reported that the structure of grain and the polyphenols influence the digestibility. Complementation of sorghum proteins with lysine and threonine is favorable from the point of view of biological value and protein retention. High-lysine sorghum is superior in comparison with normal sorghum grain.

Evidence that sorghum might not be as digestible as other cereals in children was first published 30 years ago by Kurien et al.[78] They found that the proteins in rice fed to seven boys aged 10 to 11 years were 75% digestible; replacement with sorghum lowered digestibility to 55%. Similar results were obtained by Daniel et al.[79] in young girls who were fed a sorghum diet. Mertz et al.[80] determined the digestibility of different cereals by the pepsin method. Wheat, maize, and rice were more digestible than either normal or high-lysine (P721 opaque) sorghum. High-lysine sorghum was in turn about 4% higher than normal sorghum. After extrusion the digestibility rose to 79% (in comparison to the 56.8% digestibility of raw sorghum). When this same extruded sorghum was tested in children the value was 81%.[81]

Traditionally in these developing countries sorghum is consumed as a porridge or flat bread. Both feeding studies and *in vitro* digestibility assays have shown that sorghum digestibility decreases significantly after cooking.[82-84] It has been suggested that the decrease in digestibility is connected with disulfide bond formation in the kafirin protein fraction. To prevent the formation of new disulfide bonds during cooking, different reducing agents were used. It was found that treating sorghum with 2-mercaptoethanol improved the *in vitro* protein digestibility.[85] Other reducing agents also enhanced the protein digestibility of sorghum.[86,87] Dithiothreitol, sodium bisulfite, and L-cysteine were used in these experiments.

The nutritive value of tannin-containing sorghums may be improved by several methods. They include the use of sodium bicarbonate[88,89] and supplementing the diets with orthophosphoric acid or dicalcium phosphate.[90]

The wet-milling process of sorghum results in starch and some by-products with high protein content. Gluten meal (42% protein) and germ meal (16.9% protein) may be obtained.[91] The production and composition of a protein concentrate from normal and high-lysine sorghum grains were described by Wu.[92]

REFERENCES

1. Harlan, J. R. and De Wet, J. M. J., A simplified classification of cultivated sorghum, *Crop. Sci.,* 12, 172, 1972.
2. Martin, J. H., History and classification of sorghum, *Sorghum bicolor* (L.) Moench, in *Sorghum Production and Utilization,* Wall, J.S. and Ross, W.M., Eds., AVI Publishing, Westport, CT, 1970.
3. Sooliman, A. O. G., Sorghum processing at the cross roads in South Africa, in *Cereal Science and Technology: Impact on a Changing Africa.* Taylor, J.R.N., Randall, P.G., and Viljoen, J.H., Eds., CSIR, Pretoria, 1993, 477.
4. Rooney, L. W. and Miller, F. R., Variation in the structure and kernel characteristics in sorghum, in Proc. Symp. Sorghum Grain Quality, 28-31 October, 1981, ICRISAT, Patanchern, India, 1982.
5. Salunkhe, D. K., Chavan, J. K., and Kadam, S. S., *Postharvest Biotechnology of Cereals,* CRC Press, Boca Raton, FL, 1985.
6. Hoseney, R. C., Varriano-Martson, E., and Dendy, D. A. V., Sorghum and millets, in *Advances in Cereal Science and Technology,* Vol. 4, Pomeranz, Y., Ed., American Association of Cereal Chemists, St. Paul, MN, 1981, 71.

7. Wall, J. S. and Paulis, J. W., Corn and sorghum grain proteins, in *Advances in Cereal Science and Technology,* Vol. 2, Pomeranz, Y., Ed., American Association of Cereal Chemists, St. Paul, MN, 1978, 135.
8. Hulse, J. H., Laing, E. M., and Pearson, O. E., *Sorghum and the Millets: Their Composition and Nutritive Value,* Academic Press, New York, 1980.
9. Rooney, L. W., A review of the physical properties, composition and structure of sorghum grain as related to utilization, in *Industrial Uses of Cereals,* Pomeranz, Y., Ed., American Association of Cereal Chemists, St. Paul, MN, 1974.
10. Deostahale, Y. G., Mohan, V. S., and Rao, K. V., Varietal differences in protein, lysine and leucine contents of some varieties of grain-sorghum, *J. Agric. Food Chem.,* 18, 644, 1969.
11. Virupaksha, T. K. and Sastry, L. V. S., Studies on the protein content and amino acid composition of some varieties of grain sorghum, *J. Agric. Food Chem.,* 18, 644, 1969.
12. Seckinger, H. L. and Wolf, M. J., Sorghum protein ultrastructure as it relates to composition, *Cereal Chem.,* 50, 455, 1973.
13. Sullins, R. D. and Rooney, L. W., Light and scanning electron microscopic studies of waxy and nonwaxy endosperm sorghum varieties, *Cereal Chem.,* 52, 361, 1975.
14. Adams, C. A. and Novellie, L., Composition and structure of protein bodies and spherosomes isolated from ungerminated seed of *Sorghum bicolor* (Linn.) Moench, *Plant Physiol.,* 55, 1, 1975.
15. Adams, C. A. and Novellie, L., Acid hydrolases and autolytic properties of protein bodies and spherosomes isolated from ungerminated seeds of *Sorghum bicolor* (Linn) Moench, *Plant Physiol,* 55, 7, 1975.
16. Rooney, L. W., Fryar, W. B., and Cater, C. M., Protein and amino acid contents of successive layers removed by abrasive milling of sorghum grains, *Cereal Chem.,* 49, 399, 1972.
17. Watterson, J. J., Shull, J. M., and Kirleis, W., Quantitation of α-, β-, and γ-kafirins in vitreous and opaque endosperm of *Sorghum bicolor, Cereal Chem.,* 70, 452, 1993.
18. Jones, R. W. and Beckwith, A. C., Proximate composition and proteins of three grain sorghum hybrids and their dry mill fractions, *J. Agric. Food Chem.,* 18, 33, 1970.
19. Landry, J. and Moureaux, T., Heterogenite des glutelines du grain de mais: extraction selective et composition en acides des trois fractions isolées, *Bull. Soc. Biol.,* 52, 1021, 1970.
20. Jambunathan, R. and Mertz, E. T., Relationship between the tannin levels, rat growth and distribution of proteins in sorghum, *J. Agric. Food Chem.,* 21, 692, 1973.
21. Wu, Y. V. and Wall, J. S., Lysine content of protein increased by germination of normal and high-lysine sorghums, *J. Agric. Food Chem.,* 28, 455, 1980.
22. Neucere, N. J. and Sumrell, G., Protein fractions from five varieties of grain sorghum: amino acid composition and solubility properties, *J. Agric. Food Chem.,* 27, 809, 1979.
23. Subramanian, V. and Jambunathan, R., Chemical composition and food quality of sorghum, in *Nutritional and Processing Quality of Sorghum,* Salunkhe, D.K., Chavan, J.K., and Jadlav, S.J., Eds., Oxford and IBH, New Delhi, 1982, 22.
24. Munck, L., Improvement of nutritional value in cereals, *Hereditas,* 72, 1, 1972.
25. Axtell, J. D. and Ejeta, G., Improving sorghum grain protein quality by breeding, in *Proc. Int. Conf. Sorghum Nutritional Quality,* Purdue University Press, W. Lafayette, IN, 1991, 117.

25a. Singh, R. and Axtell, J. D., High-lysine mutant gene (hl) that improves protein quality and biological value of grain sorghum, *Crop Sci.,* 13, 535, 1973.

26. Mohan, D. D. and Axtell, J. D., Diethyl sulphate-induced high lysine mutants in sorghum, in Proc. 9th Bienn. Grain Sorghum Res. Util. Conf., Lubbock, TX, March 4, 1975.
26a. Ejeta, G. and Axtell, J. D., Development of hard-endosperm high-lysine sorghums, in *Proc. Int. Conf. Sorghum Nutritional Quality,* Purdue University Press, W. Lafayette, IN, 1991, 126.
27. Mertz, E. T., Axtell, J. D., Ejeta, G., and Hamaker, B. R., Development and recent impact of quality protein maîze and sorghum, in *Cereal Science and Technology: Impact on a Changing Africa,* Taylor, J.R.N., Randall, P.G., and Viljoen, J.H., Eds., CSIR, Pretoria, 1993, 115.
28. Jambunathan, R., Mertz, E. T., and Axtell, J. D., Fractionation of soluble proteins of high lysine and normal sorghum grain, *Cereal Chem.,* 52, 119, 1975.
29. Van Scoyoc, S. W., Ejeta, G., and Axtell, J. D., Kernel characteristics and protein fraction changes during seed development of high-lysine and normal sorghum, *Cereal Chem.,* 65, 75, 1988.
30. Chavan, J. K., Ghonsikar, C. P., Kandam, S. S., and Salunkhe, D. K., Protein, tannin and starch changes in developing seeds of low and high-tannin cultivars of sorghum, *J. Food Biochem.,* 3, 13, 1979.
31. Ejeta, G. and Axtell, J., Protein and lysine levels in developing kernels of normal and high-lysine sorghum, *Cereal Chem.,* 64, 137, 1987.
32. Mazhar, H. and Chandrashekar, A., Differences in kafirin composition during endosperm development and germination in sorghum cultivars of varying hardness, *Cereal Chem.,* 70, 667, 1993.
33. Shull, S. M., Chandrashekar, A., Kirleis, A. W., and Ejeta, G., Development of sorghum (*Sorghum bicolor* L.), *Food Struct.,* 9, 253, 1990.
34. Chung, O. K., and Pomeranz, Y., Amino acids in cereal proteins and cereal fractions, in *Digestibility and Amino Acid Availability in Cereals and Oilseeds,* Finley, J.W. and Hopkins, D.T., Eds., American Association of Cereal Chemists, St. Paul, MN, 1985.
35. Mossé, J., Huet, J. C., and Baudet, J., The amino acid composition of whole sorghum grain in relation to its nitrogen content, *Cereal Chem.,* 65, 271, 1988.
36. Baudet, J., Huet, J. C., and Mossé, J., Variability and relationships among amino acids and nitrogen content of maize grains, *J. Agric. Food Chem.,* 34, 365, 1986.
37. Hassen, M. M., Mertz, E. T., Kirleis, A. W., Ejeta, G., Axtell, J. D., and Villegas, E., Tryptophan levels in normal and high-lysine sorghums, *Cereal Chem.,* 63, 175, 1986.
38. Beckwith, A. C. and Jones, R. W., Physical properties of grain sorghum prolamin fractions and components, *J. Agric. Food Chem.,* 20, 259, 1972.
39. Sastry, L. V. S. and Virupaksha, T. K., Alcohol soluble proteins of grain sorghum, *Cereal Chem.,* 46, 284, 1969.
40. Mazhar, H., Chandrashekar, A., and Shetty, H. S., Isolation and immunochemical characterization of the alcohol extractable proteins (kafirins) of *Sorghum bicolor* (L.) Moench, *J. Cereal Sci.,* 17, 83, 1993.
41. Shull, J. M., Watterson, J. J., and Kirleis, A. W., Proposed nomenclature of the alcohol soluble proteins (kafirins) of *Sorghum bicolor* L. Moench based on molecular weight, solubility and structure, *J. Agric. Food Chem.,* 39, 83, 1991.
42. Shull, J. M., Watterson, J. J., and Kirleis, A. W., Purification and immunocytochemical localization of kafirins in *Sorghum bicolor* L. Moench endosperm, *Protoplasma,* 171, 64, 1992.

43. Haikerwall, M. and Mathieson, A. R., Extraction and fractionation of proteins of sorghum kernels, *J. Sci. Food Agric.*, 22, 142, 1971.
44. Paulis, J. W. and Wall, J. S., Distribution and electrophoretic properties of alcohol soluble proteins in normal and high-lysine sorghum, *Cereal Chem.*, 56, 20, 1979.
45. Sastry, L. V. S., Paulis, J. W., Bietz, J. A., and Wall, J. S., Genetic variation of storage proteins in sorghum grain: studies by isoelectric focusing and high-performance liquid chromatography, *Cereal Chem.*, 63, 420, 1986.
46. Watterson, J. J., Shull, J. M., and Kirleis, A. W., Quantitation of α-, β- and γ-kafirins in vitreous and opaque endosperm of *Sorghum bicolor, Cereal Chem.*, 70, 452, 1993.
47. Taylor, J. N. and Schussler, L., Sorghum cultivar verification by electrophoresis, *J. Sci. Food Agric.*, 35, 1, 1984.
48. Kirleis, A. W., Crosby, K. D., and Housley, T., A method for quantitatively measuring area in sectioned sorghum grain, *Cereal Chem.*, 61, 556, 1984.
49. Abdelrahman, A. A. and Hoseney, R. G., Basis for hardness in pearl millet, grain sorghum, and corn, *Cereal Chem.*, 61, 232, 1984.
50. DeRose, R. T., Din-Powma, In-Sook Kwon, Hasnain, S. E., Klassy, R. C., and Hall, C., Characterization of the kafirin gene family from sorghum reveals extensive homology with zein from maize, *Plant Mol. Biol.*, 12, 245, 1989.
51. Bietz, J., Cereal prolamin evolution and homology revealed by sequence analogy, *Biochem. Genet.*, 20, 1039, 1982.
52. Shewry, P. R. and Miflin, B. J., Seed storage proteins of economically important cereals, in *Advances in Cereal Science and Technology,* Vol. 7, Pomeranz, Y., Ed., American Association of Cereal Chemists, St. Paul, MN, 1985, 1.
53. Tatham, A. S., Shewry, P. R., and Belton, P. S., Structural studies of cereal prolamins, including wheat gluten, in *Advances in Cereal Science and Technology,* Vol. 10, Pomeranz, Y., Ed., American Association of Cereal Chemists, St. Paul, MN, 1990, 1.
54. Argos, P., Pedersen, K., Marks, M. D., and Larkins, B. A., A structural model for maize zein proteins, *J. Biol. Chem.*, 257, 9984, 1982.
55. Spena, A., Viotti, A., and Pirrotta, V., A homologous repetitive block structure underlies the heterogeneity of heavy and light chain zein genes, *EMBO J.*, 1, 1589, 1982.
56. Spena, A., Viotti, A., and Pirrotta, V., Two adjacent genomic zein sequences: structural organization and tissue specific restriction pattern, *J. Mol. Biol.*, 169, 799, 1982.
57. Geraghty, D. E., Messing, J., and Rubinstein, I., Sequence analysis and comparison of cDNAs of the zein multigene family, *EMBO J.*, 1, 1329, 1982.
58. Taylor, J. R. N. and Schussler, L., The protein compositions of the different anatomical parts of sorghum grain, *J. Cereal Sci.*, 4, 361, 1986.
59. Bright, S. W. J. and Shewry, P. R., Improvement of protein quality in cereals, *Crit. Rev. Plant Sci.*, 1, 49, 1983.
60. Beckwith, A. C., Grain sorghum glutelin: isolation and characterization, *J. Agric. Food Chem.*, 20, 761, 1972.
61. Taylor, J. R. N., Von Benecke, R., and Carlsson, F. H. H., Distribution, purification and N-terminal amino acid sequence of sorghum reduced-soluble protein, *J. Cereal Sci.*, 9, 169, 1989.
62. Wilson, C. M., Shewry, P. R., and Miflin, B. J., Maize endosperm proteins compared by sodium dodecyl sulfate gel electrophoresis and isoelectric focusing, *Cereal Chem.*, 58, 275, 1981.
63. Evans, D. J., Schussler, L., and Taylor, J. R. N., Isolation of reduced-soluble-protein from sorghum starchy endosperm, *J. Cereal Sci.*, 5, 61, 1987.

64. Taylor, J. R. N., Schussler, L., and Liebensberg, N. V. D. W., Location of zein-2 and crosslinked kafirin in maize and sorghum protein bodies, *J. Cereal Sci.,* 2, 249, 1984.
65. Jambunathan, R. and Mertz, E. T., Amino acid composition of whole kernel and endosperm fractions of sorghum, in *Research Progress Report on Inheritance and Improvement of Protein Quality in* Sorghum bicolor *L. Moench,* Axtell, J.D. and Oswald, D.L., Eds., Purdue University Press, West Lafayette, IN, 1972.
66. Kruger, J. E., Lineback, D. R., and Stauffer, C. E., Eds., *Enzymes and Their Role in Cereal Technology,* American Association of Cereal Chemists, St. Paul., MN, 1987.
67. Hill, R. D. and McGregor, A. W., Cereal α-amylases in grain research and technology, in *Advances in Cereal Science and Technology,* Vol. 9, Pomeranz, Y., Ed., American Association of Cereal Chemists, St. Paul, MN, 1988.
68. MacGregor, A. W., Marchylo, B. A., and Kruger, J. E., Multiple α-amylase components in germinated cereal grains determined by isoelectric focusing and chromatofocusing, *Cereal Chem.,* 65, 326, 1988.
69. Taylor, J. R. N., Sorghum malt: its current use and future potential for brewing in South Africa, in *Cereal Science and Technology: Impact on a Changing Africa,* Taylor, J.R.N., Randall, P.G., and Viljoen, J.H, Eds., CSIR, Pretoria, 1993, 413.
70. Mushonga, J. N. and Muza, F. R., Genetic variability for diastatic activity in sorghum (*Sorghum bicolor* L. Moench), in *Cereal Science and Technology: Impact on a Changing Africa,* Taylor, J.R.N., Randall, P.G., and Viljoen, J.H., Eds., CSIR, Pretoria, 1993, 433.
71. Munck, L. and Mundy, J., Sorghum malting studies, in *Proc. Symp. Processing of Sorghum and Millets,* ICC, Vienna, 1984, 56.
72. Mundy, J., Isolation and characterization of two immunologically distinct forms of α-amylase and a β-amylase from seeds of germinated *Sorghum bicolor* L. Moench, *Carlsberg Res. Commun.,* 47, 264, 1982.
73. Weselake, R. J., MacGregor, A. W., and Hill, R. D., Endogenous α-amylase inhibitor in various cereals, *Cereal Chem.,* 62, 120, 1985.
74. Wall, J. S. and Bietz, J. A., Maximizing use of normal and high-lysine sorghums in foods, in Proc. 10th Congr. ICC Symp. Sorghum and Millet for Human Food, Vienna, 1980, 120.
75. Paulis, J. W. and Wall, J. S., Albumins and globulins in extracts of corn grain parts, *Cereal Chem.,* 46, 265, 1969.
76. Hori, O. J. and Conrad, J. H., Nutritive value of protein selected sorghum lines as measured by rat performance, *Nutr. Rep. Int.,* 13, 307, 1976.
77. Hahn, D. H., Faubion, J. M., Ring, S. H., Doherty, C. A., and Rooney, L. W., Semiautomated in vitro analysis of sorghum protein availability via pronase hydrolysis, *Cereal Chem.,* 59, 132, 1982.
78. Kurien, P. P., Narayanarao, M., Swaminathan, M., and Subrahamayan, V., The metabolism of nitrogen, calcium and phosphorus in undernourished children. VI. The effect of partial or complete replacement of rice in poor vegetarian diets by kaffir corn *(Sorghum vulgare), Br. J. Nutr.,* 14, 339, 1960.
79. Daniel, V. A., Leela, R., Doraiswamy, T. R., Rajalakshmi, D., Rao, S. V., Suminathan, M., and Parpia, H. A. B., The effect of supplementing a poor kafirin corn *(Sorghum vulgare)* diet with l-lysine and dl-threonine on the digestibility coefficient, biological value and net utilization of proteins and retention of nitrogen in children, *J. Nutr. Diet.,* 3, 10, 1966.

80. Mertz, E. T., Hassen, M. M., Cairns-Whittern, C., Kirleis, A. W., Tu, L., and Axtell, J. D., Pepsin digestibility of proteins in sorghum and other major cereals, *Proc. Natl. Acad. Sci. U.S.A.,* 81, 1, 1984.
81. McLean, W. C., Lopez de Romana, G., Gastanaday, A., and Graham, G. G., The effect of decortication and extrusion on the digestibility of sorghum by preschool children, *J. Nutr.,* 113, 2071, 1983.
82. Eggum, B. O., Monowar, L., Bach Knudsen, K. E., Munck, L., and Axtell, J., Nutritional quality of sorghum and sorghum foods from Sudan, *J. Cereal Sci.,* 1, 127, 1983.
83. Hamaker, B. R., Kirleis, A. W., Mertz, E. T., and Axtell, J., Effect of cooking on the protein profiles and in vitro digestibility of sorghum and maize, *J. Agric. Food Chem.,* 34, 647, 1986.
84. Mitaru, B. N. and Blair, R., Comparative effects of cooking and high moisture storage of sorghums on protein digestibility in rats, *Nutr. Rep. Int.,* 30, 397, 1984.
85. Hamauer, B. R., Kirleis, A. W., Butler, L. G., Axtell, J. D., and Mertz, E. T., Improving the in vitro digestibility of sorghum with reducing agents, *Proc. Natl. Acad. Sci. U.S.A.,* 84, 626, 1987.
86. Mertz, E. T., Axtell, J. D., Ejets, G., and Hamaker, B. R., Development and recent impact of quality protein maize and sorghum, in *Cereal Science and Technology Impact* on a Changing Africa, Taylor, J.R.N., Randall, P.G., and Viljoen, J.H., Eds., CSIR, Pretoria, 1993, 115.
87. Rom, D. L., Shull, J. M., Chandrashekar, A., and Kirleis, A. W., Effects of cooking and treatment with sodium bisulfite on in vitro protein digestibility and microstructure of sorghum flour, *Cereal Chem.,* 69, 178, 1992.
88. Mundi, P. J., Thomke, S., and Ekman, R., The effect of Magadi soda treatment on the tannin content and nutritive value of grain sorghums, *J. Sci. Food Agric.,* 32, 25, 1981.
89. Drinah, B. C., Banda, N., and Vohre, P., Nutritional improvement of tannin-containing sorghums *(Sorghum bicolor)* by sodium bicarbonate, *Cereal Chem.,* 67, 533, 1990.
90. Ibrahim, S., Fisher, C., Alaily, H. E., Soliman, H., and Anwar, A., Improvement of nutritional quality of Egyptian and Sudanese sorghum grains by the addition of phosphates, *Br. Poult. Sci.,* 29, 721, 1988.
91. Reiners, R. A., Hummel, J. B., Pressich, J. C., and Morgan, R. E., Composition of feed products from wet milling of grain sorghum, *Cereal Sci. Today,* 18, 378, 1976.
92. Wu, Y. V., Protein concentrate from normal and high lysine sorghums: preparation, composition and properties, *J. Agric. Food Chem.,* 26, 305, 1978.
93. Sunitha Kumari, R. and Chandrashekar, A., Isolation and purification of three antifungal proteins from sorghum endosperm, *J. Sci. Food Agric.,* 64, 357, 1994.
94. Sunitha Kumari, R. and Chandrashekar, A., Antifungal proteins from sorghum endosperm and their effect on fungal mycelium, *J. Sci. Food Agric.,* 66, 121, 1994.
95. Dendy, D. A. V., Ed., *Sorghum and Millets: Chemistry and Technology,* American Association of Cereal Chemists, St. Paul, MN, 1994.
96. Mazhar, H. and Chandrashekar, A., Quantification and distribution of kafirins in the kernels of sorghum cultivars varying in endosperm hardness, *J. Cereal Sci.,* 21, 155, 1995.

8 Rice Proteins

I. INTRODUCTION, GENERAL CHARACTERIZATION OF RICE PROTEINS

Although world production of wheat is greater than that of rice, the latter serves as the main staple food for the greater part of the world population. The structure of the rice grain is similar to that of other cereals. The rice grain (rough rice) consists of an edible portion, the rice caryopsis, and its covering structures, the hull and the husk. The rice hull constitutes from 18 to 28% of the rough-rice weight. The caryopsis is also called brown rice because of its brownish pericarp. Technologically, the most important parts of the brown rice are the pericarp, aleurone layer, embryo (germ), and the starchy endosperm. The pericarp constitutes from 1 to 2% of the caryopsis weight, the aleurone layer 4 to 6%, the germ 2 to 3%, and the starchy endosperm 89 to 94%. The germ is relatively small in comparison with other cereals. The aleurone layer may have from one to seven cell layers and is thicker on the dorsal surface than along the lateral and ventral surfaces. The cells of the aleurone layer are filled with small, protein-rich aleurone grains enclosed in a sheath of fat-staining material. The starchy endosperm consists of walled parenchyma cells, usually radially elongated and heavily loaded with compound starch granules and some protein bodies. Ordinary rice is nonglutinous and has vitreous endosperm. Another type of rice, known as glutinous, sweet, or waxy rice, has chalky opaque endosperm. The differences in the physical properties of the endosperm are connected with the different characters of the starches of the two rice types. Abrasive milling removes the outer layers (pericarp, greater part of aleurone layer, part of embryo and endosperm), producing milled or polished rice and the by-products bran and polish. Usually 10% of the brown rice is removed during milling.

Reviews about general problems of rice chemistry and technology, including the structure of the rice kernel, were published by Juliano[1,2] and Salunkhe et al.[3]

The protein content of brown rice varies from 7.1 to 15.4% (calculated as N × 5.95),[1-7] depending on the variety and on climatic and agrotechnical conditions. The milling process for rice results in white milled rice (40 to 55%) plus three major by-products: husks (20%), bran (10%), and brokens (10 to 22%).[9] Protein content of commercial milling fractions can be categorized as follows: milled rice, 8%; husks, 3%; bran, 17%; and brokens, 8.5%. Milled rice contains lower quantities of protein because during the milling some of the protein-rich aleurone cells are removed. The data reported by other authors vary from 5.6 to 13.3%.[1-7]

As with other cereal grains, the protein contents of the embryo and the aleurone layer are higher (up to 20 to 25%) than that of the endosperm. Nevertheless, the greatest part of the total protein is located in the endosperm, and the main characteristics of the protein are determined by the properties of the endosperm storage proteins.

Up to 95% of the endosperm proteins are observed to be in the form of discrete particles called protein bodies.[10-14] These range in size from 1 to 4 μm. Protein bodies are mostly concentrated in peripheral-lateral and in peripheral-dorsal cells. Electron micrographs of isolated protein bodies indicate a layer structure such as is present in starch granules.[25] Another type of protein body having uniformly electron-dense structure was also found.[24,26,27] An investigation of these protein bodies showed that those with layered structure are composed mainly of prolamin-type proteins and the others contain glutelin polypeptides.[2,26,27,118]

Osborne's classification of proteins based on solubility has been widely used in rice protein chemistry. The data reported in the literature concerning the protein solubility fractions vary within a wide range (see Table 1). The differences between the data reported by different research workers depend on the rice variety, but the uncertainties of the extraction procedure may also play a role. Nevertheless, it is clear from all determinations that the most important fraction is glutelin (oryzenin). It is also characteristic that the prolamin content of rice is low. The distribution of the different solubility fractions in the rice grain is uneven. Albumins and globulins are concentrated in the embryo and aleurone layer. The storage proteins (oryzenin, prolamin) occur in the highest amount in the endosperm. Generally the proportion of albumin and globulin is highest in the outer layers of the milled rice and decreases toward the center of the grain. The distribution of the protein fractions is also different in the milling fractions. Bran contains high amounts of albumins and globulins, and more than 90% of the oryzenin is located in the milled rice. Some high-protein varieties of rice contain 45% more protein than ordinary brown rice, and the high-protein starchy endosperm contains 49% more protein than ordinary starchy endosperm, as reported by Bradbury et al.[13] The major increase in protein was observed in the starchy endosperm. Morphological studies[13] showed that the high-protein variety had a greater number of round protein bodies that stained blue with aniline blue black. The increase of the lysine content is smaller: when the total protein content increased 49% the lysine content of the milled rice increased only about 28%.[13] Slightly lower digestibility was also observed.[24]

The amino acid composition of the total protein of the rice grain is generally characterized by a higher lysine content and lower glutamic acid (glutamine) content in comparison with other cereals. The varietal differences in gross amino acid composition are probably connected with the different solubility fraction distributions. The differences between brown rice and milled rice are also related to changes in the distribution of protein fractions. Some data are summarized in Table 2.

Due to the differences in the protein fraction distribution, the amino acid compositions of the different morphological parts of the rice grain as well as those of the milling products are also different. Some data are summarized in Tables 3 and 4. The by-products contain mostly germ and aleurone proteins, which are rich in lysine and poor in glutamic acid. The gross amino acid composition of the rice

TABLE 1
Protein Solubility Fractions of Brown and Milled Rice (% of Extracted Protein)

Albumin	Globulin	Prolamin	Glutelin	Ref.
		Brown Rice		
9.8–15.3	9.8–15.3	3.3–7.1	77.8–84.5	16
5.84	14.17	9.17	70.9	17
4.4–11.6	7.9–13.4	1.6–4.8	74.3–83.3	18
3.0–18.7	0–12.2	2.9–20.6	55.0–88.1	19
13.0	14.5	9.9	62.6	20
5.0	10.0	5.0	80.0	28
		Milled Rice		
2.9–9.9	6.6–11.0	1.9–4.2	73.6–87.0	18
6.5	12.7	8.9	71.9	20
0.85–3.36	7.24–8.97	5.60–8.66	82.06–84.16	21
0–2.6	4.7–19.9	0.4–10.3	61.8–89.7	19
0.9–1.0	1.4–2.8	5.5–8.4	89–91	22,23

protein changes very slightly if proteins of waxy and normal rice grains are investigated. Some differences were observed between the gross amino acid compositions of the total protein of low- and high-protein cultivars.[2,13,18] It was reported that low- and high-protein milled-rice samples of eight cultivars showed a negative correlation between protein and lysine content. The negative correlations may be explained — as with other cereals — by the fact that the increase in protein content is highest in the starchy endosperm[13] and lower in the germ and aleurone layer. This suggests that the increased biosynthesis of the proteins mainly produces storage proteins and that the quantity of metabolically active cytoplasmic proteins changes only slightly.

The changes in the amino acid composition due to development of the rice kernel were also investigated.[33,34] A decrease in the content of several free amino acids, including lysine, was observed. This observation may also be explained by the fact — known from other cereals — that in the last stage of grain development about the only proteins synthesized are storage proteins. The changing protein fraction distribution is reflected by the changing amino acid composition. The correlation between protein content, amino acid composition, and the thickness of the rough-rice kernel was investigated by Matthews et al.[36] and Wadsworth et al.[37] Higher protein content was observed in the thin kernels; nevertheless, the amino acid composition of the fractionated lot containing thin kernels did not differ significantly from that of the unfractionated lot. Some data are summarized in Table 5 which show the amino acid profiles of two unfractionated rough rices (A and B) and those of the thin fractions obtained from these rough rices.

TABLE 2
Amino Acid Composition of Milled Rice (g/16.8 g N)[a]

	Milled Rice				
Amino Acid	**Baldi[16]**	**Hussein[29]**	**Bressani et al.[30]**	**Nesterin and Skurychin[31]**	**Brown Rice (Baldi[16])**
Isoleucine	3.7–4.2	3.6	4.8–5.3	4.6	3.4–4.0
Leucine	7.8–8.8	9.3	7.8–9.6	8.9	6.5–8.5
Lysine	2.6–3.2	3.9	3.4–4.3	3.6	3.2–3.9
Methionine	1.9–2.2	2.3	1.8–3.5	1.8	1.5–2.1
Phenylalanine	4.8–5.6	4.7	5.6–6.3	5.1	5.1–5.7
Threonine	2.8–3.4	3.9	3.8–4.1	3.1	3.1–3.9
Tryptophan	ND	1.5	1.0–1.4	1.1	ND
Valine	5.6–6.1	5.0	6.2–7.3	4.9	4.0–6.2
Alanine	5.1–6.0	6.1	5.7–6.2	4.8	5.3–6.5
Arginine	7.2–8.0	8.7	7.4–8.8	7.4	7.4–9.3
Aspartic acid	8.6–9.7	10.0	9.5–10.4	8.0	8.5–9.5
Cystine	1.9–2.4	2.1	1.4–1.8	1.7	1.7–2.4
Glutamic acid	18.3–19.8	20.7	18.3–21.1	16.6	16.5–19.4
Glycine	4.0–4.3	4.7	4.5–4.8	4.9	4.3–1.7
Histidine	1.8–2.2	2.0	2.5	2.3	2.0–2.5
Proline	3.9–4.7	5.0	4.7–5.0	4.4	4.1–1.6
Serine	3.6–5.0	5.6	5.7–6.9	4.0	4.6–5.2
Tyrosine	1.6–4.5	4.3	5.0–5.9	3.4	3.0–4.4

Note: ND, not determined.

[a] Some data recalculated from g/16 g N.

The amino acid composition of rice grain as a function of nitrogen content was studied by Mossé et al.[38] Brown rice grains with nitrogen contents ranging from 1.27 to 2.07% of grain dry matter were subjected to accurate amino acid analysis. The amino acids in grain protein changed as a hyperbolic function of nitrogen content. While significantly decreased lysine, methionine, and cysteine concentrations were noted, little or no variation was observed for glycine, alanine, threonine, phenylalanine, tryptophan, histidine, and arginine, and the relative amounts of other amino acids increased. Rice proteins, as compared to other cereals, were richer in lysine than wheat, maize, and sorghum proteins for any N value, poorer than rye and triticale proteins for $N < 2.15$, and always poorer than those of oats. The changes in the N-to-protein conversion factor were also studied. It was stated that the usual coefficient of 5.95 was an overestimate (for investigated rice samples a factor of 5.5 to 5.6 seems more realistic). The amino acid compositions of rice samples are shown in Table 6.

TABLE 3
Amino Acid Composition of Rice Milling Products (g/16.8 g N)

Amino Acid	Germ[a]	Bran[b]	Bran[a]	Polish[a]	Polish[b]
Lysine	4.5	4.9	4.3	4.4	4.3
Histidine	1.6	2.8	1.4	1.6	2.7
Arginine	6.6	7.7	6.1	7.2	8.5
Aspartic acid	9.5	9.2	9.6	9.4	9.4
Glutamic acid	15.3	14.3	16.8	17.2	16.5
Serine	5.2	4.6	5.2	4.8	5.0
Threonine	3.7	3.8	3.3	3.7	3.6
Cystine	1.2	2.2	1.2	1.3	2.2
Methionine	3.0	2.2	2.7	2.6	2.4
Glycine	4.6	5.2	4.1	5.3	5.0
Alanine	5.5	6.6	7.1	6.0	5.8
Valine	5.5	5.7	5.6	5.7	5.4
Isoleucine	3.7	3.9	4.9	4.5	3.7
Leucine	8.1	7.2	9.2	8.3	7.8
Phenylalanine	5.2	4.4	6.1	6.7	4.7
Proline	8.1	4.5	5.2	5.9	5.0
Tyrosine	4.9	3.3	5.0	6.0	4.5
Tryptophan	1.5	1.4	1.4	1.5	1.5

[a] From Ronda Lain and Soto Rodriguez.[32]
[b] From Barber and Barber.[4]

II. STORAGE PROTEINS OF RICE

A. Low Molecular Weight Storage Proteins (Prolamins)

The low molecular weight storage proteins (prolamins) of rice (like prolamins of other cereal grains) may be extracted with 70% (v/v) ethanol. Propanol (50%, v/v) also may be used. Extraction with ethanol (or propanol) and a reducing agent is also used; however, in experiments described in this chapter the prolamin fractions are always extracted without a reducing agent. A fractionation of rice prolamins may be realized by physical separation of protein bodies of the kernel. As mentioned earlier, rice storage proteins are located in two types of protein bodies.[26,27] The spherical protein bodies contain the prolamins, which may be solubilized. The mean prolamin content of seven International Rice Research Institute (IRRI) milled rices (8.8% mean protein content) was 3.0% of the total protein when extracted with 70% (v/v) ethanol and 6.5% when extracted with 60% propanol.[2] On the other hand,

TABLE 4
Amino Acid Composition of Some Morphological Parts of Rice Grain (g/16.8 g N)

Amino Acid	Embryo[a]	Embryo[b]	Endosperm[a]	Aleurone Layer + Cell Coats[a]	Rice Protein Bodies[c]
Lysine	7.1	6.5	4.3	5.7	1.2
Histidine	3.4	3.5	2.6	3.0	1.9
Arginine	12.0	9.2	8.0	8.4	5.8
Serine	4.8	4.6	3.8	4.0	5.9
Cysteine	0.5	2.2	0.5	0.5	4.6
Valine	6.9	4.9	7.0	7.3	6.2
Methionine	1.3	1.9	1.4	0.8	4.8
Isoleucine	3.3	3.6	3.9	3.6	4.9
Leucine	7.0	6.8	9.5	8.6	12.1
Phenylalanine	5.1	4.5	5.9	5.9	6.6
Tryptophan	—	1.5	—	—	0.6
Glutamic acid	16.0	15.2	20.1	15.3	—
Aspartic acid	9.5	8.8	9.8	11.0	—
Proline	4.4	4.7	6.3	5.6	—
Alanine	6.8	6.2	6.3	7.1	—
Glycine	7.9	5.5	5.1	4.3	—
Tyrosine	2.6	3.2	3.4	3.2	—
Threonine	4.4	3.8	3.4	3.8	—

Note: Some values recalculated from residues per 100 g residues.

[a] From Bradbury et al.[12]
[b] From Barber and Barber.[4]
[c] From Juliano.[35]

Hibino and coworkers[39] reported that prolamin constitutes 20% of milled japani rice protein and 30% of milled India rice protein. Taking into account all available literary data it seems that the values between 5 and 10% are the most realistic. In comparison with wheat, barley, and maize prolamins, this protein fraction of the rice has been relatively poorly investigated. This is probably due to the low quantity of this fraction and its relative lack of importance in determining the quality of rice.

The prolamin fraction of rice, like prolamins of other cereals, may be separated into different components. Results of early investigations were reviewed by Houston[40] and Juliano.[41] Mandac and Juliano[42] analyzed fractions from developing and mature grain by SDS-PAGE. The prolamin fraction showed a major band of 17 kDa and a minor one of 23 kDa. Other workers (for review see References 43 and 35) also detected several components in the same range.

TABLE 5
Amino Acid Composition (mg/g) of Unfractionated Lots and Combined Thin Fractions of Two Brown Rice Lots[36]

Amino Acid	Unfractionated Lot A	Unfractionated Lot B	Thin Fractions Lot A	Thin Fractions Lot B
Alanine	59	58	58	59
Valine	56	62	60	63
Glycine	47	49	44	50
Isoleucine	37	42	40	44
Leucine	77	79	83	81
Proline	45	45	46	46
Threonine	35	35	36	37
Serine	52	49	54	50
Methionine	23	21	22	21
Phenylalanine	61	53	54	52
Aspartic acid	94	95	90	95
Glutamic acid	177	168	183	163
Tyrosine	42	38	41	41
Lysine	44	39	41	41
Histidine	38	33	36	32
Arginine	86	86	78	83
Cystine	17	25	17	20
Tryptophan	15	25	18	23

More recent studies of Kim and Okita,[44] Ogawa et al.,[45] Sugimoto et al.,[46] and Resurrection et al.[47] revealed three different prolamin classes — occurring in protein bodies of lamellar structure — using electrophoresis; they had molecular weights of 10, 13 to 15, and 16 kDa. Horikoshi et al.[48] separated five bands by isoelectric focusing of rice prolamin. The bands had pI values of 5.6, 7.1, 7.3, 7.6, and 8.0. The pI 7 component was the major one.

Savich[49] and Savich and Peruansky[50] separated the prolamin fraction into four subgroups. The total number of bands was 19.

The success in variety identification of other cereals based on gel electrophoresis spectra of prolamin (storage) proteins has stimulated research on biochemical identification of rice varieties. The first methods were published by Park and Stegemann[51] and du Cros et al.[52] Guo et al.[53] examined the prolamin fractions of 25 varieties of Chinese rice by electrofocusing. They observed as many as 20 protein bands in the prolamin fractions. Based on the pI values and staining intensities of the protein bands, the 25 varieties of Chinese rice could be divided into four groups. Two bands (pI 5.3 and 7.7) were constitutive. Four major bands allow differentiation of Indica,

TABLE 6
Amino Acid Compositions of Rice Samples (g/16 g N)

Variety[a]	BO1	Cig	Mar	Bal	Arl	BO2	BO3	BO4
N[b]	1.27	1.42	1.45	1.48	1.60	1.70	1.79	2.07
Gly	4.4	4.5	4.5	4.4	4.5	4.4	4.4	4.5
Ala	5.3	5.3	5.2	5.4	5.5	5.5	5.4	5.5
Val	5.6	5.9	5.8	5.8	6.2	6.0	5.9	6.1
Leu	7.5	7.9	7.8	7.9	8.1	8.0	7.9	8.1
Ile	3.8	4.2	4.1	3.9	4.3	4.0	4.2	4.3
Ser	4.6	5.0	4.9	5.0	5.0	5.2	5.0	5.3
Thr	3.3	3.5	3.4	3.5	3.5	3.5	3.5	3.5
Tyr	4.8	4.9	4.9	5.1	5.1	5.0	5.1	5.3
Phe	4.8	5.1	5.0	5.0	5.1	5.1	4.9	5.2
Trp	1.2	1.2	1.2	1.2	1.2	1.2	1.2	1.2
Pro	4.0	4.5	4.4	4.3	4.5	4.3	4.5	4.6
Met	2.3	2.4	2.6	2.3	2.6	2.2	2.3	2.1
Cys/2	2.4	2.3	2.6	2.5	2.4	2.3	2.2	2.1
Lys	3.8	3.7.	3.8	3.8	3.8	3.6	3.7	3.6
His	2.3	2.4	2.3	2.3	2.4	2.3	2.3	2.3
Arg	8.0	8.5	8.2	8.4	8.5	8.2	8.1	8.3
Asx[c]	8.5	8.5	8.6	8.8	8.6	8.7	8.6	8.6
Glx–	15.1	16.6	16.4	16.8	16.9	16.7	17.3	17.6
Amide[d]	2.2	1.9	1.9	1.9	2.1	2.2	2.21	2.2
R[e]	90.6	93.1	92.1	92.6	95.2	93.7	93.8	95.4

[a] Arl: Arlésienne; Bal: Balilla; BO1 to BO4: varieties derived from Balilla; Cig: Cigalen; Mar: Mara 136.
[b] *N*: grain N content (g/100 g dry matter).
[c] Asx and Glx were evaluated in terms of grams of Asp and Glu.
[d] Amide: amide N from Asn and Gln, expressed as NH_3.
[e] R: N recovered as amino acids (including amide N) as % of total grain N.

From Mosse, J., Huet, J. C., and Baudet, J., *Cereal Sci.,* 8, 165, 1988. With permission.

Japonica, and glutinous rices and their hybrids and also indicate the application of physicochemical treatment. Minor bands allow further differentiation within each group. Some correlation was found between electrophoretic spectra and quality of rice. Differences in storage proteins between round and long rice seeds were found by SDS-PAGE analysis.[54]

Huebner et al.[55] developed methods for identification of genetically diverse rice varieties. The method was applied to semidwarf rice varieties from the IRRI derived from the same cross, which are especially difficult to differentiate. Acid PAGE of 5 *M* acetic acid extracts of brown and milled rice differentiated sister lines IR 36 and IR 42 (but not sister lines IR 28 and IR 29); IR 32, IR 38, and IR 40; IR 52 and IR 54; and IR 56 and IR 60. Rice varieties from Vietnam and Hungary were studied for variety identification by Kárpáti et al.[56] and Le Truong et al.[57] using PAGE. Difficulties in identification of some rice cultivars by PAGE and successful use of RP-HPLC in separation of cereal proteins stimulated the application of the latter technique in rice variety identification. Several workers reported successful use of this technique in studies of rice storage proteins.[55,58-60] Not only were the commercial long-, medium-, and short-grain types separated, but all investigated samples were differentiated by their prolamin HPLC patterns and grain type[59] (Figure 1). Use of capillary electrophoresis was also reported.[119]

The amino acid composition of rice prolamin is similar to other prolamins extracted from cereal grains (see Table 7). The lysine content is very low and the amount of glutamic acid is high. A low tryptophan concentration is also characteristic. It must be noted that the so-called total prolamin fraction (extracted in the presence of a reducing agent) is somewhat different. The biggest difference is observed in cystine content. The authors (Shewry and Miflin[43]) explained this difference by the lower degree of purity of their preparation, the more complete extraction (due to the use of 2-mercaptoethanol together with 1-propanol), and the efficient protection of cysteine from oxidation during hydrolysis. Comparison of the data with the amino acid compositions published by different authors for the alcohol-insoluble glutelin (oryzenin) fraction of rice (Table 8) seemed to indicate that high-sulfur polypeptides of the oryzenin fraction were included in the total protein fraction.

The amino acid sequences of rice prolamins have not been as intensively studied as the sequences of prolamins of wheat, barley, and maize. Bietz[61] attempted to determine the N-terminal amino acid sequence of total rice prolamins by automated Edman degradation. This gave initial yields of only 1 to 2% with no major amino acids at each cycle. It was concluded that these were derived from nonspecific cleavage and that most if not all of the rice prolamins had blocked N-termini. More recently Horikoshi et al.[48] published the complete amino acid sequence of a major prolamin of rice endosperm. The major component had a pI of 7.1; it was purified by ion-exchange chromatography and RP-HPLC. The N-terminal amino acid residue of this protein was not detected by Edman degradation analysis. The blocked N-terminal peptide was isolated from the acidic fraction of a peptic digest of the protein. The N-terminal amino acid was identified as pyroglutamic acid after digestion of the peptide with carboxypeptidase A. The complete amino acid sequence of the polypeptide is shown in Figure 2. The protein consists of 131 amino acid residues and has a molecular weight of 14,930. The polypeptide is rich in glutamine (22%), leucine (13%), and alanine (7%) residues. Lysine, cysteine, and methionine residues were not detected. The sequence was similar to that deduced from cDNA clones by Kim and Okita[44] for the mature protein. Only 13 of the 131 amino acids were different, and 90% homology was maintained. On the basis of HPLC analysis and amino acid composition the authors showed that there are several homologous prolamins in rice. They purified another prolamin from the rice endosperm which was very similar to the major prolamin. The two showed 92% homology of amino acid sequence. This suggests that there are several homologous prolamins encoded

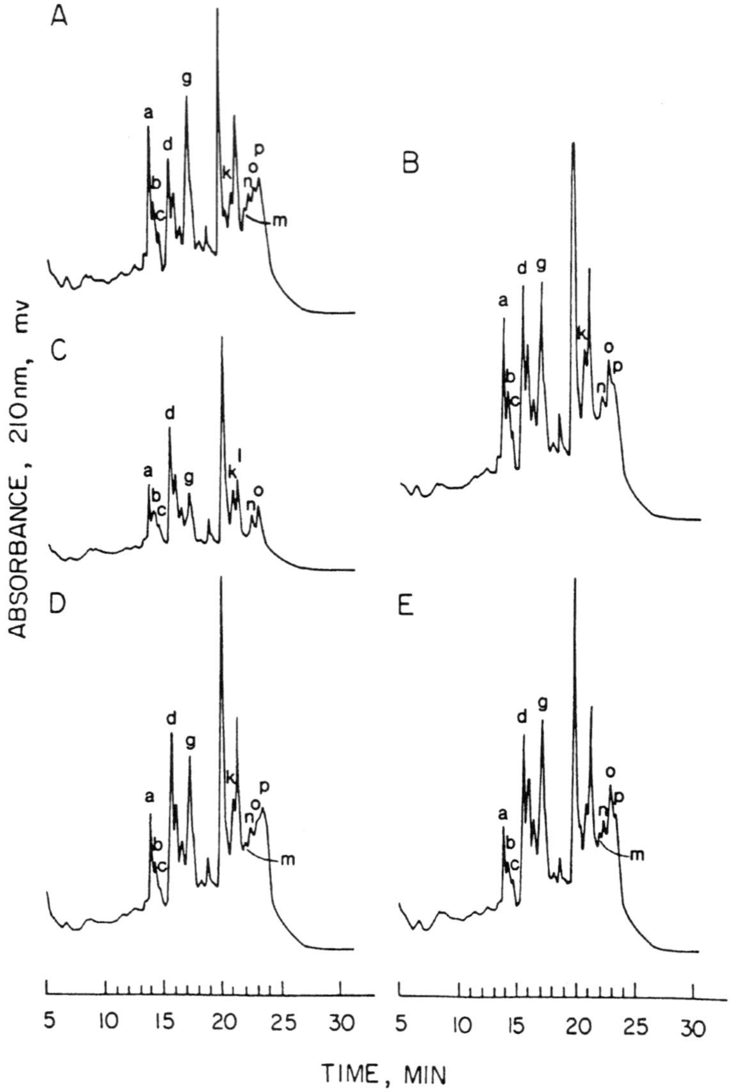

FIGURE 1 High-performance liquid chromatography prolamin patterns of long-grain rice cultivars L-201 (A), Leah (B), Lebonnet (C), Lemont (D), and Skybonnet (E). (From Lookhart, G.L., Albers, L.E., Pomeranz, Y., and Webb, B.D., *Cereal Chem.,* 64, 199, 1987. With permission.)

by multigene families. They have common features such as high levels of glutamine, leucine, and alanine and low levels of lysine, histidine, cysteine, and methionine. The purified prolamin was shown to be very hydrophobic. The N- and C-terminal regions are hydrophilic, while the central region contains many hydrophobic amino acid residues.

TABLE 7
Amino Acid Compositions of Rice Prolamins (g/16.8 g N)

Amino Acid	Lindner et al.[19]	Shewry and Miflin[43] [a]	Tecson et al.[82]	Tamura et al.[83]
Lysine	0.6	0.8	Trace–1.1	0.5
Histidine	ND	1.4	0.9–1.5	1.1
Arginine	4.7	4.7	5.3–6.6	7.0
Aspartic acid	6.9	6.4	7.9–8.3	5.4
Glutamic acid	18.3	19.0	20.8–23.3	31.8
Serine	6.5	6.3	4.7–6.9	7.3
Threonine	2.3	3.4	2.2–3.1	1.7
Methionine	0.2	3.1	Trace–0.6	3.6
Cystine	ND	4.2	Trace–1.0	0.6
Glycine	5.5	6.1	2.6–3.8	4.0
Alanine	5.0	8.6	6.6–6.9	ND
Isoleucine		4.1–6.5	4.6	
Leucine	ND	10.3	10.6–13.3	11.4
Valine	5.2	6.0	5.6–7.0	7.5
Proline	7.3	6.2	4.0–4.6	6.7
Phenylalanine	4.1	4.4	5.7–6.6	6.2
Tyrosine	5.3	5.4	7.7–9.8	8.7
Tryptophan	ND	ND	0.9	1.1

Note: ND, not determined.

[a] Total prolamin extracted in the presence of reducing agent.
[b] Isoleucine and leucine.

B. High Molecular Weight Storage Proteins (Glutelins)

The high molecular weight storage protein of rice (rice glutelin, oryzenin) is the most important protein in the rice kernel. This protein fraction may be extracted with dilute alkali. Gel filtration chromatography on Sepharose columns demonstrated both the heterogeneity of this fraction and also the high molecular weight of its components.[41,62]

The molecular weights ranged from 10^5 to the millions. Reduction of oryzenin with 2-mercaptoethanol and alkylation with acrylonitrile drastically reduced the molecular weight. Early work on gel electrophoresis investigation of oryzenin (and subunits obtained with reduction of disulfide bonds) was summarized by Juliano.[41] These investigations revealed that native oryzenin consists of several polypeptides bound by disulfide bonds. The presence of different subunits was confirmed by other authors also.[62-64] Using SDS-PAGE it was shown by Juliano and Boulter[63] that oryzenin consists of three major subunits having molecular weights of 38, 25, and

TABLE 8
Amino Acid Composition of Oryzenin (g/16 g N)

Amino Acid	Iwasaki et al.[68]	Juliano[35]	Juliano and Boulter[63]	Le Xoan Xien et al.[69]	Takeda et al.[62]
Ala	5.0	—	8.1	6.5–6.7	4.8
Arg	10.6	7.4	6.2	8.8–9.1	10.3
Asp	10.6	—	10.7	11.5–12.0	8.7
Cys	1.3	0.5	2.0	0.7	—
Glu	20.2	—	12.5	19.8–20.0	18.1
Gly	4.5	—	7.2	6.0–6.1	4.6
His	2.5	2.0	1.9	3.0–3.1	4.0
Ile	4.7	4.1	4.3	5.3–5.4	4.4
Leu	7.9	8.6	8.5	9.3–9.5	10.0
Lys	3.5	1.9	3.0	5.0–5.2	5.6
Met	1.4	2.4	2.0	1.5	1.0
Phe	6.2	5.1	4.4	6.0–6.2	5.8
Pro	4.2	—	5.0	2.5–2.6	8.3
Ser	6.9	6.1	6.3	5.8–6.0	6.1
Thr	3.7	—	4.0	4.0–4.1	3.3
Tyr	5.1	—	3.7	3.2	2.9
Trp	—	—	—	1.7–1.8	ND
Val	6.5	6.2	7.4	7.0–7.1	6.0

Note: ND, not determined.

16 kDa. Tanaka et al.[118] studied the crystalline protein bodies of endosperm containing mainly glutelins. Five components were found, with molecular weights of 22, 26, 37, 38, and 39 kDa. Comparing the results with those of Juliano and Boulter[63] they concluded that the 16-kDa polypeptide probably belongs to the prolamin fraction. The groups of 37, 38, and 39 kDa may be identical with the 38 kDa component being heterogeneous. Zhao et al.[65] extracted the glutelin fraction from grain meals of rice *(Oryza sativa)* with TRIS-HCl buffer (pH 8.8) containing 6 *M* urea and 2-mercaptoethanol. Polypeptides of glutelin were separated and purified by ion exchange chromatography under denaturing conditions. The scheme of the fractionation is shown in Figure 3. Two-dimensional SDS-PAGE (under nonreducing and reducing conditions) showed that two major glutelin subunits (22 and 36 kDa) were linked by disulfide-bonded pairs containing one 36-kDa and one 22-kDa component. The 22-kDa component was purified by preparative RP-HPLC and the peptides were sequenced. A partial amino acid sequence was determined. A homology of the 22-kDa rice glutelin subunit and the β-subunit of pea legumin was detected. It was proposed that the major component of rice glutelin was a legumin-like protein. This confirmed the results of Yamagata et al.,[66] who studied *in vivo* and *in vitro* synthesis of these proteins. Homology of the 12S globulins of oat and rice proteins was studied also by Robert et al.[72]

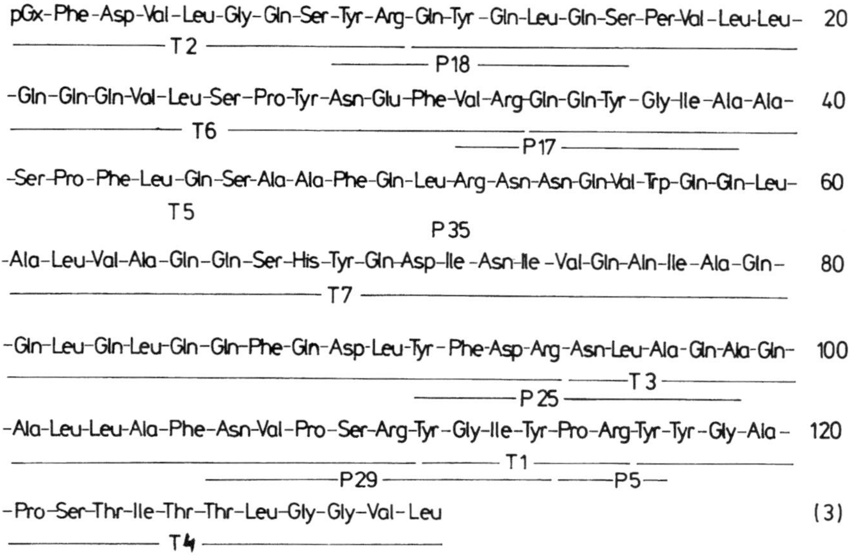

FIGURE 2 Complete amino acid sequence of major prolamin of rice endosperm. The restriction enzyme map and sequencing strategy are shown. T 1-7, tryptic peptides; P 1-35, peptic peptides. (From Horikoshi, M., Kobayashi, H., Yamazoe, Y., Mikami, B., and Morita, Y., *J. Cereal Sci.,* 14, 1, 1991. With permission.)

Electrophoretic spectra (SDS-PAGE) of rice cultivars from Vietnam and Hungary were studied by Le Trong Ha.[57] Five to seven major bands and up to 20 minor bands were observed. The spectra were suitable for variety identification.

Changes of disulfide bonds during storage were recently studied by Chrastil and Zarins.[67] An increase in disulfide bond content and a decrease of thiol groups were observed in the glutelin fraction.

The amino acid composition of oryzenin is similar to those of glutelins of other cereals. Higher lysine, methionine, cysteine, and histidine content is characteristic in comparison with the prolamin fractions. Some data reported by different research workers are summarized in Table 8. The amino acid compositions of three oryzenin subunits are shown in Table 9.

III. CYTOPLASMIC (METABOLICALLY ACTIVE) PROTEINS

A. Albumins and Globulins

The water- and salt-soluble proteins belong to the more intensively investigated groups of rice proteins. Both fractions are highly heterogeneous and contain a number of biologically important components. Subfractions may be obtained by salt precipitation and dialysis, gel chromatography, and electrophoresis.

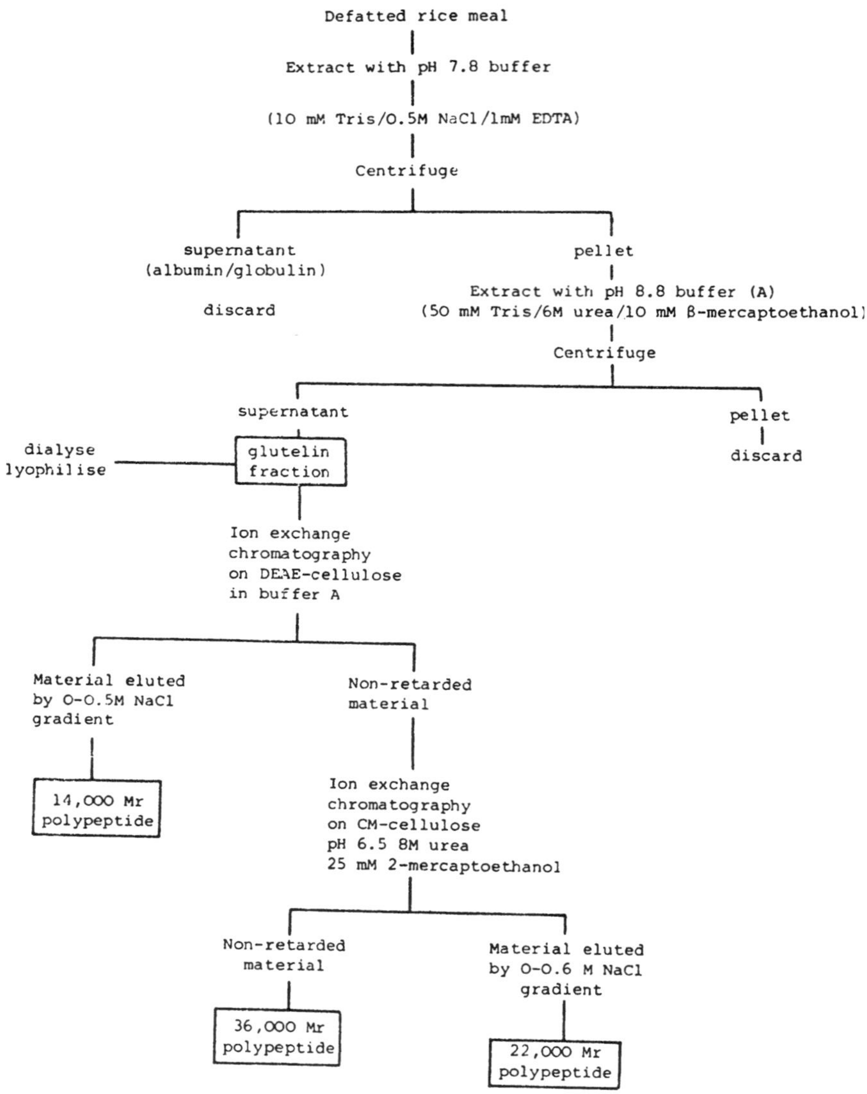

FIGURE 3 Flow diagram for purification of rice glutelin polypeptides. (From Zhao, W.-M., Gatehouse, J.A., and Boulter, D., *FEBS Lett.*, 162, 96, 1983. With permission.)

Albumins of rice were separated into three to four subfractions using gel filtration chromatography on Sephadex G-100 columns.[34,70] The molecular weights of the subfractions ranged from 10 to 200 kDa. In an early work Silayev et al.[71] reported on the separation of 9 to 11 albumin components with polyacrylamide gel electrophoresis. Other early work using electrophoretic and other techniques was reviewed by Juliano.[41] In a more recent work Iwasaki et al.[70] separated about 20 components using starch gel electrophoresis. Albumins of three types of rice showed many

TABLE 9
Amino Acid Compositions of Some Oryzenin Subunits[43] (g/16 g N)

Amino Acid	Subunit 38 kDa	25 kDa	16 kDa
ASP	10.2	13.3	11.3
THR	3.7	2.7	3.8
SER	7.0	6.7	6.4
GLU	18.7	14.1	15.9
PRO	4.7	3.9	4.8
GLY	8.2	8.7	6.7
ALA	6.1	8.7	8.2
CYS	1.5	1.1	1.0
VAL	6.9	7.7	7.1
MET	0.7	1.3	1.5
ILE	3.7	4.5	5.8
LEU	7.5	8.2	8.7
TYR	3.3	3.5	4.1
PHE	5.4	4.2	4.6
HIS	2.1	2.1	2.0
LYS	2.3	3.5	2.2
ARG	7.9	6.1	6.3

similarities and some clear differences. Sometimes only one band was found in one variety, and in some cases significant differences were observed in the intensities of several bands. The results of the investigations support the view that albumins may be used in electrophoretic variety identification.

Guo et al.[53] examinated albumin fractions of Chinese rice varieties by electrofocusing. More than 50 bands appeared, spread fairly evenly throughout the pH range 3.5 to 9.5. Because of the complexity of the patterns they considered the albumin fraction to be unsuitable for variety identification of Chinese rices.

Houston and Mohammed[73] isolated α-globulin from milled rice by precipitation from a 1% acid solution of crude globulin adjusted to pH 4.5 with sodium hydroxide. More recently the α-globulin of rice was characterized by Perdon and Juliano.[74] Gel chromatography gives a molecular weight of about 25 kDa. Glutamic acid and arginine are the main amino acid components of this protein fraction. The sulfur-containing amino acid content is also quite high (over 10%), the tryptophan content is low, and histidine and lysine are practically absent.

Iwasaki et al.[70,75,76] investigated the albumins and globulins of rice endosperm. Subunits were separated by gel electrophoresis. It was stated that the globulins of rice are highly heterogeneous and have a complicated structure. Morita and Yoshida[77] studied the properties of globulins from bran, embryo, and outer and inner endosperm. Using gel filtration chromatography on Sephadex G-200 columns they separated the globulins into three subfractions. The middle fraction, named α-globulin, a major component in bran and embryo, had a molecular weight of about 150 kDa. Later this protein was purified and characterized.[78-81,84] Three major globulin components (α-1, α-2, and α-3), which were found to be homogeneous by electrophoresis as well as by sedimentation, were isolated by DEAE-Sephadex A-50 chromatography. α-1 globulin contains small amounts of carbohydrates (hexose, pentose, hexosamine) and hydroxyproline. It is a slightly basic protein and is composed of 10 subunits. A high-purity α-globulin was isolated and characterized by Pan and Reeck.[85]

The globulins of rice endosperm may be separated by gel filtration chromatography into four subfractions; molecular weights range from 16 to 130 kDa. The amino acid compositions of rice albumins and globulins are presented in Tables 10 and 11. The albumins of rice have the highest lysine content and the lowest content of glutamic acid. High amounts of glutamic acid and arginine and a relatively high concentration of methionine are characteristic for the globulin fraction.

TABLE 10
Amino Acid Composition of Rice Albumins (g/16.8 g N)

			Iwasaki[a] et al[70]		
Amino Acid	**Lindner et al.[19]**	**Tecson et al.[82]**	**Long[a]**	**Short[a]**	**Tamura et al.[83]**
Alanine	6.0	8.7	7.02	7.19	ND
Arginine	7.8	8.4	7.74	8.40	5.7
Aspartic acid	7.6	10.8	8.36	9.04	7.7
Cystine	ND	2.9	2.91	2.64	3.0
Glutamic acid	18.4	12.5	10.14	10.50	18.5
Glycine	5.2	6.9	5.83	6.10	4.6
Histidine	ND	2.6	2.64	2.72	2.3
Isoleucine	—	4.1	2.97	3.17	6.2
Leucine	14.3[b]	7.9	6.96	7.25	10.4
Lysine	5.0	4.9	4.40	4.33	7.0
Methionine	3.0	2.5	2.29	1.68	2.0
Phenylalanine	4.6	3.0	3.46	3.58	4.1
Proline	9.3	6.6	5.46	5.83	6.2
Serine	7.0	5.2	3.81	3.86	7.3
Threonine	4.4	4.6	3.78	3.86	3.5
Tryptophan	1.6	1.9	ND	ND	1.5
Tyrosine	5.6	3.9	4.32	4.34	3.7
Valine	9.8	8.7	6.67	6.87	8.2

Note: ND, not determined.

[a] g/100 g N.
[b] Isoleucine and leucine.

TABLE 11
Amino Acid Composition of Rice Globulins

Amino Acid	Lindner et al.[19] [a]	Tecson et al.[82] [b]	Iwasaki et al.[68] Long[c]	Iwasaki et al.[68] Short[c]	(α-Globulin)[d]
Alanine	4.7	9.1	4.64	4.99	—
Arginine	7.5	11.0	15.00	15.99	15.2
Aspartic acid	7.3	7.8	4.29	4.32	—
Cystine	ND	0.0	3.50	3.62	3.0
Glutamic acid	24.5	11.8	21.11	19.91	—
Glycine	6.0	5.9	5.43	5.66	—
Histidine	ND	1.6	0.59	0.39	0.4
Isoleucine	—	3.0	2.09	1.94	1.8
Leucine	11.8[e]	6.52	7.14	6.6	—
Lysine	3.7	2.5	1.10	1.42	1.1
Methionine	4.5	2.3	4.11	4.55	4.0
Phenylalanine	4.1	3.3	3.37	3.51	3.4
Proline	7.0	5.5	4.68	5.69	—
Serine	8.0	5.5	6.48	4.75	8.8
Threonine	3.7	2.9	2.20	1.91	—
Tryptophan	1.3	1.3	ND	ND	0.6
Tyrosine	6.6	5.0	6.27	6.20	—
Valine	6.3	6.2	4.38	4.85	4.0

Note: ND, not determined.

[a] g/16.8 g N.
[b] g/16.8 g N.
[c] g/100 g protein.
[d] g/16 g N.
[e] Leucine and isoleucine.

Differences in electrophoretic patterns of globulins of different rice cultivars may be used for variety identification, as reported by several authors.[86-88]

B. Enzymes and Enzyme Inhibitors

Rice seed, like seed of other cereals, contains enzymes. From a practical point of view, amylases, lipases, proteases, and oxidoreductases are the most important. A review of earlier work on rice enzymes was given by Akazawa.[89]

The mature sound rice grain has low α- and β-amylase activity. Gel electrophoresis studies revealed multiple forms of rice seed β-amylases. Several bands showing β-amylase activity were observed, suggesting the presence of isoenzymes. The α-amylases, particularly those in germinating seeds, were more intensively studied.[91-93]

A review about cereal α-amylases was published by Hill and MacGregor.[94] Isoelectric focusing showed that rice, in contrast to wheat, rye, barley, and triticale, does not contain high-pI α-amylases; only low-pI α-amylases are present.[92] The changes in diastatic activity of milled rice during storage were also studied.[95,96] A decrease in activity was observed, influencing gelatinization conditions of rice starch during cooking.

The lipid-splitting enzymes of rice were also studied by several workers.[98-100] The heat inactivation of the lipases in the bran was studied by Martovschuk et al.[101] A review article on lipoxygenases was published by Gardner.[97] As for other enzymes, studies on rice proteases,[95,96] glutamate dehydrogenases,[102] and cytochrome oxidases[103] may be mentioned.

In rice seeds, as in other cereal grains, protease inhibitors are found.[104,105] The rice bran trypsin inhibitor is a basic protein with a molecular weight of 14,500, and its amino acid composition (and sequence) is similar to that of other trypsin inhibitors in cereal seeds.[106] A cysteine protease inhibitor[107-109] and a serine protease inhibitor[110] have also been isolated from rice seeds.

Saunders and Yetter[111] and Baker[112] detected low levels of inhibitory activity from rice endosperm extracts toward insect α-amylases. Feng et al.[113] fractionated the rice albumins using RP-HPLC; 13 of the HPLC fractions contained inhibitors of one or more of the α-amylases (insect, mammalian, bacterial). Like wheat α-amylase inhibitors, all the rice inhibitors were very stable.

C. Other Proteins

The complex proteins of the rice kernel have not yet been investigated. Nevertheless, they are present in the different parts of the seed. A nucleohistone of the rice embryo was isolated.[114] The histone was fractionated using carboxymethylcellulose chromatography. The histone preparation is high in arginine, in contrast to the wheat embryo, which is rich in lysine. Limas et al.[115] reported that rice contains low molecular weight salt-soluble proteins that inhibit protein biosynthesis and bind immunoglobulins.

IV. NUTRITIVE VALUE OF RICE PROTEINS

Due to its high lysine content, rice protein has one of the highest nutritive values among the cereal proteins. Some observations indicate poor availability of threonine. Using white rats, the biological values range from 67 to 89 for brown rice and from 61 to 81 for milled rice. From the protein fractions the albumins have the highest value and the prolamins have the lowest value. The high-protein rice cultivars have advantages from the point of view of nutrition. The slight decrease in protein quality is overcompensated by the increase in protein content. Breeding efforts to improve the nutritional value of the rice grain have concentrated on improving the protein content. The true digestibility of rice protein in man is about 85% compared with 90% for wheat flour.[35]

Because of the relatively low protein content, protein concentrates were not prepared from rice. Some interest exists for producing concentrates from rice bran.[116]

REFERENCES

1. Juliano, B. O., *Rice Chemistry and Technology,* 2nd ed., American Association of Cereal Chemists, St. Paul., MN, 1986.
2. Juliano, B. O., Structure, chemistry and function of the rice grain and its fractions, *Cereal Foods World,* 37, 772, 1992.
3. Salunkhe, D. K., Chavan, J. K., and Kadam, S. S., *Postharvest Biotechnology of Cereals,* CRC Press, Boca Raton, FL, 1985.
4. Barber, S. and Barber, C. B., Chemical and biological data of rice proteins for nutrition and feeding, in *Amino Acid Composition and Biological Value of Cereal Proteins,* Lásztity, R. and Hidvégi, M., Eds., Reidel, Dordrecht, 1985, 481.
5. Sotelo, A., Sousa, V., Montalvo, I., Hernandez, M., and Hernandez-Aragon, L., Chemical composition of different fractions of 12 Mexican varieties of rice obtained during milling, *Cereal Chem.,* 67, 209, 1990.
6. Mossé, J. and Baudet, D., Crude protein content and amino acid composition of seeds: variability and correlations, *Qual. Plant. Plant Foods Hum. Nutr.,* 32, 225, 1983.
7. Tabekhia, M. M. and Toma, R. B., Crude protein and amino acid compositions of three California rice varieties, *Nutr. Rep. Int.,* 23, 805, 1981.
8. Skurichin, J. M. and Volgarev, M. N., *Chimitcheskiy Sostav Pistchevych Produktov,* Agropromizdat, Moscow, 1987.
9. Barber, S., Barber, C. B., and Tortosa, E., Theory and practice of rice by-products utilization, in *Cereals, a Renewable Resource,* Pomeranz, Y. and Munck, L., Eds., American Association of Cereal Chemists, St. Paul, MN, 1981, 471.
10. Bechtel, D. B. and Pomeranz, Y., Ultrastructure of the mature ungerminated rice *(Oryza sativa)* caryopsis. The germ, *Am. J. Bot.,* 65, 75, 1978.
11. Bechtel, D. B. and Pomeranz, Y., Ultrastructure of the mature ungerminated rice *(Oryza sativa)* caryopsis. The starchy endosperm, *Am. J. Bot.,* 65, 684, 1978.
12. Bradbury, J. H., Collins, J. G., and Pyliotis, N. A., Methods of separation of the major histological components of rice and characterization of their proteins by amino acid analysis, *Cereal Chem.,* 57, 133, 1980.
13. Bradbury, J. H., Collins, J. G., and Pyliotis, N. A., Amino acid analysis of the proteins of the major histological components of a high-protein rice, *Cereal Chem.,* 57, 343, 1980.
14. Mitsuda, H., Yasumoto, K., Murakami, K., Kusano, T., and Kishida, H., Studies on the proteinaceous subcellular particles in rice endosperm: electron microscopy and isolation, *Agric. Biol. Chem.,* 31, 293, 1967.
15. Bechtel, D. B. and Pomeranz, Y., Ultrastructure of the mature ungerminated rice *(Oryza sativa)* caryopsis, the caryopsis coat and the aleurone cells, *Am. J. Bot.,* 64, 966, 1979.
16. Baldi, G., Studi sulle proteine del riso, *Riso,* 18, 3, 1969.
17. Kozmina, N. P. and Kretovich, V. L., *Biochimya Zerna i Produktov Jego Pererabotky,* Pishtshe-promizdat, Moscow, 1951.

18. Cagampang Gloria, B., Cruz Lourdes, J., Espiritus, G., Santiago Remedios, G., and Juliano, B. O., Studies on the extraction and composition of rice proteins, *Cereal Chem.,* 43, 145, 1966.
19. Lindner, K., Korpáczy I., Jaschik, S., and Szöke, K., Der Nahrwert der in Ungarn angebauten Reissorten, *Qual. Plant Mater. Veg.,* 8, 25, 1961.
20. Vu Van Ky and Lásztity, R., Recent results of cereal protein research, *Period. Polytech.,* (Tech. Univ. Budapest), 16, 331, 1972.
21. Albert, L., Hazai rizsek fehérjefrakcióinak vizsgálata, *Agrokém. Talajtan,* 2, 147, 1953.
22. Padmoyo, M. and Högl O., Papierelektrophoretischer Nachweis von Prolamin in Reiseiweiss, *Mitt. Geb. Lebensmittelunters. Hyg.,* 52, 29, 1961.
23. Padmoyo, M. and Högl, O., Beitrage zu der Papierelektrophorese der Getreide-Eiweisses, *Mitt. Geb. Lebensmittelunters. Hyg.,* 53, 290, 1962.
24. Roxas, B. V., Inteugan, C. L., and Juliano, B. O., Protein quality of high-protein and low-protein milled rices in preschool children, *J. Nutr.,* 109, 832, 1979.
25. Mitsuda, H., Murakami, K., Kusano, T., and Yasumoto, K., Fine structure of protein bodies isolated from rice endosperm, *Arch. Biochem. Biophys.,* 130, 678, 1969.
26. Bechtel, D. B. and Juliano, B. O., Formation of protein bodies in the starchy endosperm of rice (*Oryza sativa* L.). A reinvestigation, *Ann. Bot.,* 45, 503, 1980.
27. Ogawa, M., Kumamaru, T., Satoh, H., Omura, T., Park, T., Shintaku, K., and Baba, K., Mutants of rice storage proteins. Isolation and characterization of protein bodies from rice mutants, *Theor. Appl. Genet.,* 783, 306, 1989.
28. Chavan, J. K. and Duggal, S. K., Studies on the essential amino acid composition, protein fractions and biological value of some new varieties of rice, *J. Sci. Food Agric.,* 29, 325, 1978.
29. Hussein, M. A., Plant Proteins and Their Role in the Solving of the Protein Problem in the Arab Republic of Egypt., D. Sci. thesis, Technical University, Al-Mansoura, Egypt, 1979.
30. Bressani, R., Elias, L. G., and Juliano, B. O., Evaluation of the protein quality of milled rices differing in protein content, *J. Agric. Food Chem.,* 19, 1028, 1971.
31. Nesterin, M. F. and Skurychin, I. M., *Chimitcheskij Sostav Pishtchevych Produktov,* Pishtde-Promizdat, Moscow, 1979.
32. Ronda Lain, E. and Soto Rodriguez, E., Subproductos de arroz, I to III, *Rev. Nutr. (Madrid),* 3, 92, 1965.
33. Palmiano, E. P., Almazan, A. M., and Juliano, B. O., Physicochemical properties of protein of developing and mature rice grain, *Cereal Chem.,* 45, 1, 1968.
34. Cagampang, G. B., Perdon, A. A., and Juliano, B. O., Changes in salt soluble proteins of rice during grain development, *Phytochemistry,* 15, 1425, 1976.
35. Juliano, B. O., Rice: recent progress in chemistry and nutrition, in *Cereals for Food and Beverages, Recent Progress in Cereal Chemistry,* Inglett, G.E. and Munck, L., Eds., Academic Press, New York, 1980, 409.
36. Matthews, J., Wadsworth, J. I., and Spadero, J. J., Chemical composition of Starbonnet variety rice fractionated by rough-rice kernel thickness, *Cereal Chem.,* 58, 331, 1981.
37. Wadsworth, J. I., Matthews, J., and Spadero, J. J., Physical and physicochemical properties of Starbonnet variety rice fractionated by rough-rice kernel thickness, *Cereal Chem.,* 56, 499, 1979.
38. Mossé, J., Huet, J. C., and Baudet, J., The amino acid composition of rice grain as a function of nitrogen content as compared with other cereals: a reappraisal of rice chemical stores, *J. Cereal Sci.,* 8, 165, 1988.

39. Hibino, T., Kidzu, T., Masumura, T., Ohtsuki, K., Tanaka, K., Kawabata, K., and Fujii, S., Amino acid composition of rice prolamin polypeptides, *Agric. Biol. Chem.,* 55, 513, 1989.
40. Houston, D. F., Ed., *Rice: Chemistry and Technology,* American Association of Cereal Chemists, St. Paul, MN, 1972.
41. Juliano, B. O., The rice caryopsis and its composition, in *Rice: Chemistry and Technology,* Houston, D.F., Ed., American Association of Cereal Chemists, St. Paul, MN, 1972, Chapter 2.
42. Mandac, B. and Juliano, B. O., Properties of prolamins in mature and developing rice grain, *Phytochemistry,* 17, 611, 1978.
43. Shewry, P. R. and Miflin, B. J., Seed storage proteins, in *Advances in Cereal Science and Technology,* Vol. 7, Pomeranz, Y., Ed., American Association of Cereal Chemists, St. Paul, MN, 1985.
44. Kim, W. T. and Okita, T. W., Structure, expression and heterogeneity of the rice seed prolamins, *Plant Physiol.,* 88, 649, 1988.
45. Ogawa, M., Kumamaru, T., Satoh, H., Iwata, N., Omura, T., Kasai, Z., and Tanaka, K., Purification of protein body I of rice seed and its polypeptide composition, *Plant Cell Physiol.,* 28, 1517, 1987.
46. Sugimoto, T., Tanaka, K., and Kasai, Z., Improved extraction of rice prolamins, *Agric. Biol. Chem.,* 50, 2409, 1986.
47. Resurrection, A. P., Xingxiang, L., Okita, T. W., and Juliano, B. O., Characterization of poorly digested protein of cooked rice protein bodies, *Cereal Chem.,* 70, 101, 1993.
48. Horikoshi, M., Kobayashi, H., Yamazoe, Y., Alikami, B., and Morita, I., Purification and complete amino acid sequence of a major prolamin of rice endosperm, *J. Cereal Sci.,* 14, 1, 1991.
49. Savich, I. M., Prolamine composition of rice grain, *Physiol. Kult. Rast.,* 12, 404, 1980.
50. Savich, I. M. and Peruansky, Y. V., Identification of rice variety forms according to electrophoretic spectra of prolamins, *Vestn. Skh. Nauki Kaz.,* 6, 92, 1989.
51. Park, W. M. and Stegemann, H., Rice protein patterns. Comparison by various PAGE techniques in slabs, *Z. Acker Pflanzenbau,* 148, 446, 1979.
52. du Cros, D. L., Wrigley, C. W., and Blakeney, A. B., Fractionation of rice-grain proteins by gradient gel electrophoresis and gel isoelectric focusing: characterization of rice genotypes, *Riso,* 28, 275, 1979.
53. Guo, Y. J., Bishop, R., Fernhstrom, H., Yu, G. F., Lyan, Y. N., and Huang, S. D., Classification of Chinese rice varieties by electrofocusing, *Cereal Chem.,* 63, 1, 1986.
54. Zhao, W. and Boulter, D., Differences in the storage protein composition of different varieties of rice, *Shyan Shengwu Xuelhan,* 18, 119, 1985.
55. Huebner, F. R., Hussain, A., Lookhart, G. L., Bietz, J. A., Bushuk, W., and Juliano, B. O., Discrimination of sisterline IR rice varieties by polyacrylamide gel electrophoresis and reserved-phase high-performance liquid chromatography, *Cereal Chem.,* 68, 583, 1991.
56. Kárpáti, M., Le Truong, H., and Lásztity, R., Variety identification of rice varieties from Vietnam and Hungary using PAGE, *Acta Aliment.,* in press.
57. Le Truong, H., Kárpáti, M., and Lásztity, R., Investigation of rice glutelins, *Period. Polytech,* in press.
58. Hussain, A., Scanlon, M. G., Juliano, B. O., and Bushuk, W., Discrimination of rice cultivars by polyacrylamide gel electrophoresis and high-performance liquid chromatography, *Cereal Chem.,* 66, 353, 1989.

59. Lookhart, G. K., Albers, L. D., Pomeranz, Y., and Webb, B. D., Identification of U.S. rice cultivars by high-performance liquid chromatography, *Cereal Chem.,* 64, 199, 1987.
60. Huebner, F. P., Bietz, D. A., Webb, B. D., and Juliano, B. O., Rice cultivar identification by high-performance liquid chromatography of endosperm proteins, *Cereal Chem.,* 67, 129, 1990.
61. Bietz, J. A., Cereal prolamin evolution and homology revealed by sequence analysis, *Biochem. Genet.,* 20, 1039, 1982.
62. Takeda, M., Namba, Y., and Nunokawa, Y., Heterogeneity of rice glutelin, *Agric. Biol. Chem.,* 34, 473, 1970.
63. Juliano, B. O. and Boulter, D., Extraction and composition of rice endosperm glutelin, *Phytochemistry,* 15, 1601, 1976.
64. Villareal, R. M. and Juliano, B. O., Properties of glutelin from mature and developing rice grain, *Phytochemistry,* 17, 177, 1978.
65. Zhao, W.-M., Gatehouse, J. A., and Boulter, D., The purification and partial amino acid sequence of a polypeptide from glutelin fraction of rice grains; homology to pea legumin, *FEBS Lett.,* 162, 96, 1983.
66. Yamagata, H., Sugimoto, T., Tanaka, K., and Kasai, Z., Biosynthesis of storage proteins in developing rice seeds, *Plant Physiol.,* 70, 1094, 1982.
67. Chrastil, J. and Zarins, Z. M., Influence of storage on peptide subunit composition of rice oryzenin, *J. Agric. Food Chem.,* 40, 927, 1992.
68. Iwasaki, T., Chikubu, S., and Watanabe, T., Summarized report about the research work done on rice in the National Food Research Institute of Japan in 1975, in *Rice Report 1975,* Barber, E., Ed., National Institute of Rice Investigations, Valencia, Spain, 1976.
69. Le Xoan Xien, Safonov, V. I., and Silaev, A. B., Isolation and investigation of glutelins of Vietnam rice (in Russian), *Dokl. Akad. Nauk SSSR,* 1976, 951, 1967.
70. Iwasaki, T., Shibuya, N., Suzuki, T., and Chikubu, S., Gel filtration and electrophoresis of soluble rice proteins extracted from long, medium and short grain varieties, *Cereal Chem.,* 59, 192, 1982.
71. Silayev, A. B., Lieh, S. H., and Safonov, V. I., Issledovanye belkov vietnamskogo risa elektroforezom na poliakrilamidnom gele, *Prikl. Biochim. Mikrobiol.,* 1, 150, 1965.
72. Robert, L. S., Nozzolillo, C., and Altosaar, I., Homology between rice glutelin and oat 12S globulin, *Biochim. Biophys. Acta,* 829, 19, 1985.
73. Houston, D. F. and Mohammed, A., Purification and partial characterization of major globulin from rice endosperm, *Cereal Chem.,* 47, 5, 1970.
74. Perdon, A. A. and Juliano, B. O., Properties of major alpha-globulin in rice endosperm, *Phytochemistry,* 17, 351, 1978.
75. Iwasaki, T., Shibuya, A. N., and Chikubu, S., Studies on rice protein. I. Albumin and globulin in rice endosperm: their heterogeneity and differences in subunits among stored heated and fresh rice, *J. Jpn. Soc. Food Sci. Technol.,* 19, 70, 1972.
76. Iwasaki, T., Shibuya, N., Suzuki, T., and Chikubu, S., Studies on rice protein. II. Albumins and globulins of regular rice and waxy rice, *J. Jpn. Soc. Food Sci. Technol.,* 22, 113, 1975.
77. Morita, Y. and Yoshida, C., Studies on gamma-globulin of rice embryo. I. Isolation and purification of gamma-globulin from rice embryo, *Agric. Biol. Chem.,* 32, 664, 1968.

78. Morita, Y., Sawai, H., and Namaguchi, K., Studies on γ-globulin of rice embryo. V. Secondary structure of γ-globulin, *Agric. Biol. Chem.,* 35, 1231, 1971.
79. Sawai, H. and Morita, Y., Studies on γ-globulin of rice embryo. II. Separation of three components of γ-globulin by ion-exchange chromatography, *Agric. Biol. Chem.,* 34, 53, 1970.
80. Sawai, H. and Morita, Y., Studies on γ-globulin of rice embryo. III. Molecular dimension and chemical composition of γ-globulin, *Agric. Biol. Chem.,* 34, 61, 1970.
81. Sawai, H. and Morita, Y., Studies on γ-globulin from rice embryo. IV. Some aspects of subunit structure of globulin, *Agric. Biol. Chem.,* 34, 771, 1970.
82. Tecson, E. M. E., Esmana-Bernadotta, V., Lontok, L. P., and Juliano, B. O., Studies on the extraction and composition of rice endosperm proteins, *Cereal Chem.,* 48, 168, 1971.
83. Tamura, G., Tsunoda, T., Kirimura, J., and Miyazawa, S., The microbiological determination of amino acids in various rice proteins and "sake", *Nippon Nogeikagaku Kaishi,* 26, 480, 1952.
84. Pascual, C. G., Juliano, B. O., and Tanaka, Y., Fractionation of globulins of milled rice, *Phytochemistry,* 20, 2471, 1981.
85. Pan, J. S. and Reeck, G. R., Isolation and characterization of rice α-globulin, *Cereal Chem.,* 65, 316, 1988.
86. Sarkar, R. and Bose, S., Electrophoretic characterization of rice varieties using single seed (salt soluble) proteins, *Theor. Appl. Genet.,* 68, 415, 1984.
87. Hauhan, J. S. and Nanda, J. S., Varietal identification in rice (*Oryza sativa* L.) by physicochemical characters of grain and electrophoretic variants of salt soluble seed proteins, *Seed Res.,* 12, 78, 1984.
88. Kusama, T., Yanag, S. O., and Iwamoto, M., Comparison of rice (*Oryza sativa* L.) seed proteins from several varieties, *Agric. Biol. Chem.,* 48, 1649, 1983.
89. Akazawa, T., Enzymes of rice, in *Rice: Chemistry and Technology,* Houston, D.F., Ed., American Association of Cereal Chemists, St. Paul, MN, 1972, 75.
90. Okamoto, K. and Akazawa, T., Purification of α- and β-amylase from endosperm tissues of germinating rice seeds, *Agric. Biol. Chem.,* 42, 1379, 1978.
91. Okamoto, K. and Kazawa, T., Enzymic mechanism of starch breakdown in germinating rice seeds. I. Amylase formation in the epithelium, *Plant Physiol.,* 63, 336, 1979.
92. MacGregor, A. W., Marchylo, B. A., and Kruger, J. E., Multiple α-amylase components in germinated cereal grains determined by isoelectric focusing and chromatofocusing, *Cereal Chem.,* 65, 326, 1988.
93. Lorenz, K. and Saunders, R. M., Enzyme activities in commercially milled rice, *Cereal Chem.,* 55, 77, 1978.
94. Hill, R. D. and MacGregor, A. W., Cereal α-amylases in grain research and technology, in *Advances in Cereal Science and Technology,* Vol. 9, Pomeranz, Y., Ed., American Association of Cereal Chemists, St. Paul, MN, 1988, 217.
95. Dhaliwal, Y. S., Sekhon, K. S., and Naki, H. P. S., Enzymatic activities and rheological properties of stored rice, *Cereal Chem.,* 68, 18, 1991.
96. Beloglazova, L. K., Prudnikova, T. N., Fedorova, S. A., and Shcherbakov, V. G., Changes in the protein complex of rice grain during storage under different moisture conditions, *Izv. Vuzov Piscsevaja Technol.* No. 6, 12, 1977.
97. Gardner, H. V., Lipoxygenase pathways in cereals, in *Advances in Cereal Science and Technology,* Vol. 9, Pomeranz, Y., Ed., American Association of Cereal Chemists, St. Paul, MN, 1988, 161.

98. O'Conner, J., Perry, J. H., and Wood, J. L., A comparison of lipase activity in various cereal grains, *J. Cereal Sci.,* 16, 153, 1992.
99. Funatsu, M., Aizoro, Y., Hayasi, K., Watanabe, M., and Eto, M., Biochemical studies on rice bran lipase, *Agric. Biol. Chem.,* 35, 734, 1971.
100. Bradbury, J. H. and Collins, J. G., Lipids of the major histological components of rice studied by ^{13}C nuclear resonance spectroscopy, *Cereal Chem.,* 59, 159, 1982.
101. Martovschuk, E. V., Kopejkovskij, V. M., and Asvaturjan, L. K., Inaktivacija fermentov risowch otrubej putem kratkovremennogo vzdejstvija ostrym parom, *Maslob. Zhir. Prom.,* 9, 18, 1981.
102. Nanda, B. B., Mali, P. C., and Lodh, S. B., Glutamate dehydrogenase activity and isoenzymes, protein, and soluble amino acids in developing grains of high and low protein rice, *Cereal Chem.,* 68, 351, 1991.
103. Morita, Y. and Ida, S., Studies on respiratory enzymes in rice kernel. I. Isolation and purification of cytochrome C and peroxidase 556 from rice embryo, *Agric. Biol. Chem.,* 32, 441, 1968.
104. Maki, Z., Tashiro., M., Sugihara, N., and Kanamosi, M., Double-headed nature of a trypsin inhibitor from rice bran, *Agric. Biol. Chem.,* 44, 953, 1980.
105. Tashiro, M. and Maki, Z., Partial purification and some properties of a trypsin inhibitor from rice bran, *Agric. Biol. Chem.,* 42, 1119, 1978.
106. Garcia-Olmedo, D., Salcedo, G., Sanchez-Monge, R., Gomez, L., Royo, J., and Carbonero, P., Plant proteinaceous inhibitors of proteinases and α-amylases, in *Oxford Surveys of Plant Molecular and Cell Biology,* Vol. 4, Miflin, B., Ed., Oxford University Press, Oxford, 1987, 275.
107. Abe, K. and Arai, S., Purification of a cysteine proteinase inhibitor from rice (*Oryza sativa* L. japanica), *Agric. Biol. Chem.,* 49, 3349, 1985.
108. Abe, K., Kondo, H., and Arai, S., Purification and characterization of a rice cysteine proteinase inhibitor, *Agric. Biol. Chem.,* 51, 2763, 1987.
109. Abe, K., Emori, Y., Kondo, H., Suzuki, K., and Ara, I. S., Molecular cloning of a cysteine proteinase inhibitor of rice (oryzacystatin), *J. Biol. Chem.,* 262, 16793, 1987.
110. Tashiro, M., Hashino, K., Shiozaki, M., Ibuki, F., and Maki, Z., The complete amino acid sequence of rice bran trypsin inhibitor, *J. Biochem.,* 102, 297, 1987.
111. Saunders, R. M. and Yetter, M., α-Amylase inhibitors in rice, in *Rice Report,* Barber, S., Mitsuda, H., Desikachar, N.S.R., and Tortosa, E., Eds., Inst. Agrochem. Technol. Alim., Valencia, Spain, 1977, 148.
112. Baker, J. E., Dietary modulation of α-amylase activity in eight geographical strains of *Sicophilus orizae* and *Sitophiles zeamays, Entomol. Exp. Appl.,* 46, 47, 1985.
113. Feng, G.-H., Chen, M., Kramer, K. J., and Reeck, G. R., α-Amylase inhibitors from rice: fractionation and selectivity toward insect, mammalian, and bacterial α-amylases, *Cereal Chem.,* 68, 516, 1991.
114. Tsuchya, T., Iwai, K., and Ando, T., The histones of rice embryo, *Seikagaku,* 39, 109, 1967.
115. Limas, G., Salinas, G., Moneo, I., Fischer, S., Wittmann-Liebold, B., and Mendez, E., Purification and characterization of ten new rice NaCl-soluble proteins: identification of four protein-synthesis inhibitors and two immunoglobulin-binding proteins, *Planta,* 181, 1, 1990.
116. Connor, M. A., Saunders, R. M., and Kohler, G. O., Rice bran protein concentrates obtained by wet alkaline extraction, *Cereal Chem.,* 53, 488, 1976.
117. Matsui, H., Chiba, S., Shimomura, T., and Takahashi, N., Multiple forms of rice seeds β-amylases on zymogram, *Agric. Biol. Chem.,* 39, 2239, 1976.

118. Tanaka, K., Sugimoto, T., Ogawa, M., and Kasai, Z., Isolation and characterization of two types of protein bodies in the rice endosperm, *Agric. Biol. Chem.,* 44, 1633, 1980.
119. Lookhart, G. L. and Bean, S., Rapid differentiation of oat cultivars and of rice cultivars by capillary zone electrophoresis, *Cereal Chem.,* 72, 312, 1995.

9 Oat Proteins

I. INTRODUCTION, GENERAL CHARACTERIZATION OF OAT PROTEINS

Out of several reported oat species the most important is the common white oat *(Avena sativa),* grown primarily for grain production in the temperate regions of the world. *Avena byzanthina* (common red oat) is grown as winter oats in the southern U.S. and other warm regions. The structure of the inflorescence of the oat plant and the structure of the oat kernel are different from those of other cereals. The inflorescence is an open panicle that bears spikelets at the ends of the branches. Several florets are initiated in each spikelet, and from one to three will develop into mature kernels. The distribution of the kernels according to weight and size is more heterogeneous than in other cereals. The kernel is surrounded by a two-pan hull. When the hull is removed, the structure called the groat remains. Because the hull contains a high amount of cellulose and a very low amount of protein there is a significant difference in composition between oat kernels and oat groats. According to data obtained by research workers[1-5] through analysis of thousands of samples, the average protein content of the oat kernel varies between 11 to 15% and that of the groat ranges from 12.4 to 24.5%. The protein content of oat groats is the highest among cereals. Oat protein has some unique features in comparison with other cereal grain proteins.[6] The average amino acid composition of oat proteins is more advantageous from the point of view of nutritional value. This fact is probably related to the substantially differing distribution of the classic protein fractions (albumins, globulins, prolamins, and glutelins, classified according to Osborne) in oats and other cereal grains. The proportion of albumins and globulins is much higher.[7]

The major parts of the oat kernel which are of particular interest to the cereal chemist are the hull, bran, aleurone layer, starchy endosperm, and embryo. The embryo constitutes about 3% of the kernel weight, and the ratio of the bran and starchy endosperm is about 1:2 (~30 and ~60%). The protein content of the embryo is the highest (over 30%), and the starchy endosperm contains about 10% protein. Relatively high protein levels occur in the bran (about 20%). The protein content of the hull is generally lower than 2%.[8,9] The oat endosperm consists of a single layer of aleurone cells surrounding the starch parenchyma cells. The aleurone cells contain lipid droplets, aleurone grains, plastids, mitochondria, and endoplasmic reticulum as well as protein-carbohydrate bodies. The cells of the endosperm contain starch granules and protein bodies. In the subaleurone layer a few small starch granules and numerous protein bodies occur, whereas in the central starchy endosperm the cells are composed primarily of starch, with protein bodies interspersed. The protein bodies of the oat endosperm differ from those of other cereals.[10] The oat protein bodies of the starchy endosperm are composed of a matrix with lighter-staining inclusions. Oats lack the protein matrix which is characteristic of wheat and some other cereals. The differences between oats and other cereal grains in the structure of the proteinaceous components is consistent with the differences in the distribution of the protein fraction. In Table 1 some data about the protein content of groats, hulls, and groat fractions are shown. The protein content of oats is generally determined by analysis of the samples for nitrogen content and then multiplying the values obtained by 6.25. (According to Tkachuk[12] the use of a factor between 5.50 and 5.80 might be more valid.) Protein concentrations vary considerably among cultivars and species and even among identical cultivars exposed to different environments.

TABLE 1
Protein Concentrations in Morphological Parts of Oat Kernel (%)

Variety	Groats	Hulls	Scutellum	Bran	Starchy Endosperm
Avena sativa[a]					
Orbit	13.8	1.7	32.4	18.8	9.6
Lodi	14.6	1.6	26.2	19.6	10.7
Garland	14.8	1.4	28.9	18.5	10.9
Froker	15.5	1.4	28.0	20.7	9.7
Portal	16.5	1.9	29.1	23.0	10.3
Dal	20.8	1.5	24.2	26.5	13.5
Goodland	22.5	1.9	32.4	32.5	17.0
Commercial[b]	18.9	5.7	—	18.8	9.6
Avena sterilis[c]					
Mean of 25 selections	23.2	1.4	31.1	31.9	17.5

[a] From Youngs.[9]
[b] From Caldwell and Pomeranz.[4]
[c] From Youngs and Peterson.[10]

The effect of the level of nitrogen fertilizers on protein concentration is well known. It has been reported by several authors[13,15] that the amino acid composition of oats is not altered as extensively by the increase of nitrogen percentage in grain as that of other cereals.

Eppendorfer[13] reported slight decreases in lysine, glycine, alanine, and cystine contents with increasing grain protein content. Peterson[15] investigated amino acid compositions of the proteins in three cultivars at different protein levels (influenced by the level of nitrogen fertilization). No differences were found. It was found that the amino acid composition of oat grain is not directly affected by differential treatment with phosphorus and potassium,[14] although the effect of deficiencies of these nutrients on yield is substantial. The protein content and amino acid composition of oat groats and their fractions and some commercially milled oats, according to Caldwell and Pomeranz,[4] are given in Tables 2 and 3. The lysine content of oats is higher than that of other cereal proteins, and the glutamic acid (glutamine) and proline contents are relatively lower. The differences between endosperm proteins and proteins of embryo are also observed in oats, but they are not as extensively expressed as in other cereals. In Table 4 the protein contents of 13 oat varieties grown in Hungary are summarized as reported by Lásztity et al.[17]

TABLE 2
Amino Acid Composition of Oats and Groats (g Amino Acid/100 g Amino Acid Recovered)

	Oats[a]		Groats[b]	
Amino Acid	Heavy	Light		
Lysine	4.2	5.2	4.5	3.9
Histidine	2.4	2.7	2.4	2.3
Arginine	6.4	6.3	6.8	6.2
Aspartic acid	9.2	11.1	8.7	9.0
Threonine	3.3	4.1	3.4	3.1
Serine	4.0	4.5	4.6	3.9
Glutamic acid	21.6	20.0	21.7	22.4
Proline	5.7	3.1	5.5	6.2
Cystine	1.7	6.1	2.1	2.0
Glycine	5.1	6.0	5.2	5.0
Alanine	5.1	5.5	5.0	5.0
Valine	5.8	6.2	5.5	5.7
Methionine	2.3	1.5	2.2	2.5
Isoleucine	4.2	4.5	3.9	4.3
Leucine	7.5	7.6	7.6	7.4
Tyrosine	2.6	2.4	3.0	2.5
Phenylalanine	5.4	5.3	5.2	5.5

[a] From Pomeranz et al.[3]
[b] From Caldwell and Pomeranz.[4]

To date the endosperm proteins of oat have been classified on the basis of solubility as elaborated by Osborne. The more scientific classification on the basis of biochemical functions is not yet used. This fact may be connected with the quite different distribution of the protein fractions as compared with other cereal grains. In wheat and some other cereals the storage proteins are insoluble in salt solutions. In the case of oats a large portion of the soluble globulins also belong to the storage proteins of the endosperm. The isolation and more detailed investigation of the

TABLE 3
Amino Acid Compositions of Different Morphological Parts of Oat Kernel (g Amino Acid/100 g Amino Acids Recovered)

Amino Acid	Endosperm[a]	Hulls[a]	Embryonic Axis[b]	Scutellum[b]
Lysine	3.7	4.9	8.2	6.9
Histidine	3.7	2.4	3.9	3.6
Arginine	6.6	6.8	8.3	9.0
Aspartic acid	8.5	10.5	10.2	9.7
Threonine	3.3	4.1	5.0	4.7
Serine	4.6	4.6	4.8	5.0
Glutamic acid	23.6	20.3	14.2	14.9
Proline	4.6	2.4	3.3	3.6
Cystine	2.2	0.5	0.5	1.0
Glycine	4.7	6.1	6.3	6.2
Alanine	4.5	5.4	7.2	6.9
Valine	5.5	6.4	6.0	6.2
Methionine	2.4	1.5	2.2	2.1
Isoleucine	4.2	4.5	3.9	3.8
Leucine	7.8	7.8	7.1	7.1
Tyrosine	3.3	2.9	2.9	3.0
Phenylalanine	5.6	5.3	4.2	4.4

[a] From Pomeranz et al.[3]
[b] From Caldwell and Pomeranz.[4]

protein bodies in the starchy endosperm may help in the exact separation of the storage proteins and cytoplasmic (metabolically active) proteins.

It is generally accepted that oat endosperm contains a relatively low quantity of prolamins and a high amount of globulins. The literary data concerning protein distribution vary widely, and in some cases they are contradictory. Some of the data are summarized in the review of Youngs et al.[18]

The ratios of different protein fractions are dependent on the conditions of extraction. When water-soluble proteins are extracted with distilled water, due to the presence of small amounts of salts in the meal the extracted fraction may contain globulins, too. The solubility of globulins is dependent on the ionic strength of the salt solution used for extraction.[20] The greatest amount of globulins was extracted with a solution containing 1.0 *M* NaCl and 0.05 *M* TRIS (hydroxymethyl) aminomethane at pH 8.5.[19] Prolamins are generally extracted with 70% (v/v) ethanol; however, for optimal extraction some authors recommend 52% ethanol.[31] Complete solubilization of oat seed proteins is generally possible only with alkaline buffer

TABLE 4
Amino Acid Compositions of Oat Varieties (g Amino Acid/16 g N)

Oat Variety	Crude Protein % D.S.	ALA	ARG	ASP	CYS	GLU	GLY	HIS	ILE
Leanda	12.1	5.18	7.42	8.92	1.94	21.04	5.26	2.26	3.91
Condor	13.0	5.14	7.34	9.14	1.80	21.11	5.22	2.25	3.91
Natal	13.3	5.02	7.62	8.96	1.89	20.79	5.20	2.29	4.02
American	13.1	5.15	7.05	8.36	1.48	22.05	5.25	2.12	4.07
CS-1	11.9	5.29	6.55	8.49	1.13	20.67	5.43	1.73	3.79
CS-2	11.1	5.52	6.62	8.59	2.36	20.20	5.64	2.58	3.83
CS-3	9.8	5.13	6.96	8.51	2.16	20.76	5.48	2.79	3.75
CS-4	11.1	5.01	7.00	8.60	0.98	20.35	5.04	3.18	3.67
Early Sz.	13.8	4.85	7.49	8.30	2.49	21.43	5.14	2.19	3.95
Naked T[a]	19.6	4.87	7.35	7.83	3.38	22.45	4.95	2.21	3.80
Astor	11.8	5.60	6.53	8.11	1.83	20.44	6.10	2.04	3.89
Karin	11.1	4.34	6.73	9.47	0.74	21.27	5.51	2.61	4.04
M. Tabaret	11.5	5.23	6.40	8.71	1.94	21.52	5.45	1.49	4.02
Ave.	12.0	5.12	6.98	8.68	1.73	21.06	5.39	1.46	3.90

Oat Variety	LEU	LYS	MET	PHE	PRO	SER	THR	TYR	VAL	NH_3
Leanda	7.67	4.49	1.87	5.07	5.28	5.09	3.67	3.34	5.29	2.30
Condor	7.65	4.39	1.39	5.07	5.41	5.27	3.87	3.33	5.26	2.47
Natal	7.64	4.40	1.69	5.10	5.49	5.03	3.67	3.59	5.20	2.40
American	7.79	4.07	1.28	5.42	6.36	4.76	3.42	3.76	5.46	2.18
CS-1	7.34	4.90	1.73	4.98	6.98	4.89	3.56	3.62	5.36	2.58
CS-2	7.28	4.80	1.82	4.44	6.10	5.07	3.67	3.87	5.25	2.34
CS-3	7.37	5.05	1.46	4.63	7.70	4.75	3.47	2.91	4.80	2.42
CS-4	7.32	5.58	1.63	4.88	6.87	4.83	3.46	3.70	4.97	2.95
Early Sz.	7.69	4.14	1.63	5.20	5.77	5.02	3.55	3.69	5.13	2.33
Naked T[a]	7.66	4.06	1.02	5.11	5.50	4.97	3.57	3.84	5.14	2.35
Astor	7.29	3.89	2.51	4.78	5.04	6.75	3.90	3.75	5.48	2.06
Karin	7.83	4.02	1.57	4.75	5.40	5.21	3.82	4.02	5.31	2.37
M. Tabaret	7.85	4.44	1.17	4.83	6.01	4.96	3.63	3.77	5.36	2.21
Ave.	7.55	4.51	1.65	4.93	6.03	5.14	3.64	3.61	5.24	2.38

Note: D.S. = dry substance.

[a] Not included in the average.

solutions containing detergents. Addition of reducing agents (e.g., 2-mercaptoethanol) is also common.[22,23] Generally water-soluble proteins and glutelins represent about 30% of the total oat protein, the remainder being distributed in approximately a 2:1 ratio between globulins and prolamins.

The amino acid compositions of the fractions show significant differences. In Table 5 the average composition of the fractions isolated from oats grown in Hungary is summarized. The lysine content of albumin is the highest. Oat prolamins are characterized by a low content of basic amino acids and a high amount of glutamic acid (glutamine), as are prolamins of other cereals.

TABLE 5
Average Amino Acid Compositions of the Different Protein Fractions Isolated from Oats Grown in Hungary (g Amino Acid/100 g Protein)

Amino acid	Albumins	Globulins	Prolamins	Glutelins
Lysine	8.3	4.9	3.1	5.2
Histidine	3.1	3.3	1.6	3.1
Arginine	5.3	8.5	5.0	9.1
Aspartic acid	12.5	9.8	4.2	10.8
Threonine	5.5	3.8	2.3	4.8
Serine	6.3	4.3	3.2	4.7
Glutamic acid	15.1	19.5	36.1	19.1
Proline	5.8	5.4	11.3	8.1
Glycine	6.5	5.8	3.0	4.0
Alanine	7.1	6.5	3.8	4.1
Cystine	1.7	1.8	3.1	1.4
Valine	7.3	5.1	5.5	4.4
Methionine	2.2	1.9	3.3	1.5
Isoleucine	4.1	4.7	3.8	4.3
Leucine	8.9	7.0	10.3	7.1
Tyrosine	2.6	2.4	2.1	4.8
Phenylalanine	7.8	6.1	7.5	7.1
Tryptophan	1.7	1.4	1.6	1.9

II. STORAGE PROTEINS OF OAT

A. Globulins

As mentioned earlier, oat is the only cereal in which the major proportion of the grain protein is soluble in salt and thus classified as globulin. Quantitative data published on the proportion of globulins vary widely (from 40–50% to 70–80%).[24,25] The globulin fraction of oats (called avenalin) is a mixture of different polypeptides as revealed by ultracentrifugation, electrophoresis, RP-HPLC, and other techniques. Burgess et al.[26] have identified and separated globulins of 3, 7, and 12S from extracts of oat grain made with 1 *M* NaCl. The major component, the 12S globulin, is an oligomeric protein with a quaternary structure very similar to that of legumins. The first detailed characterization of this protein was by Peterson,[19] who showed that the 12S fraction has a molecular weight of 322 kDa. Separation by SDS-PAGE under reducing conditions revealed the presence of two major subunits with molecular weights of about 32 and 22 kDa, called the α- and β-subunits. The α- and β-subunits are disulfide bonded in the native globulin, forming a dimer with a molecular weight of about 54 kDa. The 12S globulin is a hexamer consisting of six 54-kDa subunits. Different authors[22,23,26-29] reported a broader molecular weight range for α,β-dimer (from 50 to 70 kDa), α-polypeptide (from 32 to 43 kDa), and β-polypeptide (from 19 to 25 kDa).

Isoelectric focusing (IEF) has demonstrated that the smaller polypeptides are basic, with pIs between 8 and 9, whereas the larger polypeptides are more acidic, with pIs of 5 to 7; the α-polypeptides are therefore called acidic and the β-polypeptides basic.[30] IEF studies indicate that heterogeneity exists within each of the two polypeptide groups. Walburg and Larkins[31] reported that 20 to 30 components were present in the α-fraction and 5 to 15 components were in the β-fraction of oat globulins. The various components have been purified and their amino acid compositions determined (Table 6). The content of basic amino acids (histidine, arginine, and lysine) is higher in β- than in α-polypeptides. Moreover, β-polypeptides contain more aspartic and glutamic acid than α-polypeptides. The group of large subunits is low in methionine.[26,27] The 12S oat globulin is compositionally and structurally related to 11S globulins in legumes.[19,27,32] Shotwell et al.[33] predicted an amino acid sequence from 12S oat globulin cDNA and compared it to that of soybean glycinin and rice globulin. Oat globulin was found to be 30 to 40% homologous with storage globulins of legumes and about 70% homologous with those of rice. The homology is supported by studies of *in vitro* synthesis. These showed that the 12S globulins of oats are synthesized as precursor molecules and that the latter are cleaved post-translationally to give subunit pairs.[27,31,34]

Oats also contain minor amounts of 3S and 7S globulins. Burgess et al.[26] purified the 7S globulin of oats and determined some of its properties. The major components were 55-kDa polypeptides. Some minor components (of molecular weight 65 kDa) were also detected. A 3S fraction was also separated from oats,[26] and it was found to consist of at least two major components, with molecular weights of about 15 and 21 kDa. Some data about amino acid composition are summarized in Table 6.

Characteristic of the 3S and 7S globulins is a relatively high glycine content but a lower glutamine + glutamic acid content than that found in 12S globulins.

The 3S and 7S globulins of oats and barley have been shown to have immunological and structural similarities to corresponding proteins in legumes and cotton seed.[35,36] However, it must be noted that studies comparing the thermal coagulation of oat globulin with that of soy glycinin have revealed a significant difference between these two proteins, although the two proteins have similar molecular structures.[37]

TABLE 6
Amino Acid Composition of Some Oat Globulins[26]

Amino Acid	12S Globulin	12S Globulin Subunits 40 kDa	12S Globulin Subunits 20 kDa	7S Globulin	3S Globulin
ASP	9.9	8.3	12.4	7.6	8.7
THR	4.0	3.3	4.4	3.4	5.0
SER	6.5	6.6	7.0	8.9	9.2
GLU	18.9	23.7	14.9	15.8	12.6
PRO	4.8	5.1	5.2	4.3	4.3
GLY	8.2	9.9	8.3	12.5	12.5
ALA	6.6	6.1	7.5	7.0	8.2
CYS	1.2	0.8	1.0	1.3	1.9
VAL	5.9	5.8	6.1	6.4	5.4
MET	0.5	0.0	0.2	0.3	0.9
ILE	4.8	4.2	5.3	3.1	3.9
LEU	7.9	7.7	7.5	6.3	7.1
TYR	3.4	3.0	3.1	2.3	3.0
PHE	5.3	5.5	4.4	4.6	3.5
HIS	2.5	2.1	3.0	2.8	3.0
LYS	3.2	2.5	3.7	4.4	5.2
ARG	6.4	5.5	6.0	9.0	5.6
TRP	N.D.	N.D.	N.D.	N.D.	N.D.

Note: N.D., not determined.

B. Oat Prolamins (Avenins)

In the present chapter the oat prolamins (avenins) are classically defined as those proteins that are soluble in ethanol-water mixtures without reduction of disulfide bonds. Total avenins are generally isolated by extraction with 70% (v/v) ethanol. The prolamin fraction of oats accounts for about 15% of the total protein of oat flour. Avenin is a mixture of different polypeptides, as revealed by various separation techniques (gel filtration,[21,37] HPLC,[38] RP-HPLC,[39,40,47,93] cation exchange chromatography,[21] SDS-PAGE,[38,39] IEF,[37] two-dimensional electrophoresis[24]). The most powerful separation technique, two-dimensional gel electrophoresis, has shown that avenin is composed of more than 20 components with molecular weights ranging from 20 to 34 kDa.

Studying the patterns on starch gel electrophoresis of avenin fractions from a range of diploid, tetraploid, and hexaploid species, Kim et al.[41] and Kim and Mossé[42] observed a total of 17 bands. Not all bands were present in any one species. The number of bands increased with ploidy level. Gel electrophoresis (SDS-PAGE) may be used in oat variety identification.[43-46] Like other cereal prolamins, the avenin polypeptides may be grouped according to electrophoretic mobility into α-, β-, γ-, and δ-avenins.[21,48] Isoelectric focusing revealed three main groups of components at pH ~6, 7.6, and 9.[37] Wieser and Belitz,[39] using RP-HPLC, separated crude avenin (oat variety Flamingsregent) into 30 components. The first group, consisting of minor components (peak 1–14), was composed of nonavenin proteins. The second group (peak 15–30) was the predominant group and corresponded to avenin proteins. These were classified into three subgroups differing mainly in their content of hydrophobic amino acids (Leu, Ile, Val, Phe). High-performance liquid chromatography of avenins was successfully used for oat variety identification.[49,50] The amino acid composition of total avenin and those of different components of avenin are generally similar to each other. Amino acid composition closely reflects the intermediate position of oats in cereal taxonomy. The high degree of amidation of glutamic and aspartic acids corresponds to that of wheat, rye, and barley. On the other hand, the fairly low content of proline (about 10 mol%) and the fairly high contents of leucine (11 mol%) and valine (8 mol%) are similar to those of rice, millet, and maize prolamins. Some data on amino acid composition of major avenin components separated by preparative RP-HPLC and amino acid composition of the subgroups of these components are shown in Table 7 and Table 8.

The amino acid sequence studies on avenin and its components started in the 1980s.[51,52] Bietz[52] subjected total avenin to automated Edman degradation and found a single unambiguous sequence for the first 23 residues. This was

1	2	3	4	5	6	7	8	9	10	11
THR–	THR–	THR–	VAL–	GLN–	TYR–	ASN–	PRO–	SER–	GLU–	GLN
12	13	14	15	16	17	18	19	20	21	22
TYR–	GLN–	PRO–	TYR–	PRO–	GLU–	GLN–	GLN–	GLU–	PRO–	PHE
23										
VAL										

The author concluded that all avenin polypeptides probably have a homologous N-terminal amino acid sequence, but that nonspecific N-terminal blocking occurs. Studies of Pernollet et al.[38] confirmed that half of the isolated oat prolamins were blocked to Edman degradation. The determined N-terminal sequences were fairly homologous. The N-terminal amino acid sequence of avenin is not related to any reported for other cereal prolamins. It is unusual in that the first three residues are threonine. Egorov and Odintsova[53] studied the N-terminal amino acid sequences of three avenin components separated by ion exchange and HPLC. The sequences of all three proteins were identical as for the first 40 amino acids. The complete amino acid sequence of one of the avenin components (designated N9), which migrates faster than others (except one minor component) when examined by sodium lactate PAGE and which is present in the majority of oat varieties, has been published by Egorov.[47] The primary structure is shown in Figure 1. Avenin N9 consists of 182 amino acids residues. Its calculated M_r of 21 kDa is in good agreement with its amino acid composition and electrophoretic mobility. It contains 30.7 mol% glutamine, 11.5 mol% proline, 4 mol% cysteine, 1.6 mol% methionine, and 60 mol%

TABLE 7
Amino Acid Compositions of Major Avenin Components Separated by RP-HPLC[39]

Fraction No. Retention Time (min)	15 50.7	16 53.0	17 54.2	18 56.0	19 58.0	20 62.6	21 63.9	22 65.3	23 82.7	24 85.8	25 87.9	26 89.2	27 91.0	28 93.9	29 96.8	30 97.7
Asx	2.2	2.1	2.2	1.9	2.3	2.0	1.9	1.9	1.7	1.7	1.6	1.7	1.5	1.4	1.5	1.5
Thr	2.3	2.2	2.1	2.1	2.1	2.0	2.1	1.9	2.1	1.9	1.8	1.7	1.3	1.1	1.1	1.1
Ser	3.2	2.7	2.4	2.1	2.4	2.2	2.1	1.9	3.8	3.6	3.6	3.5	3.4	3.6	3.7	3.7
Glx	37.0	37.1	37.9	38.1	37.4	39.3	39.6	40.1	37.5	37.9	38.2	39.0	40.1	40.4	40.3	40.1
Pro	11.6	11.8	11.6	11.5	11.2	11.5	11.7	11.6	10.8	10.7	10.4	10.6	9.8	10.2	10.1	9.7
Gly	2.5	2.0	1.8	1.6	1.7	1.8	1.6	1.5	3.3	2.9	2.4	2.0	1.0	0.7	0.8	0.7
Ala	5.8	5.8	5.7	5.8	6.2	5.3	5.1	5.1	5.1	5.2	5.2	5.2	5.5	5.6	5.6	5.7
Val	9.8	10.4	10.7	10.6	10.1	9.7	10.0	10.0	7.6	7.4	7.2	7.3	7.4	7.4	7.3	7.8
Met	0.8	1.1	0.8	1.3	1.5	0.8	0.8	1.0	1.7	2.2	2.5	2.2	1.6	1.1	0.8	1.0
Ile	3.0	3.5	3.0	3.1	3.3	2.5	2.4	2.4	4.1	3.8	3.7	3.7	2.9	2.8	2.7	2.7
Leu	7.7	7.8	7.8	7.7	8.1	8.8	9.1	9.3	10.4	11.4	12.6	12.8	16.0	16.5	16.5	16.6
Tyr	2.0	1.7	1.8	1.9	2.0	1.7	1.7	1.6	1.4	1.5	1.5	1.4	1.4	1.4	1.5	1.5
Phe	7.0	7.3	7.7	7.9	7.0	7.9	7.9	7.9	5.2	5.3	4.9	4.6	4.1	4.0	4.2	4.3
His	1.0	0.8	0.8	0.9	1.0	1.0	0.8	0.8	1.4	1.0	0.9	1.0	0.9	0.9	0.9	0.8
Lys	1.0	0.8	0.8	0.7	0.6	0.7	0.6	0.5	1.0	0.6	0.7	0.7	0.9	1.0	1.0	0.9
Arg	3.1	2.9	2.9	2.8	3.1	2.8	2.6	2.5	2.9	2.9	2.8	2.6	2.2	1.9	2.0	1.9
Yield[a]	1.5	3.2	3.6	13.4	11.7	1.9	2.7	7.5	1.1	3.5	5.6	4.6	8.1	8.7	2.5	6.4

Note: Values in mol%; the values of Thr, Ser, Glx, Val, and Ile were corrected using the factors 1.05, 1.09, 0.95, 1.08, and 1.07, respectively; Cys and Trp were not determined.

[a] %, based on total protein recovered from the column. The protein content was derived from amino acid analysis.

TABLE 8
Range of Amino Acid Compositions[a] and Yields[b] of Subgroups from Crude Avenin

Fractions Retentin Time (min)	1–14 12.2–44.0	15–22 50.7–65.3	23–26 82.7–89.2	27–30 91.0–97.7
Asx	2.7–8.2	1.9–2.3	1.6–1.7	1.4–1.5
Thr	3.0–6.1	1.9–2.3	1.7–2.1	1.1–1.3
Ser	4.0–6.7	1.9–3.2	3.5–3.8	3.4–3.7
Glx	14.7–32.0	37.0–40.1	37.5–39.0	40.1–40.4
Pro	6.5–10.6	11.2–11.8	10.4–10.8	9.7–10.2
Gly	4.9–10.6	1.5–2.5	2.0–3.3	0.7–1.0
Ala	3.4–8.2	5.1–6.2	5.1–5.2	5.5–5.7
Val	3.6–8.8	9.7–10.7	7.2–7.6	7.3–7.8
Met	1.7–4.4	0.8–1.3	1.7–2.5	0.8–1.6
Ile	4.5–6.2	2.4–3.5	3.7–4.1	2.7–2.9
Leu	7.4–9.1	7.7–9.3	10.4–12.8	16.0–16.6
Tyr	1.9–5.2	1.6–2.0	1.4–1.5	1.4–1.5
Phe	1.6–4.9	7.0–7.9	4.6–5.3	4.0–4.3
His	1.0–2.1	0.8–1.0	0.9–1.4	0.8–0.9
Lys	1.6–6.4	0.5–1.0	0.6–1.0	0.9–1.0
Arg	3.6–10.9	2.5–3.1	2.6–2.9	1.9–2.2
Yield[a]	12.6	45.5	14.8	25.7

[a] See Table 7 note and footnote.

hydrophobic amino acids. It has a unique N-terminal amino acid sequence and contains three conserved regions — A (residues 43 to 67), B (residues 86 to 121), and C (residues 150 to 174) — which are present in all the S-rich prolamins of cereals. In more recent publications,[94,95] Egorov et al. reported about sequences of avenin components. It has three sequence repeats of the type $PFVQ^n$, where n = 3, 4, or 5. Chesnut et al.[54] sequenced three oat prolamin cDNA clones. The polypeptides encoded by the prolamin clones had deduced molecular weights of 23,538, 23,376, and 18,441. The sequences confirmed the high degree of homology of avenin components and the presence of repetitive units: –PRO–PHE–VAL–$(GLN)_4$.

C. Oat Glutelin (Residue Protein)

Generally the glutelin fraction is defined as the protein fraction extracted with basic or acidic solutions after removal of water-soluble albumins, salt-soluble globulins, and alcohol-soluble prolamins.[51,55,56] Unfortunately, these extractions are generally incomplete and some nitrogen remains in the residue.

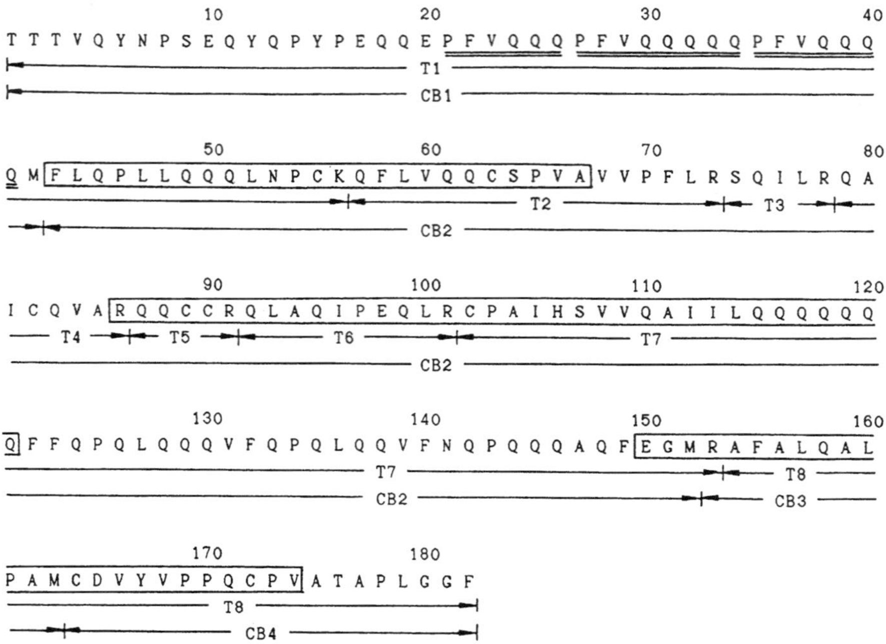

FIGURE 1 The amino acid sequence of the fast avenin component (avenin N9). Arrows show the alignment of tryptic and CCBr peptides. Conserved regions A (residues 43–67), B (residues 86–121), and C (residues 150–174) are in boxes; repetitive sequences are above double lines. The single letter code for amino acids is used. (From Egorov, T.A., *J. Cereal Sci.*, 8, 289, 1988. With permission.)

and 18,441. The sequences confirmed the high degree of homology of avenin components and the presence of repetitive units: –PRO–PHE–VAL–$(GLN)_4$.

C. Oat Glutelin (Residue Protein)

Generally the glutelin fraction is defined as the protein fraction extracted with basic or acidic solutions after removal of water-soluble albumins, salt-soluble globulins, and alcohol-soluble prolamins.[51,55,56] Unfortunately, these extractions are generally incomplete and some nitrogen remains in the residue.

Total solubilization may be achieved with alkaline solutions containing 2-mercaptoethanol and sodium dodecyl sulfate.[22] After the albumins, globulins, and prolamins have been removed, such a solution completely solubilizes the remaining proteins, which necessarily include the glutelins. However, this fraction may contain non-storage proteins, too. In addition, the quantity of glutelins observed is often directly related to the efficiency of the preceding extractions of the albumins, globulins, and prolamins. So it is understandable that values ranging from 5% to 66% have been reported.

or globulins, and these minor proteins likely were oat glutelins. Western blot analysis of residual proteins using anti-oat 21S immunoglobulin G has demonstrated conclusively that the major proteins of the oat residue are globulins. The results mentioned above confirm the view that glutelin accounts for less than 10% of oat protein.

III. METABOLICALLY ACTIVE PROTEINS

A. Enzymes

Most of the metabolically active proteins of oat are in the water-soluble albumin fraction. Nevertheless, it cannot be excluded that the globulin fraction and probably the glutelin (residue) fraction contain this type of protein. Oat albumins account for 1 to 12% of the total protein.[20,29,58,59] Major albumin components have been determined to have molecular weights of 14 to 17, 20 to 27, and 36 to 47 kDa.[20,29,30,37,60] Most of albumin components have isoelectric points between pH 4 and pH 7.5.[28]

From a practical point of view the most important metabolically active proteins of oat are the enzymes. The oat groat, like other cereal grains, contains numerous enzymes. Early investigations revealed the presence of proteases, maltase, α-amylase, lichenase, phenoxyacetic acid hydroxylase, phosphatase, tyrosinase, and lipase, as summarized by Caldwell and Pomeranz[61] and Youngs et al.[62] Results of more recent investigations are summarized by Kruger et al.[63]

In the production of oat products for human consumption it is generally considered necessary to inactivate lipase activity by means of various hydrothermal or other treatments before processing.[64-67] Otherwise, a degradation of the fat due to hydrolysis and oxidation will lead to rancidity, which is the main limiting factor in the storage and handling of oat products. Lipase activity and its distribution were studied by several authors.[68-70] It was found that lipase activity is not evenly distributed in the oat kernel. It is associated with the parts located close to the surface of the caryopsis, in the aleurone layer. In accordance with the lipase distribution found in the oat kernel, the lipase activity is higher in flour fractions close to the superficial bran layer and is lowest in the internal endosperm fractions. The development of lipase activity during maturation and during germination was also studied.[68,69]

Concerning other enzymes it may be mentioned that tyrosinase forms the basis of a convenient colorimetric method of determining whether rolled oats have had sufficient heat treatment to inactivate lipase. The isoenzymes of different enzymes occurring in oat were also investigated.[44] Characteristic differences were observed between varieties. α-Amylases of germinated oats were studied by McGregor et al.[71] Oat α-amylase components were similar to those of maize, sorghum, millet, and rice and differed from those of wheat, barley, and rye.

Low activity of phytase was found in oats using ^{31}P-nuclear magnetic resonance (NMR) spectroscopy.[72] Due to heat treatment practically no phytase activity exists in commercial products.

occurring in oat were also investigated.[44] Characteristic differences were observed between varieties. α-Amylases of germinated oats were studied by McGregor et al.[71] Oat α-amylase components were similar to those of maize, sorghum, millet, and rice and differed from those of wheat, barley, and rye.

Low activity of phytase was found in oats using ^{31}P-nuclear magnetic resonance (NMR) spectroscopy.[72] Due to heat treatment practically no phytase activity exists in commercial products.

B. Other Proteins

Recently a low molecular weight lipoprotein was isolated from oat grain. The apoprotein of this complex was named avenothionin.[73-76] Avenothionin was isolated by the method of Balls and Hale.[76] Like purothionin, it was toxic to *Saccharomyces cerevisiae* and *S. uvarum.* Raw avenothionin was fractionated by gel chromatography on Sephadex G-75 and investigated by gel electrophoresis. The low molecular weight components were separated by column chromatography on CMC-52; α- and β-avenothionins were separated. α-Avenothionin could not be separated into further subfractions. The primary structure of avenothionin was also reported,[33] as shown in Figure 2.

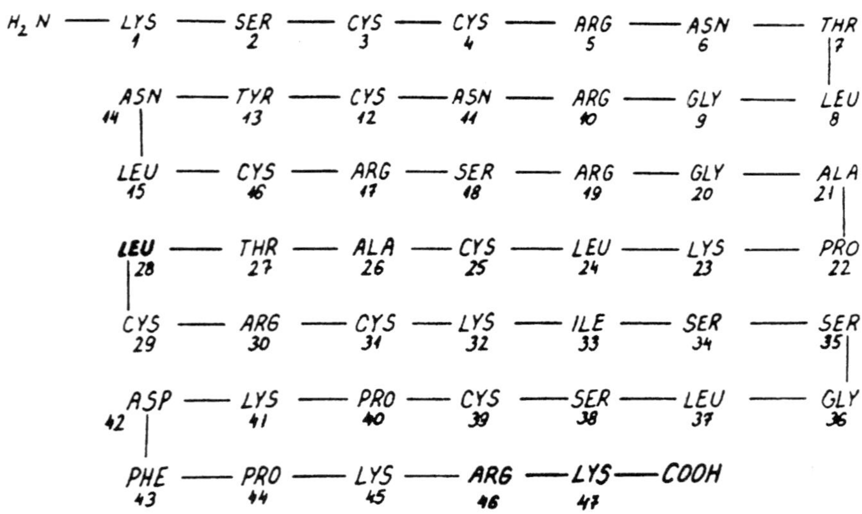

FIGURE 2 Primary structure of avenothionin.

Lipoavenothionin was also separated.[74] It was very similar to lipopurothionin. The similarity in lipid composition may be explained by the similarity of the primary structures of the apoproteins. The sites of binding of the polar lipids are the same (residues of lysine and arginine) and have practically the same location in the molecule.

B. Other Proteins

Recently a low molecular weight lipoprotein was isolated from oat grain. The apoprotein of this complex was named avenothionin.[73-76] Avenothionin was isolated by the method of Balls and Hale.[76] Like purothionin, it was toxic to *Saccharomyces cerevisiae* and *S. uvarum.* Raw avenothionin was fractionated by gel chromatography on Sephadex G-75 and investigated by gel electrophoresis. The low molecular weight components were separated by column chromatography on CMC-52; α- and β-avenothionins were separated. α-Avenothionin could not be separated into further subfractions. The primary structure of avenothionin was also reported,[33] as shown in Figure 2.

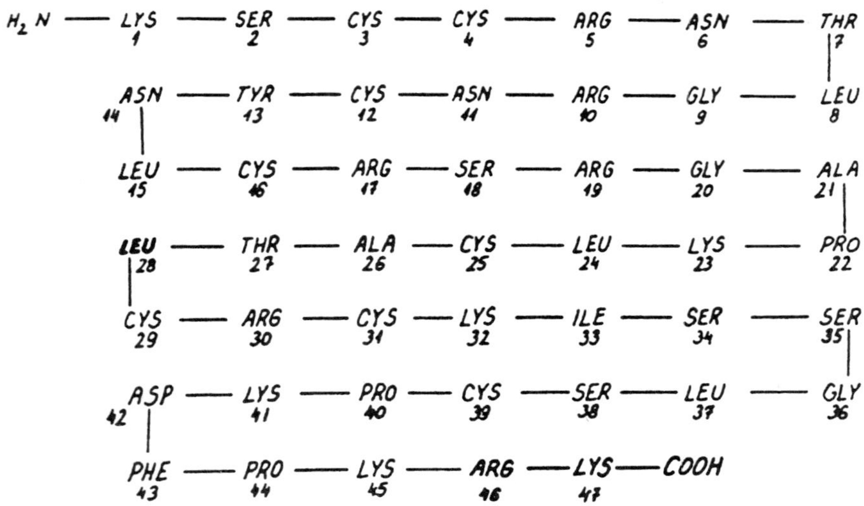

FIGURE 2 Primary structure of avenothionin.

Lipoavenothionin was also separated.[74] It was very similar to lipopurothionin. The similarity in lipid composition may be explained by the similarity of the primary structures of the apoproteins. The sites of binding of the polar lipids are the same (residues of lysine and arginine) and have practically the same location in the molecule.

IV. NUTRITIVE VALUE OF OAT PROTEINS AND PROTEIN CONCENTRATES

As was mentioned for the characterization of oat proteins, their amino acid composition is more advantageous from the point of view of nutrition than that of other cereal grain proteins. This is primarily because of the higher lysine and basic amino acid contents. In addition, some results of studies reported recently[77] suggest that oats possess some physiological properties which may have implications to man and which appear to be unique to oats among the cereal grains.

It was reported[13] that oats with increased protein concentration resulting from higher nitrogen fertility have a higher digestibility in rat feeding experiments. The biological value of the total protein declines only slightly, so that an increase in digestibility is nearly proportional to the increase in net protein utilization.

Due to the good nutritional quality of oat proteins, efforts have been made to develop oat protein concentrates. The procedures used for the production of concentrates are different. The air classification procedure may be used with high effectiveness. Although in the case of flours of other cereals the protein-rich fractions obtained by this procedure contain maximally 25% protein, the air classification of oat flours has resulted in a concentrate with an 85% protein concentration.[78]

Oat protein concentrates have been prepared by alkaline extraction and subsequent isoelectric precipitation,[60,79-81] salt extraction,[81] and density separation in aqueous[82] and non-aqueous solvents.[83] Isolation from distiller's stillage[84] and as a by-product of the oat starch process[29] has also been reported. The alkaline and salt extraction procedures result in a higher percentage of protein (over 60 to 80%) in concentrates than does density separation in solvents (50 to 70%). Oat distiller's grains and centrifuged solids have protein contents of 20 and 40%, respectively.[84]

Functional properties of oat protein preparations have also been intensively studied. High solubility of isolates was observed at pH <3 and pH >9. In the pH range from 4 to 7 the solubility is low (less than 20%).[29,85]

The emulsification properties of oat protein have been reported to be competitive with those of soy protein products.[29,80,81] Gel formation of oat globulin is restricted to a narrow pH range between 8 and 10. The hardness of the gel is comparable to that of 10% egg white gel.[29,86] Chemical modification of isolates (deamidation, acylation, tryptic digestion) are tools for modification of functional properties.[87-89]

Oat protein concentrates and isolates may be used as ingredients for protein enrichment (or substitution) in baked goods[90] and meat products.[91,92]

REFERENCES

1. Webster, F. H., Ed., *Oats: Chemistry and Technology,* American Association of Cereal Chemists, St. Paul, MN, 1986.
2. Youngs, V. L., Gilchrist, K. D., and Peterson, D. M., Protein, the current emphasis in oat quality, *Cereal Sci. Today,* 18, 409, 1973.
3. Pomeranz, Y., Youngs, V. L., and Robbins, G. S., Protein content and amino acid composition of oat species and tissues, *Cereal Chem.,* 50, 702, 1973.
4. Caldwell, E. F. and Pomeranz, Y., Industrial uses of cereal oats, in *Industrial Uses of Cereals,* Pomeranz, Y., Ed., American Association of Cereal Chemists, St. Paul, MN, 1974, 393.
5. Robert, L. S., Matlashewski, G. J., Adeli, K., Nozzolillo, C., and Altosaar, I., Electrophoretic and developmental characterization of oat (*Avena sativa* L.) globulins in cultivars of different protein content, *Cereal Chem.,* 60, 231, 1983.

6. Pomeranz, Y., Proteins and amino acids of barley, oats and buckwheat, in *Protein Nutritional Quality of Foods and Feeds,* Part 2, Friedman, M., Ed., Marcel Dekker, New York, 1975, 13.
7. Shewry, P. R. and Miflin, B. J., Seed storage proteins of economically important cereals, in *Advances in Cereal Science and Technology,* Vol. 7, Pomeranz, Y., Ed., American Association of Cereal Chemists, St. Paul, MN, 1985, 1.
8. Salunkhe, D. K., Chavan, J. K., and Kadam, S. S., *Postharvest Biotechnology of Cereals,* CRC Press, Boca Raton, FL, 1985.
9. Youngs, V. L., Protein distribution in the oat kernel, *Cereal Chem.,* 49, 407, 1972.
10. Youngs, V. L. and Peterson, D. M., Protein distribution in the oat (*Avena sterilis* L.), *Crop. Sci.,* 13, 365, 1973.
11. Bechtel, D. B. and Pomeranz, Y., Ultrastructure and cytochemistry of mature oat (*Avena sativa* L.) endosperm, *Cereal Chem.,* 58, 61, 1981.
12. Tkachuk, R., Nitrogen-to-protein conversion factors for cereals and oilseed meals, *Cereal Chem.,* 46, 206, 1969.
13. Eppendorfer, W. H., Nutritive value of oat and rye grain protein as influenced by nitrogen and amino acid composition, *J. Sci. Food Agric.,* 28, 152, 1977.
14. Eppendorfer, W. H., Effects of nitrogen, phosphorus and potassium on amino acid composition and on relationship between nitrogen and amino acids in wheat and oat grain, *J. Sci. Food Agric.,* 29, 995, 1978.
15. Peterson, D. M., Protein concentration, concentration of protein fractions, and amino acid balance in oats, *Crop Sci.,* 16, 663, 1976.
16. Völker, T., Untersuchungen über den Einfluss der Stickstoffdüngung auf die Zusammensetzung der Weizen- und Hafer-proteine, *Arch. Acker Pflanzenbau Bodenkd.,* 19, 267, 1975.
17. Lásztity, R., Berndorfer-Kraszner, É., and Huszár, M., On the presence and distribution of some bioactive agents in oat varieties, in *Cereals for Food and Beverages, Recent Progress in Cereal Chemistry,* Inglett, G.E. and Munck, L., Eds., Academic Press, New York, 1980, 429.
18. Youngs, V. L., Peterson, D. M., and Brown, C. M., Oats, in *Advances in Cereal Science and Technology,* Vol. 5, Pomeranz, Y., Ed., American Association of Cereal Chemists, St. Paul, MN, 1982, 49.
19. Peterson, D. M., Subunit structure and composition of oat seed globulin, *Plant Physiol.,* 62, 506, 1978.
20. Galle, A. M., Sallantin, M., and Petnollet, J. C., Influence of ionic strength on the extraction of oat seed storage proteins, *Plant Physiol. Biochem.,* 26, 733, 1988.
21. Kim, S. I., Charbonnier, L., and Mossé, J., Heterogeneity of avenin, the oat prolamin. Fractionation, molecular weight and amino acid composition, *Biochim. Biophys. Acta,* 537, 22, 1978.
22. Robert, L. S., Nozzolillo, C., Cudjoe, A., and Altosaar, I., Total solubilization of groat proteins of oat (*Avena sativa* L., cv. Hinoat): evidence that glutelins are minor component, *Can. Inst. Technol. J.,* 16, 196, 1983.
23. Robert, L. S., Nozzolillo, C., and Altosaar, I., Characterization of oat (*Avena sativa* L.) residual proteins, *Cereal Chem.,* 62, 276, 1985.
24. Shewry, P. R. and Miflin, B. J. Seed storage proteins of economically important proteins, in *Advances in Cereal Science and Technology, Vol. 7,* Pomeranz, Y., Ed., American Association of Cereal Chemists, St. Paul, MN, 1985, 1.
25. Lapvetelainen, A., Barley and Oat Protein Products from Wet Process. Food Use Potential, Ph.D. thesis, University of Turku, Turku, Finland, 1994.

26. Burgess, S. R., Shewry, P. R., Matlashewski, G. J., Altosaar, I., and Miflin, B. J., Characteristics of oat (*Avena sativa* L.) seed globulins, *J. Exp. Bot.,* 34, 1320, 1983.
27. Brinegar, A. C. and Peterson, D. M., Separation and characterization of oat globulin polypeptides, *Arch. Biochem. Biophys.,* 219, 71, 1982.
28. Ma, C. Y. and Harwalkar, V. R., Chemical characterization and functionality assessment of oat protein fractions, *J. Agric. Food Chem.,* 32, 144, 1984.
29. Lapveteiainen, A. and Aro, T., Protein composition and functionality of high-protein oat flour derived from integrated starch-ethanol process, *Cereal Chem.,* 71, 133, 1994.
30. Peterson, D. M. and Brinegar, A. C., Oat storage proteins, in *Oats: Chemistry and Technology,* Webster, F.H., Ed., American Association of Cereal Chemists, St. Paul, MN, 1986, 153.
31. Walburg, G. G. and Larkins, B. A., Oat seed globulin. Subunit characterization and demonstration of its synthesis as a precursor, *Plant Physiol.,* 72, 161, 1983.
32. Shotwell, M. A. and Larkins, B. A., The biochemistry and molecular biology of seed storage proteins, in *The Biochemistry of Plants, Vol. 15,* Marcus, A., Ed., Academic Press, New York, 1989, 297.
33. Shotwell, M. A., Afonso, C., Davies, E., Chesnut, R. S., and Larkins, B. A., Molecular characterization of oat seed globulins, *Plant Physiol.,* 87, 698, 1988.
34. Croy, R. D., Lycett, G. W., Gatehouse, J. A., Yarwood, J. N., and Boulter, D., Cloning and analysis of cDNAs encoding plant storage protein precursors, *Nature (London),* 295, 76, 1982.
35. Robert, L. S., Adelik, K., and Altosaar, I., Homology among 3S and 7S globulins from cereals and pea, *Plant Physiol.,* 78, 812, 1985.
36. Yupsanis, T., Burgess, S. R., Jackson, P. J., and Shewry, P. R., Characterization of the major protein component from aleurone cells of barley (*Hordeum vulgare* L.), *J. Exp. Bot.,* 41, 385, 1990.
37. Ma, C. Y. and Harwalkar, V. R., Thermal coagulation of oat globulin, *Cereal Chem.,* 64, 212, 1987.
38. Pernollet, J. C., Potier, B., Galle, A. M., Huet, J. C., Beauvais, F., and Sallantin, M., 2-D-HPLC separation, electrophoretic characterization and N-terminal sequences of oat seed prolamins, *Phytochemistry,* 28, 256, 1989.
39. Wieser, H. and Belitz, H. D., Amino acid compositions of avenins separated by reversed-phase high-performance liquid chromatography, *J. Cereal Sci.,* 9, 221, 1989.
40. Bietz, J. A., Separation of cereal proteins by reversed phase high-performance liquid chromatography, *J. Chromatogr.,* 255, 21, 1983.
41. Kim, S. I., Saur, L., and Mossé, J., Some features of the inheritance of avenins, the alcohol soluble proteins of oat, *Theor. Appl. Genet.,* 54, 39, 1979.
42. Kim, S. I. and Mossé, J., Electrophoretic patterns of oat prolamins and species relationships in *Avena, Can. J. Genet. Cytol.,* 21, 309, 1979.
43. Wrigley, C. W., Autran, J. C., and Bushuk, W., Identification of cereal varieties by gel electrophoresis of the grain proteins, in *Advances in Cereal Science and Technology,* Vol. 5, Pomeranz, Y., Ed., American Association of Cereal Chemists, St. Paul, MN, 1982, 211.
44. Almgard, G. and Clapham, D., Isoenzyme variation distinguishing 18 *Avena* cultivars grown in Sweden, *Swed. J. Agric. Res.,* 5, 61, 1975.
45. Singh, R. S., Jain, S. K., and Qualset, C. O., Protein electrophoresis as an aid to oat variety identification, *Euphytica,* 22, 98, 1973.

46. Hansen, A. E., Nassuth, A., and Altosaar, I., Rapid electrophoresis of oat (*Avena sativa* L.) prolamins from single seeds for cultivar identification, *Cereal Chem.,* 65, 153, 1988.
47. Egorov, T. A., The amino acid sequence of the 'fast' avenin component (*Avena savita* L.), *J. Cereal Sci.,* 8, 289, 1988.
48. Waldschmidt-Leitz, E. and Zwisler, O., Über die Proteine des Hafers, *Hoppe Seylers Z. Physiol. Chem.,* 322, 216, 1963.
49. Lookhart, G. L. and Pomeranz, Y., Characterization of oat species by polyacrylamide gel electrophoresis and high performance liquid chromatography of their prolamin proteins, *Cereal Chem.,* 62, 162, 1985.
50. Lookhart, G. L., Identification of oat cultivars by combining polyacrylamide gel electrophoresis and reversed-phase high-performance liquid chromatography, *Cereal Chem.,* 62, 345, 1985.
51. Wieser, H., Seilmeier, W., and Belitz, H. D., Vergleichende Untersuchungen über partielle Aminosauresequenzen von Prolaminen und Glutelinen verschiedenen Getreidearten. I. Proteinfraktionierung nach Osborne, *Z. Lebensm. Unters. Forsch.,* 170, 17, 1980.
52. Bietz, J. A., Cereal prolamin evolution and homology revealed by sequence analysis, *Biochem. Genet.,* 20, 103, 1982.
53. Egorov, T. A. and Odintsova, T. I., Microsequence analysis of prolamins with gas-phase protein sequencer, in *Gluten Proteins,* Lásztity, R. and Békés, F., Eds., World Scientific, Singapore, 1987, 434.
54. Chesnut, R. S., Shotwell, M. A., Boyer, S. K., and Larkins, B. A., Analysis of avenin proteins and the expression of their mRNAs in developing oat seeds, *Plant Cell,* 1, 913, 1989.
55. Kim, S. I., Pernollet, J. C., and Mossé, J., Evolution des proteines d'albumen et de l'ultrastructure du caryopse d'*Avena sativa* du cours de la germination, *Physiol. Veget.,* 17, 231, 1979.
56. Wieser, H., Seilmeier, W., and Belitz, H. D., Vergleichende Untersuchungen über partielle Aminosauresequenzen von Prolaminen und Glutelinen verschiedenen Getreidearten. II. Fraktionierung der Gluteline, *Z. Lebensm. Unters. Forsch.,* 171, 430, 1980.
57. Robert, L. S., Nozzolillo, C., and Altosaar, I., Characterization of oat (*Avena sativa* L.) residual proteins, *Cereal Chem.,* 62, 276, 1985.
58. Peterson, D. M. and Smith, D., Changes in nitrogen and carbohydrate fractions in developing oat groats, *Crop. Sci.,* 16, 67, 1976.
59. Lookhart, G. L., Cereal proteins: composition of their major fractions and methods for identification, in *Handbook of Cereal Science and Technology,* Lorenz, K.J. and Kulp, K., Eds., Marcel Dekker, New York, 1991, 441.
60. Ma, C. Y., Chemical characterization and functionality assessment of protein concentrates from oats, *Cereal Chem.,* 60, 36, 1983.
61. Caldwell, E. F. and Pomeranz, Y., Industrial uses of cereal oats, in *Industrial Uses of Cereals,* Pomeranz, Y., Ed., American Association of Cereal Chemists, St. Paul, MN, 1974, 393.
62. Youngs, V. L., Peterson, D. M., and Brown, C. M., Oats, in *Advances in Cereal Science and Technology, Vol. 5,* Pomeranz, Y., Ed., American Association of Cereal Chemists, St. Paul, MN, 1982, 49.
63. Kruger, J. E., Lineback, D. R., and Stauffer, C. E., *Enzymes and Their Role in Cereal Technology,* American Association of Cereal Chemists, St. Paul, MN, 1987.

64. Vorwerck, K., Hydrotermische Behandlung von Hafer, *Getreide Mehl Brot,* 42, 199, 1988.
65. Urquhart, A. A., Altosaar, I., Matlashewsi, G. J., and Sahasrabudme, M. R., Localization of lipase activity in oat grains and milled oat fractions, *Cereal Chem.,* 60, 181, 1983.
66. Ekstrand, G., Gangby, I., Akeson, G., Stöllman, U., Lingnerth, H., and Dahl, S., Lipase activity and development of rancidity in oats and oat products related to heat treatment during processing, *J. Cereal. Sci.,* 17, 247, 1993.
67. Lukkonen, K., Kaukovirta-Norja, A., and Laakso, S., Elimination of lipid hydrolysis in aqueous suspensions of oat flour, *J. Cereal Sci.,* 17, 255, 1993.
68. Matlashewski, G. J., Urquhart, A. A., Sahasrabudhe, M. R., and Altosaar, I., Lipase activity in oat flour suspensions and soluble extracts, *Cereal Chem.,* 59, 418, 1982.
69. Ekstrand, B., Gangby, T., and Akesson, G., Lipase activity in oats — distribution, pH dependence, and heat inactivation, *Cereal Chem.,* 69, 373, 1992.
70. Youngs, V. L. and Peterson, D. M., Oat lipids and lipid related enzymes, in *Oats: Chemistry and Technology,* Webster, F.R., Ed., American Association of Cereal Chemists, St. Paul, MN, 1986.
71. McGregor, A. W., Marchylo, B. A., and Kruger, E. J., Multiple alpha-amylase components in germinated cereal grains determined by isoelectric focusing and chromatofocusing, *Cereal Chem.,* 65, 32, 1988.
72. Frolych, W., Wahlgren, M., and Drankenberg, T., Studies on phytase activity in oats and wheats using ^{31}P-NMR spectroscopy, *J. Cereal Sci.,* 8, 47, 1988.
73. Békés, F. and Lásztity, R., Isolation and determination of amino acid sequence of avenothionin, a new purothionin analogue from oat, *Cereal Chem.,* 58, 360, 1981.
74. Békés, F., Study of purothionin analogues of certain cereals, *Acta Aliment.,* 10, 343, 1981.
75. Békés, F. and Lásztity, R., Comparative analysis of the primary structure of grain thionins, *Acta Aliment.,* 10, 357, 1981.
76. Balls, A. K. and Hale, V. S., A sulfur-bearing constituent of the petroleum ether extract of wheat flour, *Cereal Chem.,* 17, 243, 1940.
77. Gould, R. M., Biofunctional properties of oats, in *Cereals for Food and Beverages, Recent Progress in Cereal Chemistry,* Inglett, G.E. and Munck, L., Eds., Academic Press, New York, 1980, 447.
78. Wu, Y. V. and Stringfellow, A. C., Protein concentrates from oat flours by air classification of normal and high protein varieties, *Cereal Chem.,* 50, 489, 1973.
79. Cluskey, J. E., Wu, Y. V., Wall, J. S., and Inglett, G. E., Oat protein concentrates from a wet-milling process, *Cereal Chem.,* 50, 475, 1973.
80. Wu, Y. V., Cluskey, J. E., Wall, J. S., and Inglett, G. E., Oat protein concentrates from a wet-milling process: composition and properties, *Cereal Chem.,* 50, 481, 1973.
81. Ma, C. Y., Preparation, composition and functional properties of oat protein isolates, *Can. Inst. Food Sci. Technol. J.,* 16, 201, 1983.
82. Youngs, V. L., Extraction of a high-protein layer from oat groat bran and flour, *J. Food Sci.,* 39, 1045, 1974.
83. Cluskey, J. E., Wu, Y. V., and Wall, J. S., Density separation of protein from oat flour in nonaqueous solvents, *J. Food Sci.,* 43, 783, 1978.
84. Wu, Y. V., Recovery of protein rich by-products from oat stillage after alcohol distillation, *J. Agric. Food Chem.,* 38, 588, 1990.
85. Lapvetelainen, A., Barley and Oat Protein Products from Wet Process. Food Use Potential, Ph.D. Thesis, University of Turku, Turku, Finland, 1994.

86. Ma, C. Y., Khanzada, G., and Harwalkar, V. R., Thermal gelation of oat globulin, *Agric. Food Chem.,* 36, 275, 1988.
87. Ma, C. Y., Yiu, S. H., and Harwalkar, V. R., Rheological and structural properties of egg-white/oat globulin co-gels, *J. Food Sci.,* 55, 93, 1990.
88. Ma, C. Y. and Wood, D. F., Functional properties of oat proteins modified by acylation, trypsin hydrolysis or linoleate treatment, *J. AOCS,* 64, 1726, 1987.
89. Ma, C. Y. and Khanzada, G., Functional properties of deamidated oat protein isolates, *J. Food Sci.,* 52, 1583, 1987.
90. Puolanne, E. and Matikkala, M., Der Einfluss des pH-Wertes auf dass Wasserbindungsvermögen der Brühwurst, *Fleischwirtschaft,* 60, 1233, 1980.
91. D'Appolonia, B. L. and Youngs, V. L., Effect of bran and high-protein concentrate from oats on dough properties and bread quality, *Cereal Chem.,* 55, 736, 1978.
92. Lapvetelainen, A., Puolanne, E., and Salovaara, H., High-protein oat flour functionality assessment in bread and sausage, *J. Food Sci.,* 60, 1995.
93. Lapvetelainen, A., Bietz, J. A., and Huebner, F. R., Reversed-phase high-performance liquid chromatography of oat proteins: application to cultivar comparison and analysis of the effect of wet processing, *Cereal Chem.,* 72, 259, 1995.
94. Egorov, T. A., Musolyamov, A. K., Kochergin, A. A., Andersen, J. S., and Roepstorff, P., Isolation, characterization by mass spectrometry and partial amino acid sequencing of avenins, *J. Cereal Sci.,* 21, 107, 1994.
95. Egorov, T. A., Musolyamov, A. K., Andersen, J. S., and Roepstorff, P., The complete amino acid sequence and disulphide bond arrangement of oat alcohol soluble avenin-3, *Eur. J. Biochem.,* 224, 631, 1994.

10 Millet Proteins

I. INTRODUCTION, GENERAL CHARACTERIZATION OF MILLET PROTEINS

Of the different millet species grown in the world, pearl millet (*Pennisetum typhoides* L., *Pennisetum americanum* L. Leeke), proso or common corn millet *(Panicum milaceum),* and finger millet *(Eleusine coracana)* are the most widely grown. Foxtail millet *(Setaria italica),* little millet *(Panicum miliare),* and Kodo millet *(Paspalum sorbiculatum)* are also known.[1]

Pearl millet has been the most investigated species, therefore, in this chapter predominantly the proteins of this species will be discussed. Pearl millet kernels are generally tear shaped and have a relatively small size in comparison with other cereals. As in other cereal grains, three main morphological parts may be observed: pericarp, embryo, and endosperm.[1-3] The pericarp contains three layers: the epicarp, the mesocarp, and the endocarp. The embryo is relatively large in proportion to the rest of the kernel. A single layer of aleurone cells surrounds the periphery of the kernel and is firmly attached to the pericarp. The hard endosperm contains starch granules embedded in a protein matrix which in turn contains protein bodies ranging in size from 0.3 to 0.4 μm.[4-6] The protein bodies have a well-defined structure.

The grains of other millet species are smaller than grains of pearl millet. Finger millet grains vary in color from white, orange, red, deep brown, and purple to almost black. Kernels are covered with thin outer hulls. The internal structures are essentially similar to those of pearl millet. The starch granules are angular and polygonal in the corneous endosperm and spherical in the floury region. The seeds of common millet are flattened and white, oval or smooth. The grains of little millet are glabrous, striated, and usually brown.

The protein content of pearl millet varies widely; values from 5 to 23% have been reported, with the average being from 10 to 13%.[3,7,8] Kovács[10] investigated nine varieties of millet grown in Hungary and found an average protein content of about 13%. Delost-Lewis et al.[9] published some data for proso *(Panicum miliaceum);* an average protein content of 11.2% was reported by Nesterin and Skurichin.[11] Some data are available also on protein content of minor millet.[12-14]

Like other cereals, the protein content of millet is influenced by variety, agricultural technique (e.g., fertilization), and many other factors.[8,15]

Efforts were made to select pearl millet varieties for increased protein content. Singh et al.[16] reported the results of a breeding program designed to develop sources of high grain protein. After six generations of selection, several inbred lines consistently producing 14 to 19% grain protein (compared to 10 to 11% in normal varieties) have been developed.

The same rules concerning protein distribution between the different morphological parts of the millet kernel are valid as in other cereal grains.

Relatively few data are available concerning the fraction distribution of the millet proteins. In the early work the solubility fractionation elaborated by Osborne was used for the separation of endosperm proteins. In an early work Shawney and Naik[17] studied the protein fraction distribution in several pearl millets varieties. The storage proteins (prolamin and glutelin) predominated (>60% of the total protein). The albumin fraction averaged 15% and the globulin fraction 9%. Prolamin and glutelin were present in similar quantities. More recent investigations[7,10,12] yielded similar data, although significant differences were found between millet varieties. In the high-protein cultivars (average protein increase of about 60%) a decrease in the albumin fraction (of about 20%) was associated with an increase in the prolamin fraction (about 15%).[16] The Landry-Moureaux[18] procedure was used by Nwasike et al.[19] for the fractionation. The extraction was very effective.

The amino acid composition of millet is generally characterized by low levels of lysine, tryptophan, threonine, and sulfur-containing amino acids (Table 1). The proportion of essential amino acids in millet grown in Hungary varied from 38 to 41% of the total amino acid content (Table 2). The differences in amino acid composition between the different morphological parts of the kernel are similar to those in other cereal grains. Some data obtained by Abdelrahman et al.[20] are summarized in Table 3. The endosperm is lower in lysine, arginine, and glycine and higher in methionine than the whole grain. Bran is higher in lysine, arginine, glycine, and aspartic acid and lower in glutamic acid and sulfur-containing amino acids. In Table 4 the amino acid compositions of proso millet flours published by Lorenz et al.[21] are shown.

II. STORAGE PROTEINS

A. Low Molecular Weight Storage Proteins (Prolamins)

The prolamin (alcohol-soluble) protein fraction of millet, like storage protein of other cereals, is heterogeneous and consists of different polypeptides with similar structure. For the prolamin of foxtail millet *(Setaria italica)* the name setarin I was proposed by Ponappa Naren et al.[15,22] These authors also distinguished setarin II, a fraction obtained from the residue after removal of albumin, globulin, and prolamin (setarin I), using for extraction 70% ethanol + 0.6% sodium acetate and 0.5% mercaptoethanol (see Figure 1). SDS-PAGE of pearl millet prolamin revealed two major bands between 21 and 26 kDa.[23] The prolamins were found to be rich in glutamic acid, proline, and leucine as well as in tryptophan. Pearl millet prolamin apparently differs markedly from that of other cereals in being unusually high in tryptophan, although — like that of other cereals — pearl millet prolamin is rich in

TABLE 1
Amino Acid Composition of the Protein of Millet (g/16 g N)

Amino Acid	Hoseney and Varriano-Marston[2] Highest Value	Hoseney and Varriano-Marston[2] Lowest Value	Kovács[10]	Nesterin and Skurichin[11] (Proso)
Tryptophan	1.9	0.8	ND	1.2
Lysine	3.9	1.9	2.02	2.2
Histidine	3.1	1.6	3.22	2.4
Arginine	6.2	3.1	4.13	4.1
Aspartic acid	11.3	5.0	8.57	5.6
Threonine	4.3	2.0	5.71	2.9
Serine	5.9	3.0	6.59	5.1
Glutamic acid	25.4	11.6	15.66	17.1
Proline	11.8	3.9	10.24	4.9
Glycine	6.4	2.2	3.69	2.3
Alanine	8.8	6.4	8.26	8.0
Cystine	3.3	1.0	ND	1.2
Valine	6.2	4.4	4.72	4.2
Methionine	2.6	1.2	2.69	1.7
Isoleucine	6.0	3.1	4.16	3.5
Leucine	12.7	7.6	10.74	8.5
Tyrosine	5.9	2.4	3.67	2.8
Phenylalanine	5.9	3.9	5.92	4.1

Note: ND, not determined.

glutamic acid and proline and deficient in lysine (Table 5). The N-terminal amino acid sequence of pearl millet prolamin was studied by Bietz.[24] This sequence, and that of maize prolamin published by Esen et al.,[26] are shown in Figure 2. The degree of similarity between the sequences is consistent with the proposed evolutionary relationship of these species.

B. High Molecular Weight Storage Proteins (Glutelins)

This protein fraction of millet is also heterogeneous as revealed by gel filtration chromatography. The increase in solubility of glutelin after reduction of the disulfide bonds and the decrease in molecular weight support the view that the glutelin component consists of several polypeptide chains (subunits) linked together by disulfide bonds.

Ponappa Naren and Virupaksha,[22] using the modified cryoprecipitation procedure of Melcher and Fraij[26] (Figure 1), extracted the subunits of glutelin of foxtail millet (*Setaria italica* L.). The subunits were separated into three groups named α,

TABLE 2
Distribution of Different Classes of Amino Acids in Millet Protein (% of Total Amino Acids)[10]

Sample No.	Amino Acids				
	Acidic	Basic	Branched Chain	Aromatic	Essential
1	24.23	6.15	19.62	12.81	39.63
2	25.97	5.30	21.90	11.87	40.08
3	23.08	5.57	19.89	13.25	40.30
4	24.52	5.79	19.64	12.25	38.91
5	25.91	5.48	20.93	11.79	40.11
6	25.61	5.48	21.82	11.76	39.99
7	30.08	—	21.49	11.97	40.03
8	25.11	5.38	18.92	10.82	38.62
9	27.01	5.48	21.55	11.01	39.66
10	25.64	5.73	19.18	12.14	40.64
11	27.94	5.40	20.93	11.52	40.09

TABLE 3
Amino Acid Composition of the Whole Grain and Fractions of Pearl Millet Kernels[20] (g/100 g Protein, Dry Weight Basis)

Amino Acid	Whole Grain	Endosperm	Germ	Bran
GLU	19.57	22.83	15.12	13.49
ASP	8.82	8.12	11.36	11.38
PRO	6.36	8.02	4.96	6.84
ALA	8.22	9.42	7.99	8.69
GLY	3.28	1.89	6.14	7.32
THR	3.63	3.29	3.86	4.64
SER	5.22	5.17	5.67	5.55
VAL	3.87	3.94	3.60	3.54
LYS	3.02	1.40	5.16	4.34
MET	2.30	2.61	1.78	1.57
ILE	3.06	3.12	2.09	2.37
LEU	9.56	11.17	6.45	7.10
TYR	3.81	3.63	3.95	4.65
PHE	5.48	5.46	4.41	4.27
HIS	4.66	4.17	6.48	6.16
ARG	4.82	2.00	9.01	5.01

β-, and γ-setarin. Both α- and β-setarin are rich in methionine; α-setarin has the highest sulfur content. The amino acid compositions of setarin II, α-setarin, and β-setarin are shown in Table 6. The amino acid compositions of α- and β-setarin are similar with respect to most amino acids; however, α-setarin has significantly lower amounts of glutamic acid, proline, and lysine and higher amounts of serine, tyrosine, and cysteine, but has much higher levels of alanine, leucine, and glutamic acid.

Setarin II, α-, β-, and γ-setarin were analyzed by SDS-PAGE under reducing conditions. The electrophoretic pattern of setarin II revealed several polypeptides in the molecular weight range of 43.5 to 7.9 kDa. α-Setarin showed a single band of 7.9 kDa and appeared to be electrophoretically homogeneous in SDS-PAGE. β-Setarin also gave a major band corresponding to a molecular weight of 9.1 kDa.

γ-Setarin consisted of three components with molecular weights of 7.9, 21.8, and 36.3 kDa. The estimated molecular weights of α- and β-setarin were in good agreement with the estimates of the minimum molecular weights made from the amino acid compositions (number of residues). Compared to other methionine-rich proteins, α- and β-seratin are relatively low molecular weight polypeptides.

N-terminal analysis of α-setarin showed that methionine was present at the amino-terminal end of the polypeptide. Thus, α-setarin appeared to be a fairly homogeneous polypeptide by the criteria of N-terminal analysis..

Both α- and β-setarins have 8 methionine residues (out of a total of 63 and 71 amino acid residues, respectively). Separation of the CNBr-cleaved, performic acid-oxidized α-setarin by two-dimensional peptide mapping resulted in at least nine ninhydrin-positive spots of varying intensity on the peptide map. It appears from these results that the large number of methionine residues present in α-setarin are randomly distributed along the peptide chain and not clustered.

Alcohol-soluble reduced glutelin (ASG) was also studied.[23] Electrophoretic studies revealed some major bands in the region of 21 to 28 kDa.

III. CYTOPLASMIC (METABOLICALLY ACTIVE) PROTEINS

After early studies on water- and salt-soluble proteins, which demonstrated the heterogeneity of these fractions, this group of proteins was recently investigated by gel chromatography and gel electrophoresis.[23,27-29] At least 20 bands were observed using polyacrylamide gel electrophoresis. The high-lysine cultivars contained a higher proportion of water- and salt-soluble proteins. The amino acid compositions of albumins and globulins are demonstrated in Table 7.

Among the enzymes of millet the amylases play an important role not only in the biology of grains, but also in the determination of the end-use properties of millet. Beleia and Varriano-Marston[30,31] investigated the pearl millet amylases. The α-amylase purified by glycogen complex formation exhibited three protein bands after separation with polyacrylamide gel electrophoresis. The preparation purified

TABLE 4
Amino Acid Compositions of Wheat and Millet Flours[a]

Amino Acid	Flour								Bran	
	Wheat	Turghai	Cope	Cope	Cope	Cope	Cope[b]	Cope[b]	Cope	Cope[b]
Lysine	1.98	1.14	1.01	0.92	0.80	0.69	0.94	0.79	3.94	3.42
Histidine	1.89	1.97	1.85	1.87	1.81	1.78	1.71	1.80	1.92	2.19
Ammonia	4.69	3.25	3.35	3.38	3.41	3.31	3.30	3.40	2.91	3.29
Arginine	2.52	2.06	1.24	1.05	1.79	1.85	1.54	1.45	6.07	4.29
Aspartic acid	4.23	6.13	6.08	6.04	5.83	5.82	6.04	5.86	11.02	10.32
Threonine	2.47	2.37	2.55	2.47	2.51	2.36	2.37	2.37	3.92	3.76
Serine	5.39	7.07	6.86	7.04	7.54	7.13	7.95	7.00	6.31	7.26
Glutamic acid	35.63	24.60	24.64	26.01	24.67	25.47	25.08	25.47	18.18	19.92
Proline	14.81	9.72	9.04	8.77	8.87	9.53	9.34	9.88	8.03	6.63
Half cystine	0.60	0.27	0.31	0.33	0.25	0.31	0.25	0.14	0.55	0.30
Glycine	3.30	1.87	1.90	1.82	1.98	1.59	1.80	1.76	4.99	4.74
Alanine	2.65	12.22	12.40	12.38	12.39	12.45	12.33	12.24	9.29	10.06
Valine	2.94	3.20	3.40	3.33	3.33	3.24	3.17	3.23	3.97	3.88

Methionine	1.55	1.76	2.03	1.95	2.03	1.98	1.88	1.92	1.44	1.61
Isoleucine	2.26	2.41	3.09	2.80	2.70	2.61	2.66	2.57	2.60	2.54
Leucine	6.40	12.33	12.34	12.43	12.56	12.55	12.30	12.63	8.21	8.86
Tyrosine	2.20	2.75	3.09	2.80	2.70	2.61	2.66	2.57	2.60	2.54
Phenylalanine	4.51	4.87	5.30	4.89	4.96	4.82	4.90	5.03	4.21	4.55
Extraction (%)	73.3	78.4	87.3	79.7	78.5	77.5	77.6	69.8	19.8	19.6
Protein (%) (N × 5.7)	13.56	15.8	14.50	14.06	13.50	13.62	14.69	13.38	6.12	6.56
Moisture (%)	6.56	9.80	8.50	9.48	9.85	10.24	6.37	11.40	6.71	5.06
Recovery (Kjeldahl N basis)	96.5	105.5	98.9	110.0	108.0	110.6	108.4	105.7	74.8	68.6
Norleucine (internal standard) recovery	96.7	101.0	98.0	94.7	98.0	96.3	95.7	96.8	86.9	99.4

[a] In grams of amino acids per 100 g of protein corrected to 100% recovery protein basis.

[b] Grain heated before conditioning and milling.

From Lorenz, K., Dilsaver, W., and Bates, L., *Cereal Chem.*, 57, 16, 1980. With permission.

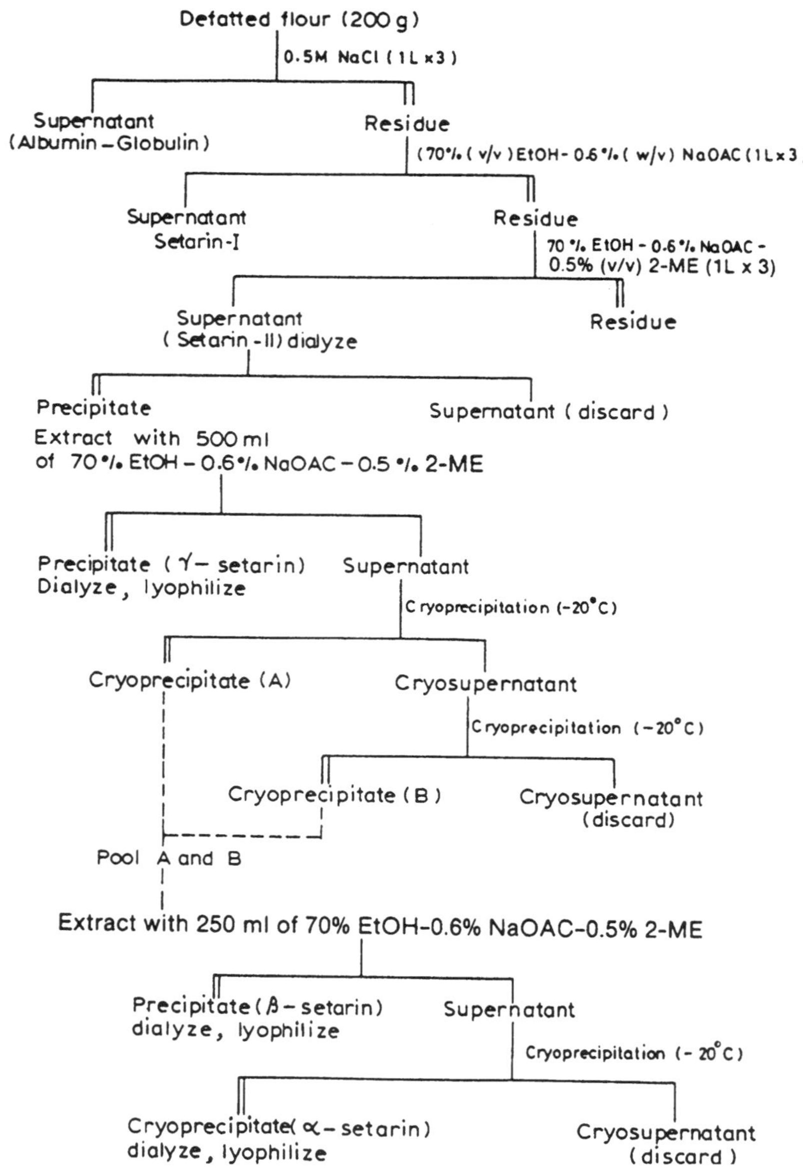

FIGURE 1 Scheme for isolation of methionine-rich proteins. EtOH, ethanol; NaOAc, sodium acetate; 2-ME, 2-mercaptoethanol. (From Ponappa Naren, A. and Virupaksha, T.K., *Cereal Chem.*, 67, 32, 1990. With permission.)

by the starch column procedure could be separated into seven components; all components showed α-amylase activity. The molecular weights of the isoenzymes ranged from 22 to 53 kDa. The pH optima were between 4.4 and 4.8; the temperature optimum was 55°C. Only low-pI (<5.5) α-amylases were found in germinated millet

TABLE 5
Amino Acid Composition of the Storage Proteins of Pearl Millet (g Amino Acid/16 g N)[11]

Amino Acid	Prolamin	Glutelin
Lysine	1.66	2.14
Histidine	2.14	1.64
Arginine	3.04	4.92
Aspartic acid	7.48	6.36
Glutamic acid	22.24	21.68
Serine	6.12	5.35
Threonine	3.46	2.92
Cystine	1.42	1.34
Methionine	1.02	1.34
Phenylalanine	3.82	4.94
Glycine	1.23	2.74
Alanine	9.41	10.42
Valine	3.24	4.12
Proline	10.23	9.42
Tyrosine	4.62	4.44
Isoleucine	3.32	3.83
Leucine	12.06	10.15
Tryptophan	2.84	0.69

```
                          5                 10
MAIZE          T  I  F  P  Q  C  S  Q  A  P
                     I
PEARL MILLET   Y  I  S  P  V  S  A  V  A  A
                          15                20
MAIZE          I  A  I  L  L  O  F  Y  L  P
                                 P     F
PEARL MILLET   T  A  S  P  L  F  W  P  Q  A
                          25                30
MAIZE          V  A  V  M  G  V  Q  Z  N  A
                     I  A  F  Y     P  L
PEARL MILLET   T  S  I  A  A  T  H  P  F  V
                     V
```

FIGURE 2 N-terminal amino acid sequences of prolamin fractions of maize and pearl millet.

by electrofocusing,[32] in contrast to wheat, rye, triticale, and barley, which contain a high-pI (>5.8) group of α-amylases.

Millet kernel also has protease and lipoxidase activities. As reported by Galyean et al.,[27] high-protein genotypes had the highest proteolytic and peroxidase activities.

TABLE 6
Amino Acid Compositions of Setarin II, α-Setarin, and β-Setarin Fractions (mol/100 mol)

Amino Acid	Setarin II	α-Setarin[a]	β-Setarin[a]
Aspartic acid	6.03	4.76 (3)	4.23 (3)
Threonine	Traces	4.76 (3)	4.23 (3)
Serine	0.05	3.17 (2)	4.23 (3)
Glutamic acid	22.27	14.29 (10)	18.31 (13)
Proline	10.85	11.11 (7)	14.08 (10)
Glycine	6.88	4.76 (3)	4.23 (3)
Alanine	16.54	11.11 (7)	9.80 (7)
1/2 Cystine[b]	Traces	4.76 (3)	4.23 (3)
Valine	5.58	3.17 (2)	2.82 (2)
Methionine[b]	1.74	12.69 (8)	11.27 (8)
Isoleucine	3.79	1.59 (1)	2.82 (2)
Leucine	16.38	9.52 (6)	7.04 (5)
Phenylalanine	5.78	7.94 (5)	5.63 (4)
Tyrosine	0.04	3.17 (2)	2.82 (2)
Histidine	1.52	1.59 (1)	1.40 (1)
Lysine	1.75	Traces	1.41 (1)
Arginine	0.80	1.59 (1)	1.40 (1)
N recovery, %	79.50	86.66	82.66

[a] Values in parenthesis indicate the number of residues based on arginine.
[b] Chomatograms did not show any cysteic acid or methionine sulfoxide in the hydrolysates. Tryptophan could not be detected by the spectrophotometric method.

Like other cereals, millet grain contains natural enzyme inhibitors, too. A bifunctional α-amylase/trypsin inhibitor of ragi (Indian finger millet, *Eleusine coracana*) was isolated by Campos and Richardson.[33]

IV. NUTRITIVE VALUE OF MILLET PROTEINS

The protein content of millet is relatively high and its nutritional value is similar to that of sorghum and corn. However, major disadvantages of millet utilization are the difficult milling properties and the development of rancidity in the whole flour.[16,17] The protein efficiency ratio values of millet alone are relatively low, but supplementation

TABLE 7
Amino Acid Compositions of the Cytoplasmic Proteins of Pearl Millet (g Amino Acid/16 g N)[17]

Amino Acid	Albumin	Globulin
Lysine	3.92	3.74
Histidine	2.18	2.22
Arginine	4.36	4.82
Aspartic acid	12.46	11.42
Glutamic acid	16.36	18.71
Serine	4.81	5.62
Threonine	2.12	2.64
Cystine	2.92	2.62
Methionine	1.94	2.12
Phenylalanine	3.82	4.14
Glycine	7.35	4.12
Proline	8.82	7.46
Alanine	8.11	6.02
Valine	5.64	7.34
Tyrosine	3.28	4.31
Isoleucine	4.12	2.48
Leucine	6.11	5.62
Tryptophan	1.52	0.54

with lysine or high-lysine proteins results in a dramatic increase in the biological value. The nutritional value of pearl millet is greatly enhanced when it is mixed with legumes because the latter complement its profile of essential amino acids.[36]

Mixtures of pearl millet and cowpea were successfully used for preparation of weaning foods of adequate nutritional value.[37-39] Although the millet grain contains a relatively high protein content, its nutritive value and its digestibility are poor (latter = 50 to 60%). The digestibility of pearl millet grain protein improved following germination.[40] The longer the period of germination, the greater the protein digestibility of sprouts. The improvement in protein digestibility during germination may be attributed to modification (degradation) of storage proteins. Furthermore, hydrolytic reduction of phytates during germination may contribute to the improvement of digestibility because phytates are known to inhibit proteases. Natural fermentation may advantageously influence *in vitro* digestibility of proteins.[41]

Protein concentrate from pearl millet was prepared and investigated by Bailey and Sumrell.[42]

REFERENCES

1. Salunkhe, D. K., Chavan, J. K., and Kadam, S. S., *Postharvest Biotechnology of Cereals,* CRC Press, Boca Raton, FL, 1985, 147.
2. Hoseney, R. C. and Varriano-Marston, E., Pearl millet: its chemistry and utilization, in *Cereals for Food and Beverages. Recent Progress in Cereal Chemistry,* Inglett, G.E. and Munck, L., Eds., Academic Press, New York, 1980, 461.
3. Hoseney, R. C. and Varriano-Marston, E., Sorghum and millet, in *Advances in Cereal Science and Technology,* Vol. 4, Pomeranz, Y., Ed., American Association of Cereal Chemists, St. Paul, MN, 1981, 71.
4. Adams, C. A., Novellie, L., and Liebenber, N. W. D. W., Biochemical properties and ultrastructure of the protein bodies isolated from selected cereals, *Cereal Chem.,* 53, 1, 1976.
5. Badi, S. M., Hoseney, R. C., and Casady, A. J., Pearl millet. I. Characterization by SEM, amino acid analysis, lipid composition, and prolamin solubility, *Cereal Chem.,* 53, 478, 1976.
6. Sullins, R. Q. and Rooney, L. W., Pericarp and endosperm structure of pearl millet, *Pennisetum typhoides,* in *Proc. Symp. Sorghum and Millet for Human Food,* Dendy, D.A.V., Ed. Trop. Prod. Inst., London, 1977, 79.
7. Hulse, J. H., Laing, E. M., and Pearson, O. E., *Sorghum and Millets. Their Composition and Nutritive Value,* Academic Press, London, 1980.
8. Rooney, L. W., Earp, C. F., and Khan, M. N., Sorghum and millets, in *Handbook of Processing and Utilization in Agriculture,* Vol. 2, Part 1, Wolf, I.A., Ed., CRC Press, Boca Raton, FL, 1982, 123.
9. Delost-Lewis, K., Lorenz, K., and Triebelhorn, R., Puffing quality of experimental varieties of proso millets *(Panicum miliaceum), Cereal Chem.,* 69, 359, 1992.
10. Kovács, B., Investigation of Proteins and Lipids of Millet (in Hungarian), Dipl. thesis, Technical University of Budapest, Budapest, Hungary, 1980.
11. Nesterin, M. F. and Skurichin, I. M., *Chimitcheskij Sostav Pishtchewych Produktov,* Pishtchevaya Prom. Publ., Moscow, 1979.
12. Indira, R. and Naik, M. S., Nutrient composition and protein quality of some minor millets, *J. Agric. Sci.,* 41, 795, 1971.
13. Ramanathan, K. M., Subbiah, S., Francis, H. J., and Krishnamurthy, K. K., A note on the nutritive value of certain minor millets, *Madras Agric. J.,* 62, 225, 1975.
14. Monteiro, P. V., Virupaskha, T. K., and Rao, D. R., Proteins of Italian millet; amino acid composition, solubility fractionation, and electrophoresis of protein fraction, *J. Sci. Food Agric.,* 33, 1072, 1982.
15. Ponappa Naren, A. and Virupaksha, T. K., Effect of sulfur deficiency on the synthesis of α-setarin, a methionine-rich protein of Italian millet, *Cereal Chem.,* 67, 136, 1990.
16. Singh, P., Singh, U., Kumar, K. A., and Andrews, D. J., Nutritional quality improvement in pearl millet *(Pennisetum americanum* L. Leeke), in *The Processing of Sorghum and Millets: Criteria for Quality of Grains and Products for Human Food,* Dendy, D.A.V., Ed., IACC, Vienna, Austria, 1984, 75.
17. Shawney, S. K. and Naik, M. S., Amino acid composition of protein fractions of pearl millet and the effect of nitrogen fertilization of its proteins, *Indian J. Genet. Plant Breed.,* 29, 395, 1969.
18. Landry, J. and Moureaux, T., Heterogenité des glutelines du grain de mais: extraction selective et composition en acides aminées des trois fractions isolées, *Bull. Soc. Biol.,* 52, 1021, 1970.

19. Nwasike, C. C., Mertz, E. T., Pickett, R. C., Clover, D. V., Chibber, B. A., and Van Scoyoc, S. W., Lysine level in solvent fractions of pearl millet, *J. Agric. Food Chem.,* 27, 1329, 1979.
20. Abdelrahman, A., Hoseney, B. C., and Variano-Marston, E., The proportions and chemical compositions of hand-dissected anatomical parts of pearl millet, *J. Cereal Sci.,* 2, 127, 1984.
21. Lorenz, K., Dilsaver, W., and Bates, L., Proso millets. Milling characteristics, proximate compositions, nutritive value of flour, *Cereal Chem.,* 57, 16, 1980.
22. Ponappa Naren, A. and Virupaksha, T. K., α- and β-setarins: methionine-rich proteins of Italian millet (*Setaria italica* L. Beauv.), *Cereal Chem.,* 67, 32, 1990.
23. Vivas, N. E., Waniska, R. D., and Rooney, L. W., Effects on proteins in sorghum, maize, and pearl millet when processed into acidic and basic to, *Cereal Chem.,* 69, 673, 1992.
24. Bietz, J. A., Cereal prolamin evolution and homology revealed by sequence analysis, *Biochem. Genet.,* 20, 103, 1983.
25. Esen, A., Bietz, J. A., Paulis, J. W., and Wall, J. S., Tandem repeats in N-terminal sequence of a proline rich protein from corn endosperm, *Nature (London),* 296, 678, 1982.
26. Melcher, U. and Fraij, B., Methionine-rich protein fraction prepared by cryoprecipitation from extracts of corn meal, *J. Agric. Food Chem.,* 29, 1134, 1980.
27. Galyean, R. D., Laney, A. J., Horden, M., and Vreig, D., Water-soluble proteins of selected pearl millet genotypes, *J. Food Sci.,* 45, 1165, 1980.
28. Hiller, A., Mlodecki, H., Kosta, B., and Wierycka, A., Tests on characterization of millet proteins by extraction with selected solvents and by molecular filtration on Sephadex G-75 gel, *Bromatol. Chem. Toksycol.,* 10, 21, 1977.
29. Gupta, D. N., Roy, M. K., Singh, T. N., Singhal, G. S., and Mehta, S. L., Changes in proteins and enzymes during grain development in pearl millet, *Biochem. Physiol. Pflanz.,* 175, 15, 1980.
30. Beleia, A. and Varriano-Marston, E., Pearl millet amylases. I. Properties of partially purified alpha amylase, *Cereal Chem.,* 58, 433, 1981.
31. Beleia, A. and Varriano-Marston, E., Pearl millet amylases. II. Activity toward intact and heated starch granules, *Cereal Chem.,* 58, 437, 1981.
32. McGregor, A. W., Marchylo, B. A., and Kruger, J. E., Multiple α-amylase components in germinated cereal grains determined by isoelectric focusing and chromatofocusing, *Cereal Chem.,* 65, 326, 1988.
33. Campos, F. A. P. and Richardson, M., The complete amino acid sequence of the bifunctional α-amylase/trypsin inhibitor from seeds of ragi (Indian finger millet, *Eleusine coracana* Gaertn.), *FEBS Lett.,* 152, 300, 1983.
34. Freeman, J. F. and Bocan, B. J., Pearl millet: a potential crop for wet milling, *Cereal Sci. Today,* 18, 69, 1973.
35. Casey, P. and Lorenz, K., Millet functional and nutritional properties, *Baker's Dig.,* 2, 45, 1977.
36. Serna-Saldivar, S. O., McDonough, C. N., and Rooney, L. W., Millets, in *Handbook of Cereal Science and Technology,* Lorenz, K. and Kulp, K., Eds., Marcel Dekker, New York, 1991, Chap. 6.
37. Almeida-Dominguez, H. D., Serna-Saldivar, S. O., Gomez, M. H., and Rooney, L. W., Production and nutritional value of weaning foods from mixtures of pearl millet and cowpeas, *Cereal Chem.,* 70, 14, 1993.

38. Guiro, A. T., Sall, M. G., Kane, O., Ndiaye, A. M., Diarra, D., and Sy, M. T. A., Protein-calorie malnutrition in Senegalese children. Effects of rehabilitation with a pearl millet weaning food, *Nutr. Rep. Int.,* 36, 1071, 1987.
39. Boeh-Ocansey, O., Developments and challenges in Africa's food industry, *Food Technol.,* 43, 84, 1989.
40. Alpana, K. and Chavhan, B. M., Effect of phytic acid on protein digestibility (in vitro) and HCl-extractability of minerals in pearl millet sprouts, *Cereal Chem.,* 70(5), 504, 1993.
41. Khetarpaul, N. and Chavnan, B. M., Effect of natural fermentation on antinutrients and in vitro digestibility of starch and protein in pearl millet flour, *J. Sci. Food Agric.,* 55, 189, 1991.
42. Bailey, A. V. and Sumrell, G., Preparation of protein concentrate from pearl millet, *J. Agric. Food Chem.,* 28, 475, 1980.

11 Nonfood Uses of Cereal Proteins

The growing interest in reducing usage of fossil raw materials, together with the big surplus of cereals, particularly in the European Community, has stimulated research work connected with nonfood uses of cereals.[1-3] Not only the seed but all components in the whole crop, including the stem and kernel, should be considered as raw materials for nonfood purposes.[4,5] Less than 100 years ago, at the beginning of this century, almost all organic chemicals were obtained through agriculture; textile and paper fibers were also of agricultural origin. After the outbreak of World War II the situation changed; fossil resources like coal, and later, crude oil and natural gas became the main raw materials for the chemical industry. Today they are totally dominant.[4] Although the reduction of environmental pollution, the search for renewable raw materials, and the maintenance or improvement of efficiency in agriculture without creating surpluses are a big argument for increasing usage of agricultural products in nonfood industries, the relatively higher price of agricultural raw materials makes these noncompetitive from an economical point-of-view. However, it may be expected that the price differential between fossil and agricultural raw materials will shift in favor of the latter. It also may be expected that the rapid development in the biotechnology sector will increase the demand for agricultural raw materials.

Returning to the subject of nonfood uses of cereal protein, we can calculate, first of all, the use of wheat gluten at the commercial level. This can be explained by two facts: (1) wheat gluten is the main byproduct of wheat starch factories, so there is a large-scale production of it already available, and (2) good progress has already been achieved in some potential fields of industrial application.

Wheat gluten may be used in its native form (vital gluten) or after such chemical modification as acylation, alkylation, reduction and oxidation, or aromatic ring substitution. Chemical modification results in changes in functional properties of gluten and increases the potential fields of application. Although chemically modified gluten may be used in the food industry too, nutritional (toxicological) problems make it more useful for nonfood purposes.

Nearly 50 years ago Reitz et al.[6] reacted wheat gluten with chlorosulfonic in pyridine or with cold concentrated sulfuric acid. This yielded a wheat gluten sulfate which absorbed 100 to 300 times its weight in water to form an odorless, tasteless, and almost water-clear gel. This "Super Slurper"-type product can be used as an absorbing agent for body fluids in cystostomes and other cases involving postoperative drainage. A high water-absorbing product from wheat gluten was also made by treatment with phosphoric acid and urea.[7]

Properties of acylated (acetylated, succinylated, citraconylated, propionylated, butylated, etc.) gluten were studied more recently by several research workers.[8-12] Generally, better solubility, better water absorption and higher water-holding capacity were observed. Succinylation leads to an increase in free carboxyl groups and net negative charge and also an increase in surface hydrophobicity.

Among potential nonfood fields of application are use in the paper and wood materials industry, as cobinders in paper coating mixtures, as fillers in urea-formaldehyde resin adhesives, use in films and coatings, and in biodegradable plastic materials.

High-grade special papers for printing are achieving a significant growth rate in the current commodity world. Such types of paper are sized and coated. In coating the raw paper, the applied pigments require binders for anchoring them to each other and to the raw paper. Wheat gluten potentially represents a valuable raw material as a possible component of so-called coating mixtures. For such uses the gluten should be chemically modified in order to be residue free and soluble and to have adequate viscosity, pigment binding power, and microbial stability.[13,14] Wheat gluten and cyanoethylated gluten were tested as fillers in urea-formaldehyde glues. Very encouraging results were obtained. Bergthaller et al.[15] have found that alkali-treated and modified gluten is the more promising. Replacement of urea-formaldehyde resins to an extent of 5% gave the best results with respect in elastomechanical and swelling properties. In addition, protein-containing extenders are capable of binding formaldehyde and so reduce the release of formaldehyde from urea-formaldehyde resins bound in a particle board.[16,17]

Major industrial markets for proteins in general are fiber, films, or adhesive compositions. In early experiments Krull and Inglett[18] found that films could be prepared from a 20% solution of gluten in a solvent mixture composed of ethanol, 20% lactic acid, and 20% water. In 1972 Anker et al.[19,21] patented a process for producing edible odor-free gluten films and coatings which could be used to wrap, package, or encase cheese, sandwiches, and hors d'oevres. In confectionery products, edible films can serve as oxygen and moisture barriers to retain crispness and inhibit oxidative and hydrolytic rancidity. Recently there has been a revival of interest in the use of wheat gluten and maize protein (zein) films and coatings to extend the shelf life of foods by offering a selective barrier against the transmission of gases, moisture, and solutes while also providing mechanical protection.[20-23] Kolster et al.,[24] Gontard et al.,[25] Kuiper et al.,[26] and Gennadios et al.[27] studied the possibility of adjusting the physical properties of gluten films to fit the specific requirements of a potential application. At room temperature gluten is in the glassy or brittle state.[23] If the temperature is increased over the Tg (glass transition temperature) gluten will change into a rubbery or elastic material. The Tg value of wheat gluten is 435 K as reported by Hoseney et al.[28] The glassy state also can be changed by addition of a plasticizer such as water or glycerol.[25,29-31] The advantageous effect of plasticizers on properties of gluten-based films is related to a decrease in the strength of the film. Oxidation or cross-linking agents such as glutaraldehyde (which establishes cross-linkages between lysine residues) increase the strength as reported by Kolster et al.[24] An important observation is that the extensibility remains practically unchanged. Gluten coatings may be used in the future to protect biodegradable starch-based polymers.

A new direction of potential industrial use of cereal proteins is the production of amino acid- or peptide-based tensides. Such compounds are known to contain hydrophilic and hydrophobic groups. Generally, benzene-sulfonic acid is used as the hydrophilic group in the majority of known and commercially produced tensides.

Protein hydrolysates (hydrolysis with hydrochloric acid) containing low level of oligopeptides may be acylated with fatty acid chlorides. As a result, a mixture of amino acid (oligopeptide)-based surface-active compounds (Figure 1) will be formed which potentially can be used in the production of cosmetics and pharmaceutical products.[32]

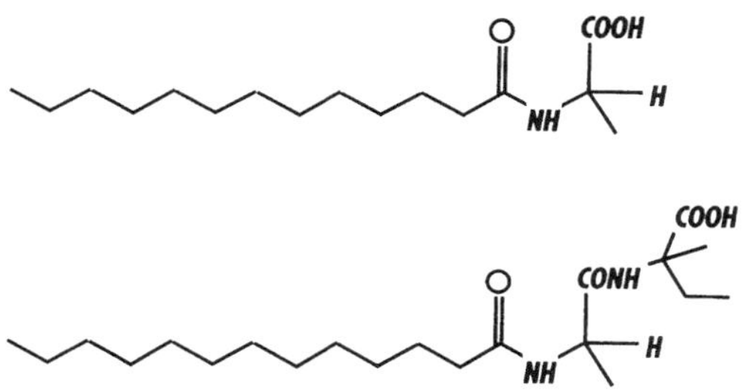

FIGURE 1 General formula of the amino acid (peptide)-based tensides.

REFERENCES

1. Rexen, F. and Munck, L., Cereal Crops for Industrial Use in Europe, Commission of the European Communities, Brussels, 1984.
2. Pomeranz, Y. and Munck, L., Eds., *Cereals: A Renewable Resource. Theory and Practice,* American Association of Cereal Chemists, St. Paul, MN, 1981.
3. Lásztity, R. and Kárpáti, M., Eds., *Proc. Int. Conf. Non Food Uses of Cereals,* MÉTE, Budapest, 1994.
4. Rexen, F., Cereals for industrial production: possibilities and constraints, in *Proc. Int. Conf. Non Food Uses of Cereals,* Lásztity, R. and Kárpáti, M., Eds., MÉTE, Budapest, 1994, 7.
5. Munck, L., A new agricultural system for Europe?, *Trends Biotechnol.,* 5, 36, 1987.

6. Reitz, H. C., Ferrel R. E., and Olcott, H. S., Gel-forming derivative of wheat gluten, *Ind. Eng. Chem.,* 36, 1149, 1944.
7. Mohammad, A., Mecham, D. K., and Olcott, H. S., Gel-forming phosphorylated derivative of gluten, *J. Agric. Food. Chem.,* 2, 136, 1944.
8. Grant, D. R., The modification of wheat flour proteins with succinic anhydride, *Cereal Chem.,* 50, 417, 1973.
9. Simmonds, D. H. and Orth, R. A., Structure and composition of cereal proteins as related to their potential industrial utilization, in *Industrial Uses of Cereals,* Pomeranz, Y., Ed., American Association of Cereal Chemists, St. Paul, MN, 1973, 51.
10. Barber, K. J. and Warthesen, J. J., Some functional properties of acylated wheat gluten, *J. Agric. Food Chem.,* 30, 930, 1982.
11. Ma, C. Y., Oomah, B. D., and Holme, J., Effect of deamidation and succinylation on some physico-chemical and baking properties of gluten, *J. Food Sci.,* 51, 99, 1986.
12. Lásztity, R., Investigation of the rheological properties of gluten. II. Viscoelastic properties of chemically modified gluten, *Acta Chem. Acad. Sci. Hung.,* 62, 75, 1969.
13. Whalen-Shaw, M., Protein pigment interactions for controlled rotograw reprinting properties. Mechanistic and structural considerations, *Tappi J.,* 67, 60, 1984.
14. Friedman, M., Wheat gluten — alkali reactions, *Proc. 10th Int. Conf. Wheat Util. Res.,* 1978, 81.
15. Bergthaller, W., Kersting, H. J., Dix, B., and Roffael, E., A technical application of modified gluten in bonding of particle board, in *Proc. Int. Symp. Non Food Uses of Cereals,* Lásztity, R. and Kárpáti, M., Eds., MÉTE, Budapest, 1984, 136.
16. Roffael, E., *Die Formaldehydabgabe von Spanplatten und anderen Werkstoffen,* DRW Verlag, Stüttgart, 1982.
17. Tinkelenberg, A., Vaessen, H., and Sven, K. W., Manufacture of Chip Board and Aminoplast Adhesive Used Therefore, *European Patent* 0025 245, 1980.
18. Krull, L. N. and Inglett, G. E., Industrial uses of gluten, *Cereal Sci. Today,* 16, 232, 1971.
19. Anker, C. A., Burchill, P. J., Foster, G. A., Jr., and Loader, M. A., Verfahren zur Herstellung von beliebig geformten Gegenstanden durch Extrusion von nicht warmekoagulierbaren einfachen Proteinen, *D.O.S. 2,045.994, Int. Cl. C.08 h 19/02,* 1972.
20. Gennadios, A. and Weller, C. L., Edible films and coatings from wheat and corn proteins, *Food Technol.,* 44, 63, 1990.
21. Anker, C. A., Foster, G. A., and Loader, M. A., Method of Preparing Gluten Containing Films and Coatings, U.S. Patent 3,653,925, 1972.
22. Gontard, A., Guilbert, S., and Cuq, J. L., Edible wheat gluten films: influence of the main process variables on film properties using response surface methodology, *J. Food Sci.,* 57, 190, 1992.
23. Aydt, T. P., Weller, C. L., and Testin, R. F., Mechanical and barrier properties of edible corn and wheat protein films, *Trans. ASAE,* 34, 207, 1991.
24. Kolster, P., Kuiper, H. J., Ric, M., Bollen, J., and Vereijken, J. M., Non-food application of coatings based on wheat gluten, in *Proc. Int. Symp. Non Food Uses of Cereals,* Lásztity, R. and Kárpáti, M., Eds., MÉTE, Budapest, 1994, 212.

25. Gontard, N., Guilbert, S., and Cuq, J. L., Water and glycerol as plasticizers affect mechanical and water vapour barrier properties of an edible wheat gluten film, *J. Food Sci.,* 58, 206, 1993.
26. Kuiper, B. J., Kolster, P., Kok, J. C., and Vereijken, J. M., Films based on wheat gluten, in *Gluten Proteins 1993,* Cereal Research Federation (Germany), Detmold, 1993.
27. Gennadios, A., Waller, C. L., and Testin, R. F., Modification of physical and barrier properties of edible, wheat-gluten-based films, *Cereal Chem.,* 70, 426, 1993.
28. Hoseney, R. C., Zeleznak, K., and Lai, C. S., Wheat gluten: a glassy polymer, *Cereal Chem.,* 6, 285, 1986.
29. Kalichevsky, M. T., Jaroszkiewicz, E. M., and Blanchard, J. M., Glass transition of gluten. I. Gluten and gluten sugar mixtures, *Int. J. Biol. Macromol.,* 14, 257, 1992.
30. Kalichevsky, M. T., Jaroszkiewicz, E. M., and Blanchard, J. M., Glass transition of gluten. II. The effect of lipids and emulsifiers, *Int. J. Biol. Macromol.,* 14, 267, 1992.
31. Huang, V. T., Significance of the food polymer science concept in cereal research: a literature review, in *Proc. '94 Int. Symp. Exhibition on New Approaches in the Production of Food-Stuffs and Intermediate Products from Cereal Grains and Oil Seeds,* Xie, G. and Ma, Z., Eds., CCOA, Beijing, 1994, 94.
32. Anon., Tenside auf Aminosa ure-Basis, *CHEManager,* 9, 1, 1994.

Index

B

C

D

E

F

H

I

J

K

L

M

R

S

T

U

V

W

Z